Delphi Methods In The Social And Health Sciences

Marlen Niederberger • Ortwin Renn
Editors

Delphi Methods In The Social And Health Sciences

Concepts, applications and case studies

Springer

Editors
Marlen Niederberger
Pädagogische Hochschule Schwäbisch Gmünd
Schwäbisch Gmünd, Germany

Ortwin Renn
Research Institute For Sustainability
Helmholtz Center Potsdam (RIFS)
Potsdam, Germany

ISBN 978-3-658-38861-4 ISBN 978-3-658-38862-1 (eBook)
https://doi.org/10.1007/978-3-658-38862-1

The translation was done with the help of artificial intelligence (machine translation by the service DeepL.com). A subsequent human revision was done primarily in terms of content.

This Springer imprint is published by the registered company Springer Fachmedien Wiesbaden GmbH, part of Springer Nature.
The registered company address is: Abraham-Lincoln-Str. 46, 65189 Wiesbaden, Germany

Preface

Delphi methods are structured group communication processes designed and facilitated by professional Delphi moderators. Delphi methods deal with complex issues and wicked problems where uncertain and incomplete knowledge exists. These issues are assessed by groups of experts in an iterative process. It is the main purpose of Delphi methods that with each new round of questioning, the aggregated group answers of the previous round are fed back and the respondents can reconsider their judgements on the basis of the received feedback and revise them if necessary. The characteristic features of Delphi methods are: (1) anonymization of responses, (2) iterative questioning with controlled feedback and (3) integration of aggregated group responses.

Delphi methods have proven themselves valid and reliable in various disciplines and fields of application around the world. The first Delphi studies were applied in the field of operations Research. To this day, they represent an important instrument for the analysis of possible future states. In addition, Delphi methods are used to record the current state of knowledge, to characterize or even resolve controversial judgements, to identify and formulate standards or guidelines, to develop instruments for assessing outcomes, to identify indicators, or to formulate recommendations for actions. In the health sciences, they have become established above all for recording a true consensus or "a consensus about dissent" among experts. Through iterative expert interviews, knowledge on an open or controversial issue can be captured, calibrated and characterized for possible divergences. Based on this, agreement and disagreement can be identified, and areas of dissent can be characterized more precisely and argumentatively substantiated. The aim is to base professional judgements on collectively available evidence, thus improving the chance of producing robust knowledge.

In recent years, numerous variants of Delphi methods have developed. Many innovative and far-reaching changes in Delphi methods have been made possible primarily by new technical possibilities in the domain of IT services. Recently, *real-time Delphis* have been carried out, in which the expert judgements are fed back online and in real time. In so-called *Delphi markets,* the Delphi method is combined with forecasting and information markets as well as with findings from big data research to improve predictive judgements. Other variants concern the objective of Delphi methods. *Policy Delphi* is not about consensus but about capturing dissent, i.e. the breadth of judgements. In *argumentative Delphi,* the focus is on the argumentative (qualitative) justification of the standardized judgements by the experts. In the *group Delphi method,* anonymity is abandoned in favour of a personal exchange and the recording of substantive reasons for dissenting judgements. During a group Delphi, the experts are invited to a joint workshop to develop a common response to complex issues and questions.

A scientific and interdisciplinary discourse on Delphi methods, in which the different variants and possible areas of application, particularly in the social and health sciences, are compared and their respective advantages and disadvantages discussed, is missing so far. The editors of the book pursue the intention to close this gap. The book focuses on the concepts, current developments, innovative procedures, methodological innovations, and examples of application of Delphi procedures in the social and health sciences. Two objectives are linked with the book: On the one hand, the book includes a long overdue overview of the multitude of variants of Delphi methods, and on the other hand, concrete examples of application are presented with a focus on methodological approaches, such as questionnaire design, expert recruitment or evaluation. The edited volume is divided into two main parts:

In the first part, several papers address the concepts of Delphi methods and different Delphi variants:

1. Kerstin Cuhls gives an insight into the concept, the different definitions, types and fields of applications. She points to the opportunities and challenges when using Delphi methods.
2. Karlheinz Steinmüller articulates practical tips for conducting Delphi methods, drawing on decades of experience in the field of futures research. He covers many topics from the development of the questionnaire to the evaluation and interpretation of the data.
3. Saskia Jünger provides an insight into epistemic potential of Delphi methods and discusses the various challenges associated with each method. In doing so, she primarily builds upon discourses from the sociology of knowledge. She

uses the field of palliative care as an example to illustrate the significance of Delphi procedures for health science research.
4. Marlen Niederberger and Ortwin Renn present the concept and the procedure of a new variant: group Delphi. This is a Delphi setting in which the experts are invited to a jointly workshop and make assessments in small groups. These assessments are then discussed together in the plenary.
5. Lars Gerhold describes the concept of Real-Time Delphi, in which experts are interviewed online and the answers are transmitted in real time. He also introduces various software programs that can be applied to real-time Delphis.
6. Simon Kloker, Tim Straub, Tobias T. Kranz and Christof Weinhardt explain Delphi markets, an innovative approach to integrate prediction markets and Delphi studies. They explain different options of integration and highlight how the combination of methods can potentially compensate for each other's weaknesses.

The second part includes papers that describe concrete Delphi methods from the health sciences. Specifically, Delphi methods from the fields of healthcare, prevention, palliative medicine, health promotion, nursing and futurology are presented. The methods illustrate the diversity of applications and the many options when applying Delphi methods. Specifically, the following case studies are presented:

1. Johannes Leinert, Alexander Rommel and Helmut Schröder present a classic Delphi study on the topic of qualification requirements in the healthcare industry. Based on a survey of about 1500 experts, it is one of the largest Delphi studies that has ever taken place in Germany. In their article, the authors focus on the composition and recruitment of the experts.
2. Hannah Gohres and Petra Kolip present a modified Delphi procedure to identify consensual recommendations for action for the further structural development of promoting physical activity in Germany. In this example, elements of a classic Delphi process were combined with those of a group Delphi. In addition, expert interviews and focus groups were part of the study.
3. Stefan Görres, Katrin Seibert and Susanne Stiefler describe a Delphi procedure to assess the healthcare situation of older people in the federal state of Bremen. This example shows the potential of Delphi methods for aggregating diverse ideas and developing corresponding strategies.
4. Nora Lämmel, Jutta Mohr and Karin Reiber conducted a Delphi survey on strategies of personnel retention and recruitment in professional nursing. In their contribution, they deal in particular with the development of the research

question, the operationalization of the theoretical concept and the creation of the questionnaire.
5. Michael M. Zwick, Marco Sonnberger, Jürgen Deuschle and Regina Schröter conducted a group Delphi to estimate health-related measures in the field of obesity prevention. This example illustrates the procedure and underlines the application potential of group Delphi methods particularly for controversial topics.
6. Clarissa Eickholt presents a Delphi study on the promotion of safety and health competence in small and medium-sized enterprises (SMEs). The aim of the Delphi study is to collect different expert opinions. The example shows how qualitative and quantitative elements can be combined or integrated in a Delphi procedure.
7. In their contribution, Marlen Niederberger, Ann-Kathrin Käfer and Laura König provide an overview of Delphi methods in health promotion. They provide a systematic review based on publications in relevant international journals. The aim is to elaborate the research practice, especially with regard to the selection of experts, the research design and the presentation of results.

With this edited volume, we would like to present an overview of Delphi methods in the social and health sciences and beyond. On the basis of concrete examples of applications and innovative procedures, we like to demonstrate what Delphi methods can contribute to knowledge generation, knowledge processing and action orientation. We would like to thank all authors for their exciting and stimulating contributions. We hope that this book will provide an important impulse for further discussions on the theory of Delphi concepts, on the structure and variants of Delphi methods, and on the various applications and cases to which Delphi methods can contribute new knowledge and to stimulate corresponding actions. We hope that this volume will encourage readers to reflect on the potential, but also limitations, of Delphi methods and its variants, especially in the health sciences.

Schwäbisch Gmünd, Germany — Marlen Niederberger
Potsdam, Germany — Ortwin Renn

Contents

About the Editors and Authors

Editors

Marlen Niederberger is professor for research methods in health promotion and prevention at the Pädagogischen Hochschule Schwäbisch Gmünd. Her expertise lies in the areas of inter- and transdisciplinary methods, participation methods and mixed-methods designs. She has specialized in particular in the group Delphi, which she uses in various fields of application and further devlops its concept and methodology. In addition, she has extensive knowledge in the field of health promotion and prevention, with a focus on the relationship level (especially municipal health promotion) and the topic of migration, integration and flight.

Ortwin Renn has been scientific director at the Research Institute for Sustainability - Helmholtz Center Potsdam (retired) and Professor emeritus of Environmental Sociology and Technolgy Assessment at the Universität of Stuttgart. In addition, Renn co-directs the DIALOGIK Research Institute, a nonprofit company for investigating and testing innovative communication and participation strategies. In addition, he holds honorary professorships in Stavanger, Beijing and Munich. His main research fields are: risk analysis (governance, perception and communication), theory and practice of citizen participation, transformation research, and social and technical change towards sustainable development.

Authors

Kerstin Cuhls has been working as a scientific project manager in the field of foresight at the Fraunhofer-Institut für System- und Innovationsforschung (ISI) in Karlsruhe since 1992. She began by conducting Delphi studies for the BMBF in international comparison. From 2007 to 2009, Kerstin Cuhls was project manager of the BMBF Foresight Process, Cycle I, and worked on follow-up projects, including Cycle II. In national, regional and international studies for very different clients, she built up an extensive repertoire of methods in foresight. From 2011 to 2012, Kerstin Cuhls was a substitute professor of Japanese studies and is since 2020 Professor at the Center for East Asian and Transcultural Studies at Ruprecht-Karls-Universität Heidelberg. She holds teaching positions at the TU Berlin (master's programme in Futures Research) and the Bundesakademie für Sicherheitspolitik. She was a member of several foresight advisory boards, the European Forum for Forward-Looking Activities (EFFLA), the Highlevel Expert Group Research, Innovation and Science Policy Experts (RISE), and the Expert Group Strategic Foresight.

Jürgen Deuschle, MA, first learned the profession of radio electronics technician and worked as a service technician in the music industry. He studied sociology and geography at the universities of Stuttgart, Tübingen and Bern. At the Akademie für Technikfolgenabschätzung Baden-Württemberg and at Universität Stuttgart, he taught and did research in projects on the topics of justice, sustainability, bioenergy and obesity, among others. His dissertation is dedicated to the questions why overweight is a stigma, why people stigmatize, and how overweight children experience and cope with stigma. In addition to his academic work, Jürgen Deuschle works as a bicycle courier and managing director of "Die Radler" in Stuttgart.

Clarissa Eickholt studied education with a focus on adult education and organizational science at Universität Cologne. After her studies, she worked as a research assistant and as divisional manager for learning and organization at systemkonzept GmbH, and has been managing director since 2010. The field of safety and health at work forms the background of her work. Her work and research focus on the transfer between science and practice, informal learning at work and media-didactic requirements for competence-oriented blended learning. Since 2014, she has been a member of the board of the Professional Association of Psychology for Occupational Safety and Health (Psychologie für Arbeitssicherheit und Gesundheit PASIG), where she heads the expert group "Training and Further Education".

Lars Gerhold is professor at the department of psychology and heads the Psychology of Sociotechnical Systems Research Group at Technische Universität Braunschweig and the Public Security Research Forum at Einstein Center Digital Future. He is also PI at the Weizenbaum Institute for the Networked Society and PI at the Einstein Center for Digital Future, Berlin. After studying political science, psychology and sociology, he earned a doctorate in psychology on dealing with uncertainty. His research focuses on security relations in sociotechnical systems and research on civil protection, security foresight, social change, perception and action research, and methods of futures research. He is founder of the journal "Zeitschrift für Zukunftsforschung" and co-editor of the "Standards of Futures Research". He teaches, among other things, the Delphi method in the master's programme in futures studies at Freie Universität Berlin.

Stefan Görres has been a professor at Universität Bremen since 1994, specializing in nursing science and gerontology; Dean of Faculty 11, Human and Health Sciences; member of the Academic Senate; and member of the Board of Directors of Instituts für Public Health und Pflegeforschung (IPP). He has numerous publications on topics such as the future of nursing, professionalization of nursing professions, future care structures, quality assurance and control models in nursing. Co-editor of scientific book series. He is member of numerous scientific societies and juries as well as scientific advisory boards of foundations and companies. Stefan provides expert opinions and consultations for ministries at the federal and state level, among others.

Hannah Gohres is a research associate and doctoral candidate in the Prevention and Health Promotion Working Group of the School of Public Health at Bielefeld University. Her expertise lies in the field of physical activity promotion, especially in childhood, as well as mixed-methods research and theory-based intervention planning.

Saskia Jünger is a health scientist with specialisation in clinical psychology. After her studies at Universität Maastricht (NL), she worked as a psychologist and research assistant in psychosomatic medicine, palliative care and general medicine. She has coordinated several national and international projects in the field of health services research; her PhD at Lancaster University (UK) focused on consensus building and knowledge production in palliative care. She has a particular interest in mental health and a sociological view of health and illness from a knowledge perspective. Since January 2021, Saskia Jünger is Professor for Research Methods with a focus on Qualitative Methods at the Department of Community Health at the University of Applied Health Sciences in Bochum, Germany.

Ann-Kathrin Käfer is a research assistant at the Pädagogischen Hochschule Schwäbisch Gmünd. She is involved in the group Delphiprocess on the topic of digital education in primary school age. She completed her master's degree at the Pädagogischen Hochschule Schwäbisch Gmünd in 2018 in health promotion and prevention.

Simon Kloker has been working on his doctorate at the Institut für Informationswirtschaft und Marketing (IISM) at the Karlsruher Instituts für Technologie (KIT) since 2015. There, he is scientifically and technically responsible for the FAZ.NET Oracle, a prediction exchange in cooperation with the Frankfurter Allgemeine Zeitung. His specific research interests relate to the topics of "manipulation and fraud on prediction exchanges", "cognitive distortions during the submission of expectations", and the "method integration of prediction exchanges and Delphi studies".

Laura König is studying for a master's degree in sustainable services and food management at Fachhochschule Münster. As part of her scientific assistant work during her bachelor's degree in health promotion at the Pädagogischen Hochschule Schwäbisch Gmünd, she dealt with Delphi methods in health promotion.

Petra Kolip is Professor of Prevention and Health Promotion at the School of Public Health of Bielefeld University. Her expertise includes quality development and evaluation in health promotion and prevention.

Tobias T. Kranz is an alumnus of Instituts für Informationswirtschaft und Marketing (IISM) at the Karlsruher Instituts für Technologie (KIT). He first came into contact with prediction methods in 2007 and wrote his diploma thesis on mobile user behaviour in prediction markets. He specialized in the design of electronic market platforms with a focus on participant support and prediction quality. He developed various prediction markets, Delphi and simulation platforms for the prediction of future events such as election outcomes, technology acceptances as well as economic, security and socio-ecological future scenarios. He received his PhD from KIT in 2015 with a thesis on continuous market design. Since 2016, he has held a senior position at a medium-sized financial services provider.

Nora Lämmel, MA Political Science, BA Social Science (HF), German Studies (NF), was a research associate in the research network ZAFH care4care in the Faculty of Social Work, Education and Nursing at Hochschule Esslingen. In addition to the project focus of ZAFH care4care "Recruitment, development and retention of skilled workers in care", another thematic focus of her work to date is co-determination in companies, especially in processes of change within companies.

Johannes Leinert holds a degree in economics. He studied economics with a focus on social security systems. After completing his studies, Mr. Leinert worked as a consultant and project manager at the Bertelsmann Foundation, Social Policy Department. He also completed his doctorate at the TU Berlin on the promotion of voluntary old-age provision. Subsequently, he worked as a research assistant at the Federal Statistical Office's health reporting department and in the thematic area of "Health Policy and System Analyses" at Wissenschaftlichen Institut der AOK (WIdO). In 2006, he moved to the infas-Institut. There he works in the thematic area of health research.

Jutta Mohr, MA Nursing Science, BSc Nursing, was a research associate in the research network ZAFH care4care in the Faculty of Social Work, Education and Nursing at Hochschule Esslingen. She has completed her doctorate on the topic of in-company training in nursing in a career-oriented perspective. Currently, she is working on the subject of further training in nursing.

Karin Reiber is Professor of Education/Didactics with a focus on nursing education/didactics at Institut für Gesundheits- und Pflegewissenschaften at Hochschule Esslingen. At the interface of nursing and healthcare research, she works, among other things, with retention studies/graduate surveys, expert interviews and Delphi studies. Her thematic focus is on nursing education, further education and training as well as the recruitment, development and retention of skilled workers.

Alexander Rommel, MA, studied sociology, political science and philosophy at the Ruprecht Karls-Universität Heidelberg. In 1999, he became research associate and project manager at the Wissenschaftliches Institut der Ärzte Deutschlands (WIAD) in the areas of health reporting, survey research and health services research. In 2012, he became research associate and project manager at the Robert Koch-Institut in the field of health reporting. In addition to conducting Delphi surveys and focus groups, his focus is on the analysis of health monitoring data at the Robert Koch-Institut as well as secondary and routine data. He has conducted research on the epidemiology of diseases and the utilization of health services.

Helmut Schröder holds a degree in educational science and a doctorate in sociology. Between 1982 and 1991, he was employed as an assistant at Universität zu Köln, of which 2 years were spent at the Seminar for General Curative Education and Sociology of the Disabled and more than 6 years at the Seminar for Social Sciences. He has been with infas since 1991, and since 2003 as one of the two heads of the Social Research Division. Mr. Schröder has been working in the field of labour market, and occupational and participation research since the mid-1980s. Mr. Schröder has many years of experience in the management and implementation of complex research projects.

Regina Schröter studied political science and sociology at Universität Stuttgart, where she received her doctorate in citizen participation in 2018. She currently works as a project communication manager for Netze BW. As a certified mediator, she also moderates public participation processes as well as teaching events and workshops. Regina Schröter publishes on various topics, currently on public participation and acceptance of large-scale and infrastructure projects.

Katrin Seibert, MSc Community & Family Health Nursing, is a nurse and research associate at Institut für Public Health und Pflegeforschung (IPP) at the Universität Bremen, Department 7 Nursing Care Research, and EBN trainer. Project work in the 'Study of the health care situation of older people in the Federal State of Bremen'. Ongoing doctoral project on the quality of care for people in need of care in their own homes.

Marco Sonnberger studied sociology and political science at the Universities of Heidelberg and Stuttgart. In 2014, he received his PhD in sociology from the University of Stuttgart. He is a senior researcher at department of sociology of technology, risk and environment of the University of Stuttgart as well as at the section for environmental sociology of the University of Jena. His research interests include sociological energy and mobility research, sustainable consumption, lifestyle research, sociology of risk, environmental sociology, and technology assessment.

Karlheinz Steinmüller is scientific director of Z_punkt GmbH The Foresight Company. He is a physicist and holds a Doctor of Philosophy, and he has been working in futurology for 25 years and deals with future studies for renowned companies and public clients. He focuses on future technologies as well as social developments. He also lectures on futurology methods at Freien Universität Berlin and at the European Business School Oestrich-Winkel. Karlheinz has published a number of books on futurology as well as science fiction. His methodological interests are especially disruptions and wild cards.

Susanne Stiefler, MA Public Health/Nursing Science with focus on prevention research and health promotion, is a research associate at Institut für Public Health und Pfl egeforschung (IPP) at Universität Bremen, Department 7 Nursing Care Research. She teaching in nursing and health science bachelor's and master's courses. Susanne has collaborations in research on ageing, quality and care mix (avoiding institutionalization, EvaQS and StaVaCare-Pilot), and is project coordinator of the "Study of the health care situation of older people in the federal state of Bremen". She is pursuing her doctoral project on predictors of institutionalization in the case of existing need for long-term care and the possibilities of counteracting this predictively.

Tim Straub is a research associate at the FZI Forschungszentrum Informatik (FZI), where he works on various projects in the field of digitalization. He is also the research group leader of the "Digital Experience & Participation" (DXP) research group of the "Information and Market Engineering" (IM) group at the Institut für Informationswirtschaft und Marketing (IISM) of the Karlsruher Instituts für Technologie (KIT). Through his PhD at IISM on the topic of "Incentive Design for Crowdsourcing" he came into contact with participation and collaboration platforms around the topic of "Wisdom of Crowds". In this context, he also developed electronic market platforms for the distribution and aggregation of scarce resources (planning game platform) as well as various prediction markets and Delphi platforms.

Christof Weinhardt is a professor at Institut für Informationswirtschaft und Marketing (IISM) at Karlsruher Instituts für Technologie (KIT). He heads the group "Information and Market Engineering" (IM). With an academic background in industrial engineering, economics and business informatics, his research focuses on interdisciplinary topics in market and engineering, and platform economics, with applications in the IT industry, the energy industry, and financial and telecom markets. In these areas, he is an editor and reviewer for numerous international journals and conferences, has published more than 150 articles in renowned journals and books, and has received a number of awards for his research and teaching. In the Enquete Commission of the German Bundestag "Internet and Digital Societ", he was active as an expert for more than 3 years, and since then, he is increasingly researching in this field (online participation).

Michael M. Zwick, sociologist, is working as a senior researcher and lecturer at the University of Stuttgart, Institute for Social Sciences. His main areas of expertise include the sociology of technology and the environment, as well as quantitative and qualitative methods of empirical social research.

Part I

Delphi Method: Concepts and Variants

The Delphi Method: An Introduction

Kerstin Cuhls

Abstract

The Delphi method has developed from a "classic" to a variety of Delphi methods or "types", which can have very different functions and are used in different subject areas. Online variants, especially the Real-time Delphi with instant feedback are becoming more and more popular. This introduction explains the different definitions, types and fields of application and shows the most important points to consider when using one of the Delphi methods. Special attention should be paid to the participants and their different backgrounds and expertise as well as to the design of the "questionnaire". For example, typical questions in a Delphi are about the importance or time horizon of realizing a statement about a future issue, e.g. a problem solution in the health care system, a technology, or an educational measure. The Delphi method will continue to have a place in the canon of methods used in Foresight and Futures Research as well as in general empirical research in various disciplines where uncertainty is an issue (e.g. business administration). The method will be integrated more and more into overall processes and is a building block in the method mix of futures sciences, e.g. coupled with scenarios.

K. Cuhls (✉)
Fraunhofer Institute for Systems and Innovation Research, Karlsruhe, Germany

University of Heidelberg, Heidelberg, Germany
e-mail: kerstin.cuhls@isi.fraunhofer.de

M. Niederberger, O. Renn (eds.), *Delphi Methods In The Social And Health Sciences*, https://doi.org/10.1007/978-3-658-38862-1_1

Writing an introduction to the Delphi method in 2018 is very presumptuous since on the one hand, there is no uniform definition, and on the other hand, different types of Delphi methods have been developed, some of which bear the name Delphi only because they ask about future topics. This is not sufficient for a definition, as discussed below. Another defining criterion common to all Delphi methods involves reassessing an issue or thesis under feedback.

In the following sections, the history of the Delphi method is briefly outlined to establish a basic understanding. An inventory of definitions is followed by an explanation of types, functions and fields of application as well as the basic questionnaire structure of a Delphi study. A short outlook summarizes the introduction.

1 The History of the Delphi Method(s)

The Delphi method was developed in the 1950s by the RAND Corporation in Santa Monica, California, as part of "operations research" (the predecessor of systems research). The name Delphi is reported to go back to the classical philologist Kaplan, who was reminded of the Greek oracle during the procedure.[1] The similarities with the ancient Delphi cannot be denied: The Oracle of Delphi predicted only action-related, subjective and individual-specific incidences. These were not given unambiguously, but in an ambiguous form by the Pythia, the medium in the temple Apollon, and passed on by the priests of the temple in interpreted, but still ambiguous form (orally or carved into slates). Since the prophecy is subjectively interpreted by the recipient, a momentum of action can lead to a (subjectively perceived) realisation as soon as it is uttered (self-fulfilling prophecy).[2] In some cases, information was obtained in advance by the oracle priests and incorporated into the interpretation of the prophecy, so that it was no longer so difficult to make an accurate statement about the person (Grupp, 1995, p. 26 ff.). Evidence for this is found in slates.

[1] On the history of the historical Delphi, see Maass (1993) or Parke (1956), but also Andronicos (1983); on the principle of self-fulfilling prophecy today, see Weaver et al. (2015) or Sternberg et al. (2011), among others.

[2] This phenomenon is also found in the very simple horoscopes (e.g. in magazines): The person who believes in the horoscope behaves accordingly and thus makes the event possible in the first place. The other possibility is that the horoscope is formulated so broadly that subjectively one of the individual events is true in any case.

The first Delphi surveys of modern times were conducted in 1953 in oral form and were devoted to military future topics, for which they had originally been developed.[3] In later times, the written form of the survey has prevailed, as it allows individual participants to easier change their mind (or not) without losing face or having to argue for it. First Delphi surveys via computer were tested early on (a first one in Germany already before 1979, Brockhoff, 1979), but it is only in the last 10 years that online variants have gained broad acceptance. An inventory shows that already in 2011, citation rates for Delphi articles were relatively high (Rowe & Wright, 2011). This suggests that the method is widely used. But let us start with the question of what is meant by the Delphi method.

2 Definition of the Delphi Method

The Delphi method is one of the subjective-intuitive methods of Foresight. The method is based on structured consultations and uses the intuitively available information of the respondents, who are usually "experts". However, the term "expert" is often defined very broadly (Cuhls, 2000, 2009, 2012). The Delphi method provides qualitative and quantitative results for Foresight and has normative as well as explorative and even prognostic elements. Since there is no single Delphi method, but diverse variations of application, there is a consensus that the "Delphi method is an expert survey in two or more rounds, in which the results of the previous round are fed back in the second or later rounds of the survey." Thus, from the second wave of the survey onwards, the experts judge under the influence of the opinions of their expert colleagues. Thus, the Delphi process is "a comparatively highly structured group communication process in which experts judge on issues about which uncertain and incomplete knowledge exists," according to Häder and Häder's (1995, p. 12; Häder, 2002, 2009, 2014) early working definition. Many use a pragmatic characteristic (see also Niederberger & Renn, 2018) similar to Wechsler's (1978, p. 23 f. translation) "standard Delphi method": "it is a monitor-group-driven, multi-round survey of a mutually anonymous group of experts for whose subjective-intuitive forecast consensus is sought. After each round of questioning, a statistical group judgement informs about the median and interquartile range of the individual forecasts and, as far as already possible, the arguments and counter-arguments of the extreme, i.e. outside the interquartile range, individual

[3] Helmer (1983), various sections. The very first Delphi surveys, however, are said to have been used for dog and horse betting since 1948, Woudenberg (1991, pp. 131–150) and Pill (1971, pp. 57–71), respectively.

forecasts are fed back in a standardised way." Whether consensus is sought or merely identified varies in each case.

Characteristic for Delphi surveys is thus:

- Contents of Delphi studies are always issues about which uncertain or incomplete knowledge exists. Otherwise, there would be more efficient methods for decision-making (Häder & Häder, 1995, p. 12).
- Delphi is a judgment process under uncertainty. The people involved in Delphi studies therefore make individual estimations (Landeta, 2006).
- Participation in Delphi studies requires experts who can make competent judgements based on their knowledge and experience (e.g. Seeger, 1979; Cuhls, 2000).
- Particular attention is given to the psychological processes taking place in the process communication of the Delphi survey, less on mathematical models (see especially Pill, 1971, p. 64; Dalkey, 1968, 1969a, pp. 541–551, 1969b; Dalkey et al., 1969; Dalkey & Helmer, 1963; Dalkey, 1967 or Krüger, 1975).
- Delphi studies attempt to harness the effects of self-fulfilling and self-destroying prophecies, each in the sense of influencing or "creating" a particular future (Cuhls, 1998).

Large scale Delphi surveys have been conducted since the 1990s (actually since 1963, see Helmer, 1966; Gordon & Helmer, 1964, or since the start of Japanese Delphi studies around 1969, Kagaku Gijutsuchô Keikakukyoku, 1971) to make use of the "wisdom of the crowd" (Surowiecki, 2004). However, it is debatable whether Surowiecki's observations are universally valid. For future topics that are in the "mainstream" and understood by many, however, more and more evidence for this joint knowledge can be found; tests in the Japanese Delphi studies also indicate this (Kanama et al., 2008; NISTEP, 2005; Kuwahara, 2001).

There is still no uniform definition of the term Delphi survey. According to Dalkey and Helmer, the procedure is suitable "to obtain the most reliable consensus of a group of experts ... by a series of intensive questionnaires interspersed with controlled feedback" (1963, p. 458). Linstone and Turoff (1975, p. 3) characterize Delphi "as a method for structuring a group communication process so that the process is effective in allowing a group of individuals, as a whole, to deal with a complex problem".

To sum up, *feedback* and *anonymity* (exception group Delphi: see Niederberger & Renn, 2018 and Schulz & Renn, 2009, respectively) are important characteristics of Delphi surveys. The Delphi technique as a Foresight tool seems to have adaptability, after all, it has "survived" the changing challenges of the last 50 years.

The procedure can be used with different understandings of Foresight and forecasting and was used by the users especially for questions concerning research, technology but also organisation, personnel or education. However, the application questions are diversifying more and more – and in practice, topics are often addressed, for which there is no need for a Delphi survey. But it sounds "fancy". Feedback is often "forgotten". The advantage of the Delphi survey is that the individual can express an opinion that is contrary to that of the other participants – and this with varying degrees of detail.

Since multiple perspectives are always required in decision-making (Linstone, 1998 or Linstone & Mitroff, 1994), the Delphi method can also be used in questions or for statements with a long-term time horizon. As has been shown in controlled scientific experiments, assessments from Delphi studies are not necessarily "better" or more accurate (especially in "predicting") than those from other consensus-based methods (Dalkey, 1969a, b or Häder & Häder, 1995, 2014). It is therefore the communicative power of Delphi approaches that enables switching from one perspective to the other.

The anonymity of the written or digital survey is an important psychological moment (Bardecki, 1984). In expert panels and other forms of group work, one of the fundamental problems is that opinion leaders emerge. "He can exert this influence because he can somehow reward or punish the influenced, e.g. by his social-emotional behaviour (friendliness), his social position or his assertiveness. He can also exert the influence if the influenced person considers him entitled to do so or identifies with him" (Becker, 1974, p. 14 f. translation). The anonymity of the Delphi procedure prevents the direct exercise of normative influence among the participants and shifts the exchange into anonymity.

This is important because there are almost always people in a group who "do not dare" to contradict or to speak out at all, especially if there are more powerful people or hierarchically higher people in the group. Thus, however, the knowledge of the influenced persons would[4] find less input into the final result compared to that of the opinion leaders (Becker, 1974, p. 52). The answer quality (in the sense of a prognosis) becomes worse, as could be proven in experiments.[5] Delphi surveys therefore involve a selection of all those who can be defined as "experts" or those affected. In order to achieve a sufficient foundation, the written form is more suitable, since in anonymous form and without "face to face" contacts, both changes

[4] Dalkey and Campbell have demonstrated that without the preservation of anonymity after the discussion, the result is not as accurate as the average opinion of the participants in the discussion before the discussion, Dalkey (1968).

[5] Dalkey (1969, p. 23 ff.). This result, however, is doubted by Sackman (1975).

of opinion, which are very difficult to admit, and insistence on one's own opinion, which may be contrary to others, are easier. Joint activity in groups is therefore not sufficient and is supported by anonymous procedures, "this further reducing the influence of certain psychological factors, such as specious persuasion, the unwillingness to abandon publicly expressed opinions, and the bandwagon effect of majority opinion" (Helmer & Rescher, 1959, p. 47).

Thus, the extent to which the expert in the interview wishes to be in cognitive dissonance (Festinger, 1978; Bardecki, 1984) with the group opinion depends on the individual. Some individuals will have a stronger desire to assimilate than others. Consequently, assenting one's own to the group opinion reduces the sense of dissonance that must otherwise be endured. For this reason, peer pressure plays a crucial role in terms of conformity (Dalkey & Helmer, 1963) and consensus-building (Woudenberg, 1991). Changing knowledge plays an equally important role (Becker, 1974, p. 54 f.).

Although the Delphi method was originally used in experiments for military purposes, it is now mainly used as a forecasting and futures research tool, in business studies but also in specific, e.g. as in this volume, nursing and health science contexts (Trevelyan & Robinson, 2015).

Users of the method particularly like the data sets "about the future", which are compiled with Delphi surveys and released for discussion (frequent feedback on BMFT 1993 and on Cuhls et al., 1998). Just writing down future topics in the form of short, concise statements seems to have an immense psychological effect, as it forces the transfer from implicit to explicit and thus "visible", transferable knowledge.

Nevertheless, there is a great danger that participants and organisers of futures studies regard the data as "the future that will be realized" – and not as working material on the way to a futures' assessment. When the media in Germany described the Delphi '98 data (see Cuhls et al., 1998) as an outlook into the next century or millennium for lack of other information about "the future", they often made the mistake of arguing that the future will be as described in Delphi '98 – without taking into account present or future decisions based on this foreknowledge. We have to be aware that decisions made today (even under a different set of information) affect things to come. So Delphi can only provide potential answers to those questions we have already identified today. Other questions or problems have yet to be identified - this requires other processes (often called "horizon scanning", see Cuhls et al., 2015).

Therefore, it can be summarized that Delphi and other surveys are tools to bring together the opinions and assessments of a certain (usually large) number of people on future issues. This type of questioning is particularly useful in processes, where the exchange of opinions and communicative effects are important, and which are particularly result-oriented. In cases, when data sets are needed for priority setting, Delphi studies provide the essential "basics", i.e. data that can also be used for subsequent roadmaps (Cuhls, 2017). In general, a Delphi process can be understood as a procedure, in which expert judgements on a specific issue are determined in an iterative procedure, with the aim of capturing and justifying consensus and/or dissent in the judgements.

3 Types of Delphi Surveys

Many different types of Delphi surveys have emerged in the meantime, and their names are often confusing. The *classic Delphi* is often referred to as the two-round or multi-round surveys that follow the basic definition mentioned above and provide feedback from the second round onwards, as well as having a strongly prognostic character (i.e. asking about the realisation period).

In addition, the *Policy Delphi* has developed, which is a classic two-round Delphi procedure, but includes policy issues or addresses solution-oriented questions (Turoff, 1970; Linstone & Turoff, 1975; Loe et al., 2016; but also Aichholzer, 2002). The aim here is to gather a wide range of opinions on a given topic. Delphi is seen here as "a tool for the analysis of policy issues" (Turoff, 1970, p. 80).

In addition to the Policy Delphi, the so-called *Decision Delphi* was developed, in which experts are called in to decide and also implement (Keeney et al,. 2011).

Mini-Delphis are studies on limited sectors or questions that are not as extensive as overview studies. However, the term is not defined. Frequently, similar approaches are found here as in the Policy Delphi, or problem- or solution-oriented statements are formulated and assessed (see e.g. Cuhls et al., 1995).

More recent developments are so-called attempts to conduct Real-Time-Delphis which run in "real time", i.e. the rounds are no longer separated, but the answers are fed back to the experts as soon as they log onto the internet platform for the second time (Gordon & Pease, 2006). These Delphi variants offer fast feedback (almost in real time) and have been further developed according to the technical possibilities, especially in recent years (for an overview of the software, see e.g. Aengenheyster et al., 2017).

The first attempts to conduct Real-Time-Delphis were promising (Friedewald et al., 2007; Zipfinger, 2007), but in practice it turns out that participants do not answer more than two or three times. The reason for this is usually time restrictions (as comments in Friedewald et al., 2007 suggest), so that the effect of having the opportunity to answer as often as desired, to change one's mind and to think about the issues again, is not so often used in the practical application of the method in the end. Real-time Delphi processes, when conducted online, also require more programming effort to enable immediate feedback, which is not complicated nowadays with ready-made tools, but it requires intense pre-testing.

The advantage of online-based methods (partly with ready-made tools) and Real-time Delphi surveys, in particular, is that the results are calculated immediately and are available at any time of the process. The disadvantage is that sample control becomes more difficult or even impossible (Aengenheyster et al., 2017). In case some people participate more often than others they theoretically have the chance to influence the results more than the less active people. In theory, they could even exert extreme influence by giving particularly strongly divergent answers, thereby misleading all other participants. However, this is only a theoretical possibility; to the author's knowledge, such behaviour has not yet been observed in reality.

A further discussion is concerns digital Delphi processes should be conducted online or offline. While the first surveys were still conducted with pen and paper surveys with the major disadvantage that they were very time-consuming (for postal or fax delivery) and printing cost-intensive, and then required further time and money to record and evaluate the results, there were already early attempts of computer-based Delphi studies (in Germany Brockhoff, 1979). Later electronic Delphi methods used e-mail or internet platforms to provide questionnaires that looked like paper questionnaires and could be printed out if necessary, only to be returned by traditional mail. In some countries, this is still the most efficient way to obtain a sufficiently large response sample[6]: conservative people or travelers without a laptop were also served in this way. In other countries, on the other hand, the Internet (online) variant has quickly become established, e.g. in Finland (Hämäläinen, 2003 or Salo & Gustafsson, 2004).

The advantages of digital questionnaires are that they allow the reflection of aggregated group responses in real-time or the integration of random variables. Real-time Delphi procedures as well as the new Argumentative Delphi surveys can only be conducted online since instant feedback is given here.

Argumentative Delphi (Gheorghiu et al., 2014; Seker, 2015): In this Delphi variant, the delivery of arguments to explain an assessment, e.g. of the realisation period or the importance of the topic, is the focus of the survey. For example, when asked about the realisation period, each participant provides one or more argu-

[6] The Japanese national Delphi of the NISTEP, for example, was for the first time conducted online in the tenth edition (published in 2015). 5 years earlier, the paper questionnaire had still been used.

ments as justification. For illustrative purposes, the first two arguments are given. The participants can now decide in favour of the given arguments (tick) or give one or two new arguments. During the course of the survey, a chain of pro and contra arguments, a ranking of the arguments, and a good understanding of the assessment are created. This can be repeated for other questions, e.g. the importance of the topic as in the EU project BOHEMIA (Andreescu et al., 2017).

Delphi Markets are an intermediate form between Delphi methods and Prediction Markets. Prediction Markets (unauthored, 2017; Luckner et al., 2005; Berg et al., 2000) are neither Delphi studies nor simple one-round surveys, and yet they can now be counted as part of the canon of surveys (with a "game-like approach") with feedback. Prediction Markets "trade" issues using fictitious "money", shares or other "currency" (chips, symbols). They are set up on a platform similar to the Real-time Delphi method, and participants can trade their "currencies" as often as they like betting on their "issues". After a certain time, a prediction market is usually terminated (for an overview of the procedure, see Luckner et al., 2005; Spann & Skiera, 2004; Berg et al., 2000).

Another variation is to use feedback with the help of special groupware in workshop discussions (e.g. Hämäläinen, 2003; Salo & Gustafsson, 2004 or Miles et al., 2004). In these cases, workshops with creativity methods or discussions are offered, and when enough statements or future topics are elaborated, they are evaluated using a certain set of criteria with the help of groupware (i.e. computers at each place in the room). Hämäläinen (2003) also describes a tool that can be used up to the decision-making stage. On the one hand, it uses anonymity for the assessments about the future and, on the other hand, it allows the participants to discuss openly and to change the opinion in the assessment of the criteria without immediately "losing face" or having to justify themselves. Consensus building is not in the forefront in these workshops – just as in other processes with Delphi procedures. Assessments can be made as often as the participants wish.

Group Delphi surveys are another alternative worth mentioning (for details, see Niederberger & Renn, 2018; Schulz & Renn, 2009; Webler et al., 1991). They consist of small, usually exclusively selected groups of participants and make use of intensive discussions. The Group Delphi was developed in the 1980s as a modification of the classic Delphi. This type of Delphi also arose from the need to obtain explanations for assessments. In the group Delphi, the questionnaire for the first round is developed at a workshop, sent to the participants before the workshop, or filled out together at the workshop. Anonymity no longer exists in these discussions. Open discussions replace the second or further rounds. For this, the focus is on consensus-building. The advantages of this face-to-face communication are mentioned by Webler et al. (1991, p. 258): immediate feedback, the justifications for differing views give insight into which deviations are accepted by the panel, and there is an internal check for the consistency of accepted opinions. Today, the procedure is mainly used when a direct exchange between experts from different disciplines seems appropriate and necessary.

Important differences exist between "one-off" surveys (also: futures surveys) and Delphi approaches (see Table 1).

4 Functions of Delphi Studies

In the early days of Delphi surveys, the improvement of the predictive ability was clearly in the forefront. However, with the use of Delphi surveys as a communication tool and the consideration that the estimation of a realisation time of the statements is "working material" instead of a classical forecast, this has changed. The focus of the investigation is more and more on the evaluation function according to the questions asked. However, in the current discussion, procedures such as "Delphi markets" are being tested, in which principles of prediction markets are combined with Delphi processes.

The main function of Delphi studies is still to look at long-term developments in order to assess and evaluate them and thus to train the handling of "uncertainty" as well as to obtain "data" (not facts!) about futures which help to deal with decisions. To achieve this, quantitative and qualitative elements are used together. Increasingly, the qualitative elements are even deliberately pushed to the fore. In an *argumentative* Delphi, for example, substantive explanations (arguments) are asked concerning the standardized quantitative judgments, and also in group Delphi or Delphi processes that are integrated into workshops (Delphi-in-workshops), substantive argumentations are combined with quantitative estimates. Delphi surveys are sometimes integrated into workshops as a building block by discussing topics and evaluating them online and instantaneously in a survey at a conceptually appropriate time. These can be conducted via an online platform and offer direct feedback, which is then either evaluated again (second round) or directly incorporated into the further discussion.

Delphi processes are increasingly combined with other research methods, as they start with theses/ statements or provide content for evaluation. Theses must be compiled in a structured process. This is done either through systematic searches in the literature, the use of standard classifications, horizon scanning (Cuhls et al., 2015) or other methods of expert inquiry such as workshops or interviews. In previous Delphi processes, the theses were often asked for and collected in a "preliminary round" (i.e. an extra survey). If the Delphi method is used in mixed-

Table 1 Differences between "one-off" futures surveys, Real-time Delphi and two-round Delphi procedures

	Futures surveys "once"	Delphi surveys	Real-time Delphi
Written or oral?	Written and oral possible	Fixed in writing	Only possible in writing online
Online or offline?	Online or offline possible	Online or offline possible	Online only
Rounds?	No correction or second assessment	Two or more "rounds": Correction and further assessment are the main component	No "rounds", but feedback and multiple requests to re-edit.
Feedback?	No feedback	Feedback (aggregated responses, anonymous)	Instant feedback (aggregated responses, anonymous)
Questions	Asking for assumptions, opinions, assessments	Asking for assumptions, assessments, opinions are usually corrected	Asking for assumptions, estimations, opinions, the possibility of correction
Number of participants	Number of participants should be statistically relevant for quantitative evaluations (minimum 20), exceptions for qualitative surveys	In the case of written quantitative assessments in the survey, the number of participants should be statistically relevant (minimum 20); in the case of group Delphi, smaller samples than 20 are also possible.	For quantitative assessments in the survey, the number of participants should be statistically relevant (minimum 20), for group Delphi also smaller samples than 20 are possible.
Background and expertise of the participants	Experts or/and non-experts, depending on the aim of the survey	Broad concept of expert ("persons who are knowledgeable about the topic")	Broad concept of expert
Representativeness	Representative survey possible, definition of what the sample should be representative for	Usually selective, not representative, since no one can be "representative" for the future	Usually selective, not representative, since no one can be "representative" for the future

(continued)

Table 1 (continued)

	Futures surveys "once"	Delphi surveys	Real-time Delphi
Anonymity	Anonymous and non-anonymous answers possible, evaluation usually anonymous	As a rule, anonymous answers, exception: Group Delphi	Anonymous answering, return of the results aggregated and anonymized
What futures?	Can be used for probable, possible or desirable futures	Can be used for probable, possible or desirable futures, but: probabilities are difficult to estimate even with two or more rounds	Can be used for probable, possible or desirable futures, but: probabilities are difficult to estimate even with two or more estimations
Alternatives	Alternatives can be asked for	Alternatives can be asked for and be evaluated in the second round	Alternatives can be asked for and included for further questioning
Comments	Comments are collected	Comments can be collected and fed back	Comments can be collected and fed back
Open questions	Explorative, open questions possible	Explorative, open questions (e.g. to complement the statements) possible	Explorative, open questions possible
Questions or statements (theses)?	Usually questions: direct, indirect, offline, online	Usually theses/ statements and questions (criteria) for the assessment of the statement	Usually theses/ statements and questions (criteria) for the assessment of the statement
Quality check	Additional quality check only via interviews	Additional quality check possible through further rounds	Additional estimations and corrections possible, but no integrated quality check

Own representation, further developed according to Cuhls (2012)

methods studies, within workshop discussions or focus groups, the actual Delphi method and its results move into the background and only make up a small (but often time-consuming) step within the overall process, but very much signify a combination of methods.

One of the functions of Delphi rounds is to enable a "consensus" to be established. However, since in some subject areas it is virtually impossible to establish a consensus (see e.g. Grupp, 1995, examples energy and biotechnology), today's Delphi surveys rather serve to determine *whether* a consensus already exists (i.e. everybody makes a similar assessment) or whether the subject is very controversial. This is also important information. If a consensus is not sought for and it is more a matter of generating information without the effect of mutual influence, it, therefore, makes sense in many cases not to conduct a Delphi survey but to set up a simple (one round) survey straight away.

One of the functions of Delphi studies is also to bring together the wisdom of the crowd (Surowiecki, 2004) into a structured process.

5 Areas of Application

The following application purposes for Delphi studies are mentioned: Delphi as

- direct means of communication
- decision-making tool
- problem-solving tool
- forecasting tool
- instrument of democratisation and participation
- planning instrument in operational or bureaucratic contexts
- evaluation and judgment tool.

In most cases, Delphi surveys simply provide information about future facts for discussion and evaluation, since there is uncertainty about these, which is to be reduced. As these facts or developments are to be assessed in a very short and, if possible, unambiguous statement form, restrictions concerning the method arise. Thus, it must first be assessed whether a multiple assessment is necessary at all or whether a simple survey is sufficient (Cuhls, 2012). Many Delphi studies are also conducted across multiple topics to generate an overview of future topics (e.g. Cuhls et al., 1998; Andreescu et al., 2017).

From the point of view of the subject areas, topics from research and technology are suitable, since these are, according to their definition, made by people and are therefore also likely to be accessible by people (always with reservations). Sometimes topics concerning educational issues are also approached with a Delphi survey (Kuwan et al., 1998; Prognos & Infratest Burke Social Research, 1998). A particularly large number of Delphi studies have been conducted in the health sector, as the contributions in this book also show. Of these, some are technology-centred, while others take the requirements of the health sector as their starting point. However, there are also studies in the area of "medical education research" (Humphrey-Murto et al., 2017), i.e., a combination with educational issues. Cross-cutting issues are often found in the topics of Delphi surveys, one example being the transfer of "private food marketing success factors to public food and health policy" (Aschemann-Witzel et al., 2012).

It is less easy to reduce societal issues to a short statement. Scenarios or other methods that work with longer descriptions are more suitable for societal and for complex issues. It is also possible to have pictorial representations assessed in a Delphi study. Images, like text, are interpreted very differently, but can also lead to a narrowing of the perspective. Which images are used must therefore be well considered – just like the question of narrowing in thinking.

Delphi studies are not only used in the academic field but are often found in applied research, for politics and ministries, associations and companies. The limits for Delphi studies lie especially in the resources (time, money, capacities), less in the topics. It should be noted, however, that very complex topics are not suitable for a survey. Complex issues have to be broken down into their components (theses, very short texts) and thus focused.

6 Questionnaire Design

The questionnaire design has all the possibilities that a classic social science survey also has - it must also meet scientific standards and it must be possible to communicate feedback and enable reassessment with the way the questionnaire is designed (see Gerhold et al., 2015).

Most questionnaires contain a set of statements to be assessed. The individual statement must be short, concise and unambiguous. Frequently, the questionnaire asks for the period of realisation of the statement in 5-year steps, the importance of the topic, the accuracy of the assessment and the expertise of the respondents (since Kagaku Gijutsuchô Keikakukyoku, 1971). Some Delphi studies also ask about the probability of occurrence, desirability (e.g. in the FAZIT project, Cuhls et al., 2007), and obstacles or problems on the way to realisation (Cuhls et al., 1995). Open questions or questions about alternative topics can also be found.

For the quantitative analyses, as in other scientific studies, the median, mean or mode are usually calculated (see Niederberger & Renn, 2018, p. 11) and fed back to the participants in the second round. For the feedback round, either distributions are presented or the median (sometimes also the average of the responses) is often fed back in a graph. Choosing a correct, non-misleading representation method that is at the same time easy to understand is the major challenge. The contributions in this book show some examples.

7 Participants

Even if Delphi studies are defined as expert surveys, they are usually dedicated to inter- and transdisciplinary research questions: The involvement of experts and practitioners in research processes plays an important role in these research questions. In overview studies, very different disciplines are addressed and the knowledge of very different expertise is combined. Therefore, the concept of expert is strongly relativized here. Delphi methods can be used for participatory knowledge production, integration or knowledge transfer. At the same time, the time between the first and second round of the survey is used to gather additional information about the topic (the brain does this by itself, it combines new information with known information - in this case, the information from the Delphi statement[7]).

In specific Delphi applications such as the Group Delphi, consensus is explicitly sought, even if it is the only consensus that there is no consensus (Schulz & Renn, 2009). However, there are also more recent attempts with dissent Delphi procedures that explicitly try to find out where the dissent lies (Steinert, 2009).

However, the most important common feature and difficulty of all Delphi methods are to attract people to participate in a survey. In a Delphi survey, the participants have to be especially motivated, because they are supposed to answer several times. This is becoming increasingly difficult, as more and more surveys are under way and it is difficult for the respondents to decide which participation is important and interesting for them personally.

The term "expert" is used very broadly for Delphi studies and now also includes people with very different backgrounds and from different sectors, who are supposed to be familiar with the topic area in each case. In most surveys, it, therefore, makes sense to carry out a self-assessment of expertise concerning the whole field or the individual topic. Often the degree of expertise is asked using a Likert scale (from "I work in the field..." to "no expertise"). A third-party assessment would be even better but is hardly feasible in practice. Over time, Foresight concepts have become more participatory, with more and more different groups of people taking part as "experts" (Cuhls, 2000).

---

[7] On the function of the brain, e.g. Burnett (2016).

The question is therefore who can be a "good" expert in the sense of good assessments of the future because particularly well-informed people are sometimes one-sided in their assessments (Grupp, 1995). For example, the experts in Delphi '98 considered the issues as "more important" when they worked in the field (Cuhls et al., 1998). Among the energy experts, particular differences were found between the supporters of solar energy and those of nuclear energy. In each case, they judged the topics from the perspective of the field, in which they worked to be more important and also realisable earlier (ibid., also Grupp, 1995; Blind & Cuhls, 2001; Blind et al., 2001). The main issue here seems to be the tendency to overestimate the own field of research (so-called "overestimation bias").

We once – in 1995 – did an involuntary test: In the second round of our Mini Delphi survey, the wrong first-round results were accidentally entered as feedback for a few theses in the second assessment round. Most of the people who rated their expertise as medium to high were surprised and expressed this surprise in the comments column – but often changed their opinion towards consensus or stuck to their previous view. Only the experts who assessed their expertise as "very high" scolded that this could not be or is a mistake, and stuck to their opinion (Cuhls et al. 1995). However, individuals working professionally in a field are better able to understand and judge complicated issues. In cases, where people with "low expertise" judge topics that they understand well, empirical evidence shows that there are hardly any differences in their judgements to those of "high-level experts" (Cuhls et al., 2002).

Therefore, for future surveys, it is usually advised to include a mixed composition of people from business, science, including non-governmental research institutions, as well as others (associations, banks, journalists, NGOs, etc.). In all studies, the number of participants must be large enough to be able to calculate and analyse the statistics properly. Further criteria should be established for the sample, such as age composition, gender, industries, etc. to find out whether older people answer differently than younger people or whether there are industry differences in the assessment of future topics. Nevertheless, in a survey of the future, the sample cannot be described as "representative", as is the case, for example, in classic opinion polls, because of the question who is representative of the future? Often women are underrepresented in surveys (especially on research and technology), this issue needs to be dealt with. Lobbying should be avoided or a solution found on how to deal with lobbyists, e.g. explicitly include the same number of people from different lobby groups. Here, however, identification is difficult.

In Foresight processes, one likes to rely on co-nomination (for details see Nedeva et al., 1996). However, these have the disadvantage that the selection of persons always remains within the relevant "circles" or "communities", i.e. no new persons or lateral thinking approaches are included, which is increasingly criticized.

Identifying addresses is becoming easier and easier: Internet, databases, online trade fair catalogues, membership lists, etc. can now be used without violating data protection guidelines. It then becomes more difficult to structure one's own database in such a way that, on the one hand, it is easy to handle to facilitate sending, recording and storing, but on the other hand, to fulfill all security requirements. However, these must be complied with.

How many people are invited to participate depends on the number of topics, statements, and questions as well as the expected response rate and other factors. If a small Delphi survey is intended in a room with computer groupware or even smartphones, the sample can be relatively small (group size of ten to twelve people). However, when it comes to a national Foresight program that requires specific representativeness, more people are asked and an attempt is usually made to get more than 100 responses per thesis. This means that up to 500 people have to be asked per field. Of course, this also depends on the country: in smaller countries, there are not so many experts in the field. In Germany, for example, finding people who are familiar with detailed questions of space travel presented us with great challenges early on (BMFT, 1993).

In some very long-term future fields, even in large countries, there are very few people working on the issues. To note this is a result in itself. The example statement "More than 20% of the EU population has coupled sensors to their brains to enhance their sense spectrum (infrared, ultraviolet, vibration, magnetic fields etc.)" certainly cannot be evaluated by many. When asked "50% of passenger transport is fully automated."[8] the ordinary citizen at least understands the statement and can assess it – perhaps differently than the expert. Involving the general public is generally possible, but then the questions must be quite easy to understand. Only then is the ordinary citizen on an equal footing with the specialist.

8 Outlook

The methods of Foresight are clearly to be selected according to their objective and the purpose of the study. In the future, online Delphi surveys will finally prevail. For all types of surveys, there will be entire modular systems, which will also enable software-supported generation of statements. However, the formulation of the questions will remain essential for the quality of the entire procedure. Even if there

[8] For examples from the BOHEMIA project, see Andreescu et al. (2017).

is now standard software for the creation and evaluation of questionnaires, the results' quality depends immensely on content of the survey and the willingness of the experts to participate.

In all cases, the Delphi method must be integrated into a larger Foresight or futures research context. Depending on the objectives and sub-steps that one wants to achieve with the survey, the methodology must be adapted. Therefore, modern Delphi studies are usually multi-methodological. To give some examples: Most Delphi surveys ask for the period of realisation in five-year steps (all Japanese Delphi studies by NISTEP, e.g. NISTEP, 2005 or 2015, predecessor: Kagaku Gijutsuchô Keikakukyoku, 1971; in Germany e.g. BMFT, 1993; Cuhls et al., 1995, 1998, 2002; Prognos et al., 1998; Andreescu et al., 2017 and many others). Simple roadmaps can be created directly from the corresponding data sets by arranging the statements and their data according to the time of realisation (Cuhls et al., 1995, 1998, 2017; Cuhls & Möhrle, 2008). If the categories and statements fit together, even limited scenarios can be elaborated (e.g. "targeted scenarios" in the BOHEMIA project, see European Commission, 2018). Such analyses can help to visualize breaks or anomalies in the assessments on survey statements or it helps to elaborate a strategy. It can be checked how plausible the results are, e.g. if one development is estimated earlier than another, it can happen that the associated technology may not have been developed yet - but the experts nevertheless estimated the development so early.

This leads to the question of plausibility. In the German Delphi '98 (Cuhls et al., 1998), we found some breaks (results that were not logical) in the sense of time jumps, especially in the field of management and production. For example, the experts expected that the salary payment systems would develop strongly in the direction of performance pay or pay in company shares (from the point of view of that time a very early median assessment, quartiles 2004 and 2010). These were bold claims at the time. However, no implausibilities could be found, it fitted that first "for the wage share no longer only the individual performance was decisive, but the group performance or the operating result" (2002–2008 expected), that in the next phase, there are "objectified evaluation keys..." and the "majority of companies remunerates performance-related with company shares..." (2003–2010).

Even if the feasibility of all surveys can be greatly simplified online, not only design, speed and manageability (as simple as possible for the users and the evaluation) are important, but the content and interpretability of the results must not be forgotten. In the case of ambiguous statements, for example, interpretation is simply impossible. If the samples and response rate are too small, a quantitative analysis cannot be carried out or can lead to a very one-sided overall result. If there are too many statistics and too many statistical tests, there is often no interpretable result left at all.

The issues of sample selection and the address database remain the same online as offline, even if it is easier to capture addresses automatically. Data protection guidelines must be observed in all cases. In online surveys, it must be taken into account to retain sample control. One experience is that response rates in online surveys are relatively low (especially in Germany), sometimes below 10% (e.g. Bioeconomy Council, 2015; El-Chichakli et al., 2016; Andreescu et al., 2017). Accordingly, more individuals need to be addressed or more incentives for participation need to be set.

Although there will be more and more modular systems for simple and multi-round surveys of all kinds in the future, each researcher must think carefully about which approach is used in which cases. Content must be precisely adapted. In recent years, many have "dabbled" in design, often failing to consider that the content is neither understandable nor evaluable. Finding the balance between design and content is an art. In the same way, some of the tools tempt you into statistical analysis that no one understands, but you have a number. This is also not helpful.

The formulation of statements is still the most important and at the same time the most time-consuming task in a Delphi survey. The questions or criteria for the theses must also be precisely coordinated and tested. Since surveys are often created under time pressure, pretests are often omitted. This is fatal because during tests the organizers of the process usually notice that the statements they thought were understandable are not at all - or even worse: ambiguous. Sometimes criteria and theses do not fit together or are simply not assessable. Sometimes also the handling of the questioning confronts the users with unsolvable problems. Therefore, time should be invested at these points.

Keys of the Delphi method, despite all the effort involved, are the feedback and the need to think about the same topic at least twice and, accordingly, to ask questions twice. In simple surveys, there is no corrective, i.e. the answer that is given once counts in the end, it cannot be corrected. Accordingly, surveys with feedback allow revising the assessment. This has advantages for estimations under uncertainty. However, the potential influence by the systems and the procedure should not be underestimated (Rowe et al., 2005, p. 396; also: involuntary test in Cuhls et al., 1995), so that it rarely becomes clear why the experts have changed their opinion and what they have allowed themselves to be influenced by. On the one hand, this can be the given assessment of other experts, but on the other hand, it can also be an external influence. For example: In the Japanese Delphi of 1997, the statements on the construction of a "nuclear fuel cycle" were strongly influenced by an accident that occurred between the first and second round of questioning (NISTEP, 1997; Cuhls, 1998, 2003).

All the questions about sample selection, generation of content, formulation of theses, and criteria that applied to written and printed questionnaires in the past have lost none of their brisance online. Even if information technology systems suggest new possibilities to us, they often reach their limits here or even limit the possibilities of the content (Aengenheyster et al., 2017).

In all Delphi variants and also in simple surveys there are still a lot of open questions. The boundaries between a Delphi, Real-time Delphi, and a one-round survey are becoming more and more blurred. This also makes the definition of a Delphi procedure "fluid". The inflationary use of the term "Delphi" is equally unhelpful here. More and more often, simple surveys without a link to the future are already called "Delphi" – and without a feedback loop, they are not Delphi either.

Delphi surveys cannot and should not be used in every case. If the topics cannot be reduced to simple statements or questions, other methods are called for in Foresight processes: scenarios, systems dynamics, discourses, time travel, more complex creative processes or other workshop-based approaches might then be the better choice.

Many surveys are "overloaded" by the new technical possibilities and designs as well as by the many topics that come to the experts' minds and the "questionnaire" is too long. Here it is still true: Less is often more and is better answered by the experts. Simple manageability is still not a matter of course.

If the goal is clear, the organizers of a survey should first consider how the results can get from one phase to the next, what form they should take, and whether the combination of methods with a Delphi procedure is, therefore, appropriate or even the right choice. Without clarifying this, the right choice cannot be made.

To carry out a Delphi study just because one "would like to do a Delphi" makes little sense. Therefore, it should be well considered at the beginning whether it should be such an elaborate approach or whether a "simple" survey would not suffice. If "facts" (in the sense of a survey) and not assumptions are asked for, Delphi methods are not necessary. The choice of methods is therefore not so easy because the repertoire of possibilities is expanding more and more. Sometimes, however, it is enough to look again and again at one's objectives and then at the differences between the methods to make the right decision.

Literature

Aengenheyster, S., Cuhls, K., Gerhold, L., Heiskanen-Schüttler, M., Huck, J., & Muszynskae, M. (2017). Real-time Delphi in practice – A comparative analysis of existing software-based tools. Technological Forecasting and Social Change https://doi.org/10.1016/j.techfore.2017.01.023.

Aichholzer, G. (2002). Das ExpertInnen-Delphi: Methodische Grundlagen und Anwendungsfeld Technology Foresight. In A. Bogner, B. Littig, & W. Menz (Hrsg.), *Das Experteninterview* (p. 133–153). VS Verlag. https://doi.org/10.1007/978-3-322-93270-9_6.

Andreescu, L., et al. or European Commission (2017). New horizons: Data from a Delphi survey in support of European Union future policies in research and innovation (Report KI-06-17-345-EN-N). 10.2777/654172 or https://ec.europa.eu/research/foresight/index.cfm. Accessed 28 April 2018.

Andronicos, M. (1983). Delphi.

Aschemann-Witzel, J., Perez-Cueto, F. J. A., Niedzwiedzka, B., Verbeke, W., & Bech-Larsen, T. (2012). Transferability of private food marketing success factors to public food and health policy: An expert Delphi survey. *Food Policy, 37*(2012), 650–660.

Bardecki, M. J. (1984). Participant's response to the Delphi method: An attitudinal perspective. *Technological Forecasting and Social Change, 25*, 281–292.

Becker, D. (1974). *Analyse der Delphi-Methode und Ansätze zu ihrer optimalen Gestaltung*. Dissertation, Mannheim.

Berg, J., Forsythe, E. R., Nelson, F., & Rietz, T. A. (2000). *Results from a dozen years of election futures markets research*. College of Business Administration, University of Iowa. http://www.biz.uiowa.edu/iem/archive/BFNR_2000.pdf. Accessed 6 Sept 2011.

Bioeconomy Council. (2015). Global visions for the bioeconomy – An international Delphi-study, durchgeführt von K. Cuhls, V. Kayser, & S. Grandt. Fraunhofer ISI. http://gbs2015.com/fileadmin/gbs2015/Downloads/GBS2015_02_Delphi-Study.pdf. Accessed 29 Sept 2018.

Blind, K., & Cuhls, K. (2001). Der Einfluss der Expertise auf das Antwortverhalten in Delphi-Studien: Ein Hypothesentest. *ZUMA-Nachrichten, 49*, 57–80.

Blind, K., Cuhls, K., & Grupp, H. (2001). Personal attitudes in the assessment of the future of science and technology: A factor analysis approach. *Technological Forecasting and Social Change, 68*, 131–149.

Brockhoff, K. (1979). *Delphi-Prognosen im Computer-Dialog. Experimentelle Erprobung und Auswertung kurzfristiger Prognosen*. Mohr.

Bundesministerium für Forschung und Technologie (BMFT) (Ed.). (1993). *Deutscher Delphi-Bericht zur Entwicklung von Wissenschaft und Technik*. BMFT.

Burnett, D. (2016). *Unser verrücktes Gehirn*. C. Bertelsmann.

Cuhls, K. (1998). *Technikvorausschau in Japan. Ein Rückblick auf 30 Jahre Delphi-Expertenbefragungen*. Physica.

Cuhls, K. (2000). Opening up foresight processes. *Économies et Sociétés, Série Dynamique technologique et Organisation, 5*, 21–40.

Cuhls, K. (2003). From Forecasting to Foresight processes – New participative Foresight Activities in Germany. Cuhls, K. & Salo, Ahti (Hrsg.), *Journal of Forecasting, Wiley Interscience, Special Issue, 22*, 93–111.

Cuhls, K. (2009). Delphi-Befragungen in der Zukunftsforschung. In R. Popp & E. Schüll (Eds.), *Zukunft und Forschung (Wissenschaftliche Schriftenreihe des Zentrums für Zukunftsstudien Salzburg): Bd.1. Zukunftsforschung und Zukunftsgestaltung. Beiträge aus Wissenschaft und Praxis*. Springer.
Cuhls, K. (2012). Zu den Unterschieden zwischen Delphi-Befragungen und "einfachen" Zukunftsbefragungen. In R. Popp (Ed.), *Wissenschaftliche Schriftenreihe Zukunft und Forschung des Zentrums für Zukunftsstudien Salzburg: Bd. 2. Zukunft und Wissenschaft: Wege und Irrwege der Zukunftsforschung* (S. 139–159). Springer.
Cuhls, K. (2017). Unternehmensstrategische Auswertung von Foresight-Ergebnissen. In M. Möhrle & R. Isenmann (Eds.), *Technologie-Roadmapping*, VDI (pp. 47–62). Springer. https://doi.org/10.1007/978-3-662-52709-2_4.
Cuhls, K., & Möhrle, M. G. (2008). Unternehmensstrategische Auswertung der Delphi-Berichte. In M. G. Möhrle & R. Isenmann (Hrsg.), *Technologie-Roadmapping, Zukunftsstrategien für Technologieunternehmen* (3. Revised and extended edition. pp. 107–135). Springer.
Cuhls, K., Breiner, S., & Grupp, H. (1995). *Delphi-Bericht 1995 zur Entwicklung von Wissenschaft und Technik – Mini-Delphi.* Karlsruhe (Druck als Broschüre des BMBF, Bonn 1996).
Cuhls, K., Blind, K. & Grupp, H. (Hrsg.). (1998). *Delphi '98 Umfrage. Zukunft nachgefragt. Studie zur globalen Entwicklung von Wissenschaft und Technik. Methoden- und Datenband, Karlsruhe.* https://doi.org/10.13140/2.1.2412.8965.
Cuhls, K., Blind, K., & Grupp, H. (2002). *Innovations for our future. Delphi '98: New foresight on science and technology. Technology, innovation and policy* (Series of the Fraunhofer Institute for systems and innovation research ISI no. 13). Physica.
Cuhls, K., von Oertzen, J., & Kimpeler, S. (2007). *Zukünftige Informationstechnologie für den Gesundheitsbereich. Ergebnisse einer Delphi-Befragung, FAZIT-Schriftenreihe.* Stuttgart. https://www.fazit-forschung.de
Cuhls, K., van der Giessen, A., & Toivanen, H. (2015). *Models of horizon scanning. How to integrate horizon scanning into European research and innovation policies.* Report to the European Commission, Brussels, also: Cuhls, K. (2019). Horizon scanning in foresight – Why Horizon Scanning is only a part of the game. *Futures and Foresight Science*. https://doi.org/10.1002/ffo2.23.
Dalkey, N. C. (1967). *Delphi*. RAND Corporation. https://www.rand.org/content/dam/rand/pubs/papers/2006/P3704.pdf. Accessed 7 April 2019.
Dalkey, N. C. (1968). *Predicting the future*. Rand Corporation.
Dalkey, N. C. (1969a). Analyses from a group opinion study. *Futures, 2*(12), 541–551.
Dalkey, N. C. (1969b). *The Delphi method: An experimental study of group opinion, prepared for United States Air Force Project Rand.* Rand Corporation.
Dalkey, N. C., & Helmer, O. (1963). An experimental application of the Delphi-method to the use of experts. *Management Science, 9*, 458–467.
Dalkey, N. C., Brown, B., & Cochran, S. (1969). *The Delphi method, III: Use of self ratings to improve group estimates*. Rand Corporation.
de Loe, R. C., Melnychuk, N., Murray, D., & Plummer, R. (2016). Advancing the state of policy Delphi practice: A systematic review evaluating methodological evolution, innovation, and opportunities. *Technological Forecasting and Social Change, 104*, 78–88.

El-Chichakli, B., Braun, J., Barben, D., Lang, C., & Philip, J. (2016). Five cornerstones of a global bioeconomy. *Nature, 535*, 221–223.

European Commission/European Union. (2018). Transitions at the horizon: Perspectives for the European Union's future research- and innovation-related policies. https://ec.europa.eu/info/research-and-innovation/strategy/support-policy-making/support-eu-research-and-innovation-policy-making/foresight/activities/current/bohemia_en

Festinger, L. (1978). *Theorie der kognitiven Dissonanz*. In M. Irle & V. Möntmann (Hrsg.), Verlag Hans Huber.

Friedewald, M., von Oertzen, J., & Cuhls, K. (2007). *European perspectives on the information society: Delphi report*. EPIS Deliverable 2.3.1. Fraunhofer ISI, Brussels: European Techno-Economic Policy Support Network (ETEPS). http://epis.jrc.es/documents/Deliverables/EPIS%202-3-1%20Delphi%20Report.pdf. Accessed 6 Sept 2011.

Gerhold, L., et al. (Eds.). (2015). *Zukunft und Forschung: Bd. 4. Standards und Gütekriterien der Zukunftsforschung. Ein Handbuch der Wissenschaft und Praxis* (S. 86–93). Springer.

Gheorghiu, R., Andreescu, L., & Curaj, A. (2014). *Dynamic argumentative Delphi: Lessons learned from two large-scale foresight exercises*. In Contribution to the 5th International Conference on Future-Oriented Technology Analysis (FTA) – Engage today to shape tomorrow, Brüssel (S. 27–28).

Gordon, T., & Pease, A. (2006). An efficient, RT Delphi: "Round-less" almost real time Delphi method. *Technological Forecasting and Social Change, 73*, 321–333.

Gordon, T. J., & Helmer, O. (1964). *Report on a long-range forecasting study*. Rand Corporation.

Grupp, H. (Ed.). (1995). *Der Delphi-report* (collaboration with S. Breiner & K. Cuhls). dva.

Häder, M. (2002). *Delphi-Befragungen – Ein Arbeitsbuch*. Springer.

Häder, M. (2009). *Delphi-Befragungen – Ein Arbeitsbuch* (Zweite Aufl.). Springer.

Häder, M. (2014). *Delphi-Befragungen: Ein Arbeitsbuch* (2. Aufl.). Springer.

Häder, M., & Häder, S. (1995). Delphi und Kognitionspsychologie: Ein Zugang zur theoretischen Fundierung der Delphi-Methode. *ZUMA-Nachrichten, 37*.

Hämäläinen, R. P. (2003). Decisionarium – Aiding decisions, negotiating and collecting. *Journal of Multi-Criteria Decision Analysis, 12*, 101–110. https://doi.org/10.1002/mcda.350

Helmer, O. (1966). *Social technology*. Rand Corporation.

Helmer, O. (1983). *Looking forward. A guide to futures research*. Sage.

Helmer, O., & Rescher, N. (1959). On the epistemology of the inexact sciences. *Management Science, 6*, 47–52.

Humphrey-Murto, S., Varpio, L., Wood, T. J., Gonsalves, C., Ufholz, L., Mascioli, K., Wang, C., & Foth, T. (2017). The use of the Delphi and other consensus group methods in medical education research: A review. Academic Medicine https://doi.org/10.1097/ACM.0000000000001812. Accessed 18 Jan 2018.

Kagaku Gijutsuchô Keikakukyoku (Hrsg.). (1971). *Gijutsu Yosoku Hôkokusho* (Bericht zur Technikvorausschau). Tôkyô.

Kanama, D., Kondo, A., & Yokoo, Y. (2008). Development of technology foresight: Integration of technology roadmapping and the Delphi method. *International Journal of Technology Intelligence and Planning, 4*(2), 184–200.

Keeney, S., Hasson, F., & McKenna, H. (2011). *The Delphi technique in nursing and health research*. Wiley-Blackwell.

Krüger, U. M. (1975). *Die Antizipation und Verbreitung von Innovationen. Entwicklung und Anwendung eines kommunikations-strategischen Konzeptes unter besonderer Berücksichtigung der Delphi-Technik*. Dissertation, Köln.
Kuwahara, T. (2001). *Technology foresight in Japan: The potential and implications of DELPHI approach* (NISTEP research material no. 77), S. 119–135.
Kuwan, H, Ulrich, J. G., & Westkamp, H. (1998). Die Entwicklung des Berufsbildungssystems bis zum Jahr 2020: Ergebnisse des Bildungs-Delphi 1997/98. *BWP, 6*, 3–8. http://www.forschungsnetzwerk.at/downloadpub/kuwan1998_bwp_06_1998.pdf. Accessed 29 Sept 2018.
Landeta, J. (2006). Current validity of the Delphi method in social sciences. *Technological Forecasting and Social Change, 73*, 467–482.
Linstone, H. A. (1998). *Multiple perspectives revisited*. In IAMOT conference, Orlando.
Linstone, H. A., & Mitroff, I. I. (1994). *The challenge of the 21st century: Managing technology and ourselves in a shrinking world*. State University of New York Press.
Linstone, H. A., & Turoff, M. (Eds.). (1975). *The Delphi method: Techniques and applications*. Addison Wesley/Advanced Book Program.
Luckner, S., Kratzer, F., & Weinhardt, C. (2005). *Stoccer – A forecasting market for the FIFA World Cup 2006*. In Proceedings of the 4th Workshop on e-Business (WeB 2005).
Maass, M. (1993). *Das antike Delphi. Orakel, Schätze und Monumente*. Wissenschaftliche Buchgesellschaft.
Miles, I., Green, L., & Popper, R. (Hrsg.). (2004). WP 4 futures forum, D4.2 Scenario methodology for foresight in the European research area, Fistera – Thematic network on foresight on information society technologies in the European research area. Manchester. http://fistera.jrc.ec.europa.eu/pages/latest.htm. Accessed 3 Dec 2010.
National Institute of Science and Technology Policy (NISTEP) (Hrsg.). (1997). *The sixth technology forecast survey – Future technology in Japan toward the year 2025* (NISTEP report no. 52). Tokyo.
National Institute of Science and Technology Policy (NISTEP) (Hrsg.). (2005). *Comprehensive analysis of science and technology benchmarking and foresight* (NISTEP report no. 99). Tokyo.
National Institute of Science and Technology Policy (NISTEP) (Hrsg.). (2015). *The 10th science and technology foresight* (Report no. 164). Tokyo. http://data.nistep.go.jp/dspace/bitstream/11035/3079/2537/NISTEP-NR164-SummaryE.pdf
Nedeva, M., Georghiou, L., Loveridge, D., & Cameron, H. (1996). The use of co-nomination to identify expert participants for technology foresight. *R&D Management, 26*(2), 155–168.
Niederberger, M., & Renn, O. (2018). *Das Gruppendelphi-Verfahren. Vom Konzept bis zur Anwendung*. Springer.
Parke, H. W. (1956). *The Delphic oracle*. Blackwell.
Pill, J. (1971). The Delphi method: Substance, context, a critique and an annotated bibliography. *Socio-Economic Planning Science, 5*, 57–71.
Prognos, A. G., & Infratest Burke Sozialforschung. (1998). *Delphi-Befragung 1996/1998 Potentiale und Dimensionen der Wissensgesellschaft – Auswirkungen auf Bildungsprozesse und Bildungsstrukturen. Integrierter Abschlussbericht*. Selbstverlag.
Rowe, G., & Wright, G. (2011). The Delphi technique: Past, present, and future prospects – Introduction to the special issue. *Technological Forecasting and Social Change, 78*, 1487–1490.

Rowe, G., Wright, G., & McColl, A. (2005). Judgment change during Delphi-like procedures: The role of majority influence, expertise, and confidence. *Technological Forecasting and Social Change, 72*, 377–399.

Sackman, H. (1975). *Delphi critique. Expert opinion, forecasting, and group process*. Rand Corporation.

Salo, A., & Gustafsson, T. (2004). Group support system for foresight processes. *International Journal of Foresight and Innovation Policy, 1*(3–4), 249–269.

Schulz, M., & Renn, O. (Eds.). (2009). *Das Gruppendelphi. Konzept und Fragebogenkonstruktion*. VS Verlag.

Seeger, T. (1979). *Die Delphi-Methode: Expertenbefragung zwischen Prognose und Gruppenmeinungsbildungsprozessen*. Hochschul.

Seker, S. E. (2015). Computerized argument Delphi technique. *IEEE Access*. https://doi.org/10.1109/access.2015.2424703

Spann, M., & Skiera, B. (2004). Einsatzmöglichkeiten Virtueller Börsen in der Marktforschung. *Zeitschrift für Betriebswirtschaft (ZfB), 74*, 25–48.

Steinert, M. (2009). A dissensus based online Delphi approach: An explorative research tool. *Technological Forecasting and Social Change, 76*, 291–300.

Sternberg, E., Critchley, S., Gallagher, S., & Raman, V. V. (2011). A self-fulfilling prophecy: Linking belief to behavior. *Annals of the New York Academy of Sciences, 1234*(1), 83–97. https://doi.org/10.1111/j.1749-6632.2011.06184.x

Surowiecki, J. (2004). *The wisdom of crowds*. Anchor: Doubleday.

Trevelyan, E. G., & Robinson, N. (2015). Delphi methodology in health research: How to do it? *European Journal of Integrative Medicine, 7*, 423–428.

Turoff, M. (1970). The design of a policy Delphi. *Technological Forecasting and Social Change, 2*(2), 149–171.

Unauthored. (2017). *Delphi*. Whitepaper Delphi Markets. https://delphi.markets/whitepaper.pdf. Accessed 15 Feb 2018.

Weaver, J., Filson Moses, J., & Snyder, M. (2015). Self-fulfilling prophecies in ability settings. *The Journal of Social Psychology*. https://doi.org/10.1080/00224545.2015.1076761

Webler, T., Levine, D., Rakel, H., & Renn, O. (1991). The group Delphi: A novel attempt at reducing uncertainty. *Technological Forecasting and Social Change, 39*(3), 253–263.

Wechsler, W. (1978). *Delphi-Methode, Gestaltung und Potential für betriebliche Prognoseprozesse (Schriftenreihe Wirtschaftswissenschaftliche Forschung und Entwicklung)*. Florentz.

Woudenberg, F. (1991). An evaluation of Delphi. *Technological Forecasting and Social Change, 40*(2), 131–150.

Zipfinger, S. (2007). *Computer-aided Delphi – An experimental study of comparing round-based with real-time implementation of the method*. Trauner.

The "Classic" Delphi. Practical Challenges from the Perspective of Foresight

Karlheinz Steinmüller

Abstract

The Delphi method is still frequently used in its original form to engage experts to assess uncertain issues. This article examines the practical challenges one is confronted with when carrying out such studies and which solutions exist: from the identification and recruitment of experts to the development of the questionnaire to the design of the survey rounds and finally to pitfalls in evaluation and interpretation. The results are largely transferable to other variants of the Delphi method.

1 Introduction

For more than half a century, the Delphi method has been one of the best-known and most frequently used tools in the repertoire of foresight methods (Popper, 2009). Accordingly, it has undergone numerous adaptions and modifications from Real-Time Delphi (Gordon, 2009b) to Group Delphi (Niederberger & Renn, 2018). With some justification, the Delphi method can be described as an almost paradigmatic procedure of futures studies. It manifests many epistemological problems

K. Steinmüller (✉)
Z punkt GmbH, Berlin, Germany
e-mail: steinmueller@z-punkt.de

M. Niederberger, O. Renn (eds.), *Delphi Methods In The Social And Health Sciences*, https://doi.org/10.1007/978-3-658-38862-1_2

and practical challenges of any foresight activity – right up to the misuse of the attractive term Delphi for surveys with only one round of inquiry. At the same time, the word Delphi still resonates with the slight irony that led the inventors of the methodology in the 1950s and early 1960s to name the procedure after the ancient oracle: We know, after all, that predictions are a difficult field and that only gods know the future from direct observation ...

The Delphi method serves to generate fairly reliable assessments of issues about which only incomplete knowledge, unsecured hypotheses or mere assumptions exist. These assessments are based on collective intelligence, the structured use of the knowledge of a community of experts - including tacit, not yet explicit knowledge – and at least to some extent through the exchange of arguments, ideally with free communication among equals. In this respect, the Delphi method is a mechanism for generating what Bertrand de Jouvenel (1967) called conjectures: reasoned speculations (hypotheses) about the future. Given its conjectural approach, it is not surprising that Delphi studies have been the subject of empirical investigation from their inception, esp. with respect to the quality of outcomes and variations in procedures (Linestone & Turoff, 1975; Rowe et al., 1991).

The Delphi method has several advantages: It allows the representation of group opinions and can therefore be regarded as a method for controlled group communication. It ensures the transfer of reputation from the participating experts to the study and its results. Above all, however, it is considered a procedure with which prejudices and biases can be contained by balancing the individual biases of the experts. Applied to future topics, the Delphi method also brings about a certain general attunement to anticipatory thinking among the participants, and generally sensitizes them to uncertainty.

In the following, after a short outline of the method, the practical challenges that have to be overcome when using the classic Delphi method will be presented. The focus here is on pitfalls in the application of the method, not on a detailed presentation of the procedure or in-depth analyses of the methodology or the philosophy of science behind it. For the former, see, for example, Häder (2009); for the latter, see, by way of example, the thematic special issue of the journal *Technological Forecasting and Social Change,* No. 78 of 2011 (Rowe & Wright, 2011). The following comments and interpretations are based on years of personal experience of the author in the field of futures research. As I see it, the insights gained here can largely be transferred to other areas and other types of Delphi studies.

2 Basic Characteristics of the Method

In general, the Delphi method serves to "obtain the most reliable opinion consensus of a group of experts by subjecting them to a series of questionnaires in depth interspersed with controlled opinion feedback" (Dalkey & Helmer, 1962, p. v). The procedure should at the same time induce and support cognitive processes and minimize negative group dynamic effects, such as pressure of opinion and groupthink, influence of social status or reputation, profiling by taking opposite stances, effects of rhetoric, ... This is guaranteed by three central characteristics of the method[1]:

1. **Anonymity:** The participants of a Delphi survey remain anonymous. They do not learn what individual assessments or estimates the other participants have made.
2. **Iteration:** Several (usually two) rounds of survey take place so that the participants can reconsider and adjust their assessments or estimates.
3. **Controlled feedback:** After each round, the responses are qualitatively and/or quantitatively (statistically) evaluated and fed back to the participants in aggregated form (frequency distribution, medians, quantiles, anonymized comments ...) so that they receive an expanded information base for renewed reflection.

The classical Delphi method is based on a series of assumptions that are generally considered plausible. For some specific cases, however, these assumptions are questioned in methodological studies (Woudenberg, 1991).

- **Expertise:** It is assumed that experts in their field, especially when they come to the same conclusions, make much more valid and better-reasoned assessments than less informed people.
- **Wisdom of the many:** It is assumed that predictions or other estimates made by a group of experts are superior to predictions or estimates made by individual experts in terms of their correctness[2] or probability of occurrence (Hill, 1982, p. 517), because a group has a broader spectrum of relevant information (Rowe

[1] For the broad spectrum of definitions and characterizations of the Delphi method, see Häder (2009, p. 19 ff.).

[2] The problems begin, however, with what is considered "valid" or "correct". In the case of items relating to the future (as with some others), agreement with the facts can only be established ex post, if at all. Grunwald points out that "equating good with correct predictions ... is meaningless" (Grunwald, 2012, p. 172 f.).

et al., 1991, p. 235). In addition, possible biases within the group may cancel each other out.

- **Convergence:** It is assumed that the assessments of the experts involved converge from round to round thanks to intermediary feedback. This convergence is expressed in a decrease of statistical measures of dispersion (variance) or comparable parameters. However, it must be emphasized that not all Delphi studies aim at consensus building.

2.1 Wide Range of Applications

Usually, the Delphi method is applied where facts are uncertain; where the question is not amenable to empirical treatment and where experts with their background experience can be relayed on. Thus, the Delphi method competes with expert interviews, surveys with only one round (Cuhls, 2012) and working group meetings or workshops. Often the Delphi method serves as a "method of last resort" (Linstone, 1978, p. 275), which is used when other approaches fail. However, it is not an "all-round method", but can only be employed usefully if certain preconditions regarding the specifics of the question and the structure of the expert community are fulfilled (Häder, 2009, p. 23). Traditional fields are in particular technology foresight and questions from the field of health care (Adler & Ziglio, 1996; Thangaratinam & Redman, 2005; Gordon, 2009a, p. 3).

Depending on purpose, different types of Delphi studies can be distinguished. Häder (2009, p. 30 f.) lists in particular Delphi surveys for the aggregation of ideas, for the prediction of future situations, for the determination of expert views and for consensus building. However, a general, overarching typology is still lacking here.

It should be taken into account that in a Delphi study, as in surveys in general, several types of items can be used. Following Gordon (2009a, p. 5), three types of questions can be distinguished in Delphi studies on technological developments:

- *Predictive type* – predictions about the occurrence of future developments: When will a certain event occur or what is the probability of occurrence within a given time horizon? What will be the value of a certain parameter (e.g. market size) at a certain future time?

- *Normative type* – items on the desirability of future developments: If a certain event occurs, would it be seen as positive (desirable) or negative (undesirable) taking into account different aspects of evaluation? Which arguments speak for or against the event?
- *Instrumental type* – items related to options of "shaping the future": What actions, strategies, or instruments can be used to ensure that a particular desired future state is achieved or an undesirable one is avoided? What are facilitating or inhibiting influences?

3 Preparatory Phase

The typical procedure of a Delphi study (Fig. 1) begins with a preparatory phase. In this phase, the objectives of the survey are defined and the procedure is planned in detail.

The first and often underestimated challenge consists in putting the research question into concrete terms and/or to define what kind of information is to be generated by the Delphi study. Experience has shown that the client's wishes regarding the type and variety of information, its granularity, the degree of detail, etc. often exceed what the study or the potentially participating experts are capable of providing. To give an almost trivial example: It would certainly be extremely useful to know when exactly and where the next wave of influenza will start and

Main steps of a Delphi

Classical Delphi studies usually follow the following basic flow chart

1. Preparation and planning of the study
2. Identification and recruitment of experts
3. Development of the questionnaire
4. First round of survey
5. Analysis of the returns of the first round and formulation of feedback
6. Second round of survey
7. Analysis of the returns of the second round
8. Further rounds of survey (if necessary)
9. Analysis of the entire survey process
10. Evaluation and reporting

Fig. 1 Typical sequence of a classical Delphi procedure. (Own representation)

how virulent the pathogen will be; but as soon as these questions become too specific (exact day, number of cases at the municipal district level in the first 72 h), even proven experts are forced into mere guesswork - or they refuse to answer "excessive" questions. It is therefore important not to fall into the trap to put all your wishes for information into the survey, but to develop realistic expectations about experts' knowledge and their willingness to provide assessments, and to formulate the items accordingly.

As with other types of studies, the time required is often underestimated. This concerns both the duration of the survey rounds (see below) and the analysis. Good project management allows for possible delays, e.g. in the recruitment of experts, in dealing with latecomers among the respondents, etc., and thus minimises friction. In general, it is advisable to think and plan from the end: How and by whom should the results be used? In what form should they be recorded? When and how should the results be presented and published?

For larger studies, it is also advisable to set up a group, often called a steering group, monitoring group or steering committee, which accompanies the project in terms of content and methodology. Such a group of experts can take on a variety of functions. It can support the project team in communication and coordination with the client, it can give methodological advice in the sense of an accompanying evaluation, it can suggest experts to be recruited or it can be involved in pre-tests. Of course, such a circle of experts is associated with additional effort, even if it is only the time for meetings.

4 Identification and Recruitment of Experts

The quality of a Delphi study stands and falls with the experts involved. Identifying them and getting them to participate is often a difficult and time-consuming task, especially if the organisers of the study do not themselves belong to the narrow specialist community – which is the rule rather than the exception in future-oriented studies.[3] The central challenge in Delphi studies is therefore, as Häder and Häder (2000, p. 18 f.) and Gordon (2009a) point out, to find those people who are most likely to be able to answer the given questions.

[3] Niederberger and Renn (2018, p. 8) point out that the Delphi team must present themselves as competent interlocutors ("quasi-experts"), i.e. they must be sufficiently familiar with the topic. This familiarity with the topic is already needed when they approach the experts,

4.1 Heterogeneity of the Panel

Ideally, the entirety of experts in a particular field would be included in the study. However, the questions of Delphi studies originate only in exceptional cases from a single discipline. As a rule, Delphi topics are interdisciplinary or transdisciplinary, they do not fall within the area of competence of a single discipline, and often enough the focus is on questions of practice, on the implementation of scientific findings, or innovations in a broad social context. The perspective of practical application – in the field of business, politics, social welfare – requires that, in addition to experts from the academic field, well-informed specialists with practical work experience also contribute their assessments: managers, politicians, representatives of social organizations – and depending on the issue, also affected citizens or, in health studies, patients.

Recruiting the panel for a survey with questions about the future cannot aim at representativeness in a socio-demographic sense. The decisive factors are expertise and diversity of perspectives. Typically, all relevant stakeholders should be included and outsider positions should also be taken into account — which entails, among other things, a great heterogeneity of the panel in terms of professional backgrounds, individual experiences, etc. Considering that the quality of the results can be controlled by the composition of the panel, this is a decisive challenge of Delphi studies. Balance and representation even of extreme positions count more than pure quantity.

4.2 Panel Size

The size of the expert group, the panel, depends on the research question. In narrowly conceived, disciplinary, monothematic studies, a size of ten to twenty responses may be sufficient; depending on the response rate, the number of persons invited to participate may be several times that. In the case of transdisciplinary questions, as they are typical for futures studies, a sufficient number of representatives from science and relevant fields of practice must be taken into account, so that thirty to fifty responses is a minimum target size. In the case of more extensive, multi-thematic Delphi studies, such as Delphi studies on several fields of technology, separate panels have to be formed, each responsible for one topical area, so that the total number of experts can quickly reach hundreds or even thousands. It is important to strike a good balance: If the number of experts is too small, extreme opinions may be given too much weight and statistical evaluation procedures will then no longer be effective. With an increasing number of experts, however, the effort - and often enough the time required - naturally increases too.

4.3 Identification and Recruitment

Within a scientific discipline, experts can be found quite efficiently based on their publications or academic positions. But where to look out for experts in business or society? Good access is offered by conferences and symposia, where practitioners from management or social organisations have their say, but you can approach also industry associations, interest groups or similar organisations. Sometimes experts attract attention through their presence in the media. Experience shows that such opinion leaders are invited more often than others to participate in studies, working groups, etc., which makes them interesting as experts with many useful connections in their field.[4]

Very often, experts are asked to recommend other experts that could be invited. Recruitment by recommendation – known as co-nomination – has, however, a certain disadvantage. It can result in a kind of selection: only experts of similar opinion (of a scientific school or of an economic or social interest group) are taken into account, which should of course be avoided. It should also be noted that although formal (academic) status and reputation are good predictors of the competence of experts, the experts with the deepest knowledge are often hidden in the hierarchical structure. Assistants often know more about a very specific subject area than their superiors.

In principle, panel recruitment is about systematically tapping into expert networks. Phone calls or individual e-mails may be time-consuming, but as a rule there is no way around them.

4.4 Motivation for Participation

The most comprehensive list of names fails to serve its purpose if the experts cannot be motivated to participate. What do they get in return for the time they invest

---

[4] In terms of content, one can rarely expect new impulses from these opinion leaders. Particularly among experts who are overrepresented in the media, there is a statistically conspicuous number of people with fixed, almost dogmatic opinions - "hedgehogs" according to Tetlock's typology (2005).

in filling out the questionnaire several times? Depending on the topic of the study and the stakeholder category, different motives come into play (Aichholzer, 2002, p. 13). Some panelists may regard it as relevant that they can influence decisions through their answers, others feel perhaps obliged to the initiators of the study or the commissioning institution, another group hopes to learn something new by participating in the study – at least they learn how colleagues assess the items. Scientists and many practitioners are usually interested in the results of the study. If only a condensed version of the results is communicated publicly, the complete package of the results or a privileged access to the results can serve as an incentive. In particular cases, book vouchers or similar material incentives can also be used. Certainly, it is essential to appreciate the commitment of the experts. Under certain circumstances, this can also include the publication of their names, e.g. in the appendix of the study.[5] Of central importance, however, is the efficient, so to speak "user-friendly" design of the questionnaire: good comprehensibility, concreteness and no excessive complexity.

5 Development of the Questionnaire

Designing questionnaires is an art of its own and an important methodological topic in empirical social research. Unclear, ambiguous formulations, missing answer options, information overload, sentences with double negatives, items that are too presuppositional or hypothetical, problems with scales are only some of the mistakes that can be observed again and again despite all warnings in textbooks. An overview of important principles of questionnaire design is given in Fig. 2. Today, more attention is often paid to an appealing visual design than to cleanly formulated items. However, we will not go into these generally known problems, but rather elaborate such challenges that are almost necessarily associated with Delphi studies, especially those on future issues.

5.1 Item Generation

Defining the items and finding the most appropriate wording is never a trivial process. Even when the specific purpose of the survey is neatly determined, e. g. in the framework of a larger research project, and the central questions are known, it

[5] If the participants agree to this. This does not set aside the anonymity of the evaluation of the individual items.

Guidelines for questionnaire design

Expertise of the experts: Ask what the experts can contribute from their experience, not everything what you wish to know.
Keep it simple: Don't overwhelm the experts with too many questions and too many response options; include only the items that are really necessary.
Clarity and specificity: Structure the questionnaire clearly and concisely and use precise, unambiguous and consistent terminology; if necessary, explain terms and concepts in a generally understandable way.
No leading questions and presuppositions: Avoid wordings that already hint to a certain answer, refrain from implicit (or explicit) judgements, e.g. through an emotionally colored choice of words.
No combined or conditional statements about the future: Avoid double negative statements. Avoid linking several aspects or hypotheses with each other, e.g. in the form of reasons, why a certain situation might occur.
Complete sets of response options: Be sure to offer all logically possible options and do not force participants to answer every question, even those where they feel absolutely incompetent. Without options of the type "don't know / no answer", a Delphi questionnaire is incomplete.

Fig. 2 Guidelines for questionnaire design. (Own representation)

makes sense to set up a specific (sub-)process for the collection, filtering and phrasing of the items. It must be clarified whether, in addition to the designated project team, (external) experts, representatives of the client or of stakeholders (associations or other organisations) should also be involved, and whether, in addition to research, brainstorming or other workshop formats may be needed to identify the items. Therefore, the formulation of the theses or items is usually preceded by a discourse with the expert community about the topics to be included and issues to be excluded, about the appropriate terminology, etc.

As with all survey methods, greatest attention should be paid to the wording of the items. Clarity, unambiguity and maximum comprehensibility should be aimed for. The Delphi method encounters the semantic difficulties inherent in futures studies (Steinmüller, 1997, p. 77): The future of society, of economy, technology, etc. is an unknown – and unnamed – field. Accordingly, there is a lack of relevant terminology for topics that are emerging and developing rapidly. Terminology is in flux, interest groups try to gain influence through their coinage of words, and, in addition, trend researchers keep feeding poorly consolidated fashionable buzzwords into debates. In the case of only recently established research fields, moreover, a uniform vocabulary has not yet emerged; various neologisms compete with each other and suffer shifts in meaning. Paraphrases and explanations are therefore often unavoidable. To formulate items concisely, precisely, without implicit value statements and at the same time meaningfully requires some experience.

On the other hand, it makes little sense to ask for facts in Delphi studies that can be determined elsewhere. This leads to an unnecessary inflation of the questionnaire. More importantly, experts in the field would not really feel appreciated, but exploited, and for participants who are not experts in the specific question, it would be a pure knowledge test.

5.2 The Challenge of Heterogeneous Panels

As mentioned above, the panels for Delphi studies are usually very heterogeneous. Terms that are trivial for experts may be new or completely unknown to practitioners – or worse, misunderstood. And vice versa, terms that are commonplace in a field of practice and understood by everyone may cause scientists to shake their heads. An explanation that puts one participant in the picture may be considered banal by another, and even the form of the items – as a thesis, as a question, a miniature scenario ... – may be received differently. Designing Delphi questionnaires can thus also imply building bridges between different knowledge cultures and doing justice to the different backgrounds and perspectives of the respondents.

As a point of orientation, one can say that the wording should be as comprehensible as a good non-fiction book. An extensive pre-test of the questionnaire with representatives of the different stakeholders or knowledge cultures is highly recommended. All too often, a very specific reading of terms, a very specific interpretation of concepts or phrasings has become ingrained in the project team. Third parties will not necessarily understand them (operational blindness of the team).

5.3 Addition of Comments

Delphi studies can include both open and closed questions. Open questions are appropriate when the range of possible answers cannot be predetermined, when the respondents' own words are important for the study, or when gaps in knowledge are to be revealed. Closed questions are appropriate when the dimensions of the responses are to be standardized and made comparable, when the frequencies and correlations of the responses are to be determined, and when only a limited number of response options are (logically) possible. As a rule, Delphi studies operate primarily with closed questions, since they have the advantage that you can base the feedback after the rounds on a statistical analysis. Quite often it is advisable to supplement closed with open questions, especially with comment fields, in which the experts can state the reasons for their assessments. Such collections of arguments – mostly pro and con – are highly relevant for the feedback between the rounds, because they allow a low-threshold discourse among the panel participants. In addition, comments often provide valuable ideas that can be evaluated and followed up.

5.4 Future-Related Items

Frequently, in Delphi studies the items are formulated as "miniature scenarios", such as "Politicians will significantly lose trust by 2030". The experts are then asked to rate the probability of occurrence according to a given scale. Alternatively, the time horizon by which such a statement could become reality is asked. To combine both would in principle make sense, because what is unlikely in the short term could become a de facto certainty in the longer run. However, a combined question - quasi as a matrix of probability and time period – might be too ambitious for most experts and, to my knowledge, is nearly never used in Delphi studies.

Of course, the items can also be formulated as questions ("Which party will have the say in the next ten years?"), refer to catchwords ("Please select adjectives that describe the jobs of the future best: flexible, multimedia ...") or include rankings ("Please sort the following arguments for the use of autonomous vehicles according to their social relevance: …").

Sometimes the experts are confronted with complex hypothetical future situations. Not everyone finds it easy to think their way into a "what if" scenario, especially if it does not correspond to their own expectations of the future. For most people it is challenging to answer questions about specific aspects of a future they regard as improbable or implausible. For example: "Imagine a world in which everyone has a digital health advisor – in the form of a smartphone app, for example - and no longer needs a GP. How will the relationship between specialist and patient change under this condition?" Not all experts are willing to engage in such hypotheses, and the question about the likelihood of the assumed future situation will influence the subsequent assessments. Nevertheless, such items may prove useful and fruitful.

5.5 Self-Assessment of Competence

Another specific feature not only of future-oriented Delphi studies are so-called subjective competence questions. They are usually included in order to let the statements of experts with specific expertise flow into the analysis with more weight than those of laypersons or only generally informed persons. The subjective competence question asks for a self-assessment of the participants with regard to an item or a group of items, e.g. whether one has specific expert knowledge for the given question, is basically informed or has no deeper knowledge.

Sometimes people are asked whether they are "very certain", "somewhat certain", "somewhat uncertain" or "very uncertain" of their assessment. The basic idea here is that experts should be very sure of their judgements. One could therefore exclude opinions of people who describe themselves as uncertain from further analysis, or at any case give them less weight. This kind of filtering does not seem justified to me. Experts are very often aware of how presuppositional their answers are, while laypersons can lull themselves into a deceptive sense of certainty. The value of such questions does not consist in their use as a filter, but in drawing conclusions - in addition to the divergence of the assessments - about the collective level of uncertainty.

6 The Rounds of Interviews

6.1 First Round

After pretesting and possible revision, the questionnaires are sent to the group of experts. In former times, this was usually done by mail or fax, today e-mail is the standard communication channel for classical Delphi studies – for real-time Delphis a website. The accompanying letter or e-mail should inform the participants about the background of the study, the clients and the intended use of the results. Equally important are details about the deadline for returns, the processing time, and that data protection and anonymity are guaranteed.

Sufficient time for the rounds should be provided for, according to experience 4–6 weeks, whereby holiday periods should be taken into account. Even if the response rate exceeds a sufficient level, it is advisable to send a reminder e-mail shortly before the deadline. In case of insufficient return rates, extensions of the deadline are not unusual. In most cases even extremly late responses are included that arrive when the team is already working on the final analysis.

The effort that has to be made to generate a sufficient number of responses is often underestimated. Follow-up campaigns, e-mails or telephone calls are nothing unusual. Often, additional participants have to be recruited, be it through recommendations from the panel (co-nominations) or further research. Well-structured participant management systems, in which every contact is recorded, are very helpful and basically indispensable for larger panels. Of course, they must comply with data protection guidelines. Subsequent incentivisation is questionable because it creates inequality.

6.2 Analysis of the Returns of the First Round

In accordance with the project objective, the responses of the first round are analysed, in the case of open questions mostly only qualitatively, in the case of closed questions quantitatively (statistically).

The feedback that is returned to the participants is meant to make them rethink their own assessments. In concrete terms, the effect of the feedback depends on the type of information given, its formulation and also the context (accompanying letter ...). Complete neutrality or objectivity of feedback information is highly desirable, but rather never perfectly achieved (Vorgrimler & Wübben, 2003, p. 766). The organisers of the study, the research team should take utmost care with the feedback, as they did in formulating the questionnaire. Sometimes a pretest of the feedback information, e. g. involving the steering committee, can be useful here. But even then vested interests might influence the wording.

Items with probabilities of occurrence and time horizons are typical for Delphi studies on future topics. In this case, frequency distribution and statistical parameters such as median and/or mean value, upper and lower quantiles are usually calculated and presented in a suitable graphical form for the feedback to the participants.

Sometimes the responses from the first round reveal shortcomings in the approach, for example when certain items have a high refusal rate or when comments point out weaknesses in the wording or missing response options that were overlooked in the pretest. Reworking the questionnaire reduces the comparability of the results of the rounds, but may be necessary in particular cases.

Sometimes first round surveys are even designed to generate additional items: Question type "Which aspects are still relevant in the context?" Indeed, the inclusion of additional items does not correspond to the pure doctrine of the Delphi method. But as long as they are only minor additions to the questionnaire, there is nothing to object to. In the analysis, however, the different genesis of the items must be taken into account.

Experience has shown that it is not very useful to work with mean values for estimated times until the occurrence of future events (e.g. until a technological breakthrough happens) – extreme assessments influence mean values too strongly. As a rule, a representation with median, lower and upper quartile is returned to the expert group. And, obviously, the comments are also fed back to the panel – at least in condensed form.

6.3 Second Round

The basic assumption of the Delphi method is that the experts replying to the second round review their assessments on the basis of the results of the first round and adjust them if necessary, so that a kind of consensus emerges. It is taken for granted that the panelists orient themselves on the assessments of the others, especially on the median, and that experts with extreme assessments that lie far from the median are more inclined to revise their judgment than those who have quasi agreed with the mainstream. However, in addition to this pull of the majority opinion, tactical counter-positions are also conceivable: one gives an even more extreme assessment in order to shift the mean or median in the direction of one's own assessment. In practice, however, this seems to happen only in exceptional cases.

The number of responses in the second round is almost always significantly lower than in the first. This so-called panel mortality can have various reasons, e. g. that individual experts have changed their job or academic position and/or can no longer be reached. Another reason may be that some experts find it annoying to fill out the same questionnaire again. In some studies on the Delphi methodology, a "dogmatic" behaviour of some experts is reported – they are not willing to deviate from their original opinion (Linstone, 1978, p. 296 f.).

Factors such as the influence of intuition, the self-assessment of experts and the size of the panels and the role of dogmatism have from the beginning been the subject of secondary studies (Linestone & Turoff, 1975; Rowe et al., 1991; Häder & Häder, 2000). The extent to which further – third and fourth – rounds contribute to more valid results has been also investigated, in particular with respect to the convergence of assessments. Closer consensus by more rounds seems to be rather an exception; the experts change their opinions only minimally (Häder, 2009, p. 120). In addition, panel mortality increases with the number of rounds. Therefore, Delphi studies with more than two rounds are a rarity.

7 Analysis of the Entire Survey Process

Numerous circumstances must be taken into account in the final analysis and interpretation. For example, higher fluctuation between rounds or relevant panel mortality can change the entire structure of the panel – composition in terms of stakeholder groups – which must of course be taken into account in the evaluation. In individual cases, especially in studies that extend over a longer period of time, recent external events (news related to the topic, new scientific findings) can influence the adjustment of expert judgements much more than the feedback within the expert community conveyed by the study.

7.1 Images of the Future

Delphi studies often provide the subject for fundamental misunderstandings in public perception, but not exclusively in public perception. The most common one is that the statements derived from the study are regarded as facts, quasi as a somehow objectively existing, real future (Cuhls, 2009, p. 214). The result of any future research, however, is always a construct, in the best case the somewhat conclusive and more or less consensual image of the future, as seen by a certain expert community (Neuhaus, 2015). A survey of a different group of experts would have produced a different picture of the future, at least in detail. Interpretations of a Delphi study must therefore emphasise that the results are the opinion of a specific panel. The Delphi procedure is designed to produce a consolidated, at least partly consensual image of the future with a higher degree of stability and validity, but it is and remains a construct that was generated in a very specific way. In addition, this image of the future can certainly be coloured by the respective zeitgeist, rather optimistic or pessimistic basic moods in the expert community – in individual cases, influences of recent news and topics covered by the media can even become visible, so that a repetition of the study with the same experts after a certain time laps would produce somewhat different results. Philosophically, this is called "the immanence of the present" (Grunwald, 2012, p. 183).

7.2 Pro-domo Assessments

The most knowledgeable expert is not able to provide absolutely objective assessments; situational aspects and biases inevitably have an effect. Delphi studies are intended to minimize these factors by way of aggregating individual assessments, but they cannot completely eliminate situational aspects or balance out biases. As a case in point, researchers frequently underestimate the time till their current or intended research efforts are successfully concluded. This may be due to exaggerated hopes or too much self-confidence, but sometimes it is clearly due to a kind of strategic positioning (pro-domo effect): Potential research sponsors or superiors would become very reluctant if they had to assume that a breakthrough would not occur within a reasonable period. On the other hand, if the time horizon is too close, experts may run the risk of being asked for their results too soon.[6] Therefore, in Delphi studies, it seems that not the experts directly involved in a topic, but the colleagues from the neighbouring laboratory or a neighbouring field give the more realistic estimates, at least with regard to the time periods necessary for a technological development or a research effort (Cuhls et al., 1995, p. 13). In addition, narrow specialisation may blur the view on important framework circumstances, so that highly specialised experts often make systematically incorrect predictions (operational blindness).

7.3 Consensus and Prediction

Consensual predictions were the primary purpose when the Delphi method was established, and they are still an important goal today. Delphi serves as tool for forecasting in peculiar, when the method is used to estimate time periods until the occurrence of a given event and/or its probability of occurrence (e. g. in the case of the realization of a miniature scenario).

The Delphi procedure is very effective in generating consensus under the condition of anonymity, it is, however, subject to similar, albeit mitigated, group pressures as other procedures. Moreover, consensus is not identical with ex post "accuracy". In general, accuracy of prediction – "hitting" exactly what will happen – should not be seen as the primary goal of Delphi studies: The results can be regarded as good (in the sense of relevant and useful) if the assessments of the items by the expert community provide new insights and useful orientation, regardless of how strongly the expert agree or disagree and whether their assessments later come true (Grunwald, 2012, p. 172 f.). Seen in this light, the Delphi method is less a procedure for generating more or less reliable forecasts or for establishing a stabilized consensus in an expert group, but rather a specific discursive procedure that triggers reflection on possible futures, on models and roadmaps and, as part of the social discourse, exerts an influence on developments. In many cases it may be therefore more productive and inspiring when dissenting opinions are upheld and justified. The communication process is the decisive factor, not the tendency towards consensus.

---

[6] One example are estimates on the time needed for a breakthrough in controlled nuclear fusion: since the first technological Delphi study in the 1960s, the breakthrough has always been expected for in about three or four decades.

In public perception, however, it is almost inevitable – even with absolutely clear and unambiguous communication – that the results of a Delphi study are misunderstood as forecasts.

7.4 Opportunities Beyond Consensus

Delphi surveys generate a wealth of information that is often not fully exploited in the analysis. A focus only on consensus or mean values and medians ignores the potential that is hidden precisely in differences, in dissent, in divergent judgements. Minority votes and extreme positions should therefore not be negated as unattractive statistical "outliers", but analysed and, if necessary, regarded as valuable indications of other points of view, especially if they are supported by comments and good arguments.

Usually, the answers to the individual items are analysed separately, which, from a statistical point of view, amounts to a marginal distribution. At most, the answers are statistically evaluated, as in representative surveys, with regard to the socio-demographic characteristics of the experts, their affiliation to professional groups, positions, etc., if these are asked for at all. Such an analysis can provide highly relevant information about differing attitudes of the mentioned groups to certain problem areas or specific questions. A much deeper opportunity offered by statistics, the analysis of correlations between items, is to my knowledge virtually never used. Cross-correlations can provide information about hidden groupings within the panel – beyond the above-mentioned characteristics – groupings that differ by certain basic attitudes, world views, perspectives, and, perhaps, by their images of the future.

7.5 Combination with the Scenario Method

Diverging expert opinions have a special value: they point to uncertainties and contingencies. Such disagreements may be based on specific experiences and different perspectives on a topic, for example that one expert rates a certain factor as an important driver, but another expert regards the same factor as driven and volatile. When using the Delphi method in the context of a scenario study (Armbruster et al., 2006), a clear and stable disagreement on an item can therefore provide a relevant hint to a key factor (a factor that has a strong impact but a high uncertainty with respect to its future development). Relevant differences in the assessments can then be translated into diverging future projections of this factor (v. d. Gracht, 2008). In this case, dissent is decidedly more productive than consensus.

8 Conclusion

The classical Delphi method has many advantages. It is a practicable and well-established way to collect expert opinions and to arrive at more or less consensual views of the future. It encourages reflection on the future and gives experts the opportunity to reconsider their own judgements. The responses of the survey rounds can be analysed in many ways: with regard to consensus and dissent, with regard to implicit and explicit images of the future, etc. Last but not least, the results of Delphi studies are easy to communicate, since they represent the wisdom of many experts.

Delphi studies can be conducted in many different ways. As a technique that is largely based on communication, the results of a Delphi are open to many influences, for example the choice of experts, the phrasing of statements, the presentation of the feedback between the rounds, etc. Methodological vigilance, a sure instinct for challenges and pitfalls as well as diplomacy in dealing with the experts are a prerequisite for the successful implementation of a study. The quality of a Delphi study stands and falls with clear research questions, a competent panel, good participant management and a well formulated questionnaire. Its usefulness, however, depends on a meaningful, differentiated interpretation of the results and preparation, presentation and documentation of the results well targeted to the research audience.

References

Adler, M., & Ziglio, E. (1996). *The Delphi method and its applications to social policy and public health*. Jessica Kingsley.

Aichholzer, G. (2002). *Das ExpertInnen-Delphi: Methodische Grundlagen und Anwendungsfeld "Technology Foresight"*. Wien: ITA – Institut für Technikfolgen-Abschätzung der Österreichischen Akademie der Wissenschaften (ITA-Manuskript 01/2002).

Armbruster, H., Kinkel, S., & Schirrmeister, E. (2006). Szenario-Delphi oder Delphi-Szenario? Erfahrungen aus zwei Vorausschaustudien mit der Kombination dieser Methoden. In J. Gausemeier (Ed.), *Vorausschau und Technologieplanung* (S. 109–137). Universität Paderborn Heinz Nixdorf Institut.

Cuhls, K. (2009). Delphi-Befragungen in der Zukunftsforschung. In R. Popp & E. Schüll (Eds.), *Zukunftsforschung und Zukunftsgestaltung. Beiträge aus Wissenschaft und Praxis* (S. 207–221). Springer.

Cuhls, K. (2012). Zu den Unterschieden zwischen Delphi-Befragungen und "einfachen" Zukunftsbefragungen. In R. Popp (Ed.), *Zukunft und Wissenschaft. Wege und Irrwege der Zukunftsforschung* (S. 139–157). Springer.

Cuhls, K., Breiner, S., & Grupp, H. (1995). *Delphi-Bericht 1995 zur Entwicklung von Wissenschaft und Technik. Mini-Delphi.* Fraunhofer-Institut für Systemtechnik und Innovationsforschung.

Dalkey, N., & Helmer, O. (1962). *An experimental application of the Delphi method to the use of experts*. RAND (RM-727/1-Abridged).

de Jouvenel, B. (1967). *Die Kunst der Vorausschau*. Luchterhand.

Gordon, T. J. (2009a). The Delphi method. In J. C. Glenn & T. J. Gordon (Eds.), *Futures research methodology version V 3.0*. The Millennium Project.

Gordon, T. J. (2009b). The real time Delphi method. In J. C. Glenn & T. J. Gordon (Eds.), *Futures research methodology version V 3.0*. The Millennium Project.

Gracht, H. A. (2008). *The future of logistics – Scenarios for 2025*. Gabler.

Grunwald, A. (2012). Ist Zukunft erforschbar? Zum Gegenstandsbereich der Zukunftsforschung. In W. J. Koschnick (Ed.), *FOCUS-Jahrbuch 2012. Prognosen, Trend- und Zukunftsforschung* (pp. 171–195). FOCUS Magazin Verlag.

Häder, M. (2009). *Delphi-Befragungen. Ein Arbeitsbuch*. VS Verlag.

Häder, M., & Häder, S. (2000). Die Delphi-Methode als Gegenstand methodischer Forschungen. In M. Häder & S. Häder (Eds.), *Die Delphi-Technik in den Sozialwissenschaften. Methodische Forschungen und innovative Anwendungen* (pp. 11–31). Westdeutscher Verlag.

Hill, G. W. (1982). Group versus individual performance: Are N + 1 heads better than one? *Psychological Bulletin, 91*(3), 517–539.

Linstone, H. A. (1978). The Delphi technique. In R. B. Fowles (Ed.), *Handbook of futures research* (pp. 273–300). Greenwood Press.

Linstone, H., & Turoff, M. (1975). *The Delphi method: Techniques and applications*. Addison-Wesley.

Neuhaus, C. (2015). Prinzip Zukunftsbild. In L. Gerhold, D. Holtmannspötter, C. Neuhaus, E. Schüll, B. Schulz-Montag, K. Steinmüller, & Karlheinz (Eds.), *Standards und Gütekriterien der Zukunftsforschung. Ein Handbuch für Wissenschaft und Praxis* (pp. 21–30). Springer.

Niederberger, M., & Renn, O. (2018). *Das Gruppendelphi-Verfahren. Vom Konzept bis zur Anwendung*. Springer.

Popper, R. (2009). *Mapping foresight. Revealing how Europe and other world regions navigate into the future*. European Commission, Directorate-General for Research (EUR 24041 EN).

Rowe, G., & Wright, G. (2011). The Delphi technique: Past, present, and future prospects – Introduction to the special issue. *Technological Forecasting and Social Change, 78*, 1487–1490.

Rowe, G., Wright, G., & Bolger, F. (1991). Delphi: A reevaluation of research and theory. *Technological Forecasting and Social Change, 39*(3), 235–251.

Steinmüller, K. (1997). *Grundlagen und Methoden der Zukunftsforschung. Szenarien, Delphi, Technikvorausschau* (SFZ-WerkstattBericht Nr. 21). Sekretariat für Zukunftsforschung.

Tetlock, P. E. (2005). *Expert political judgment. How good is it? How can we know?* Princeton University Press.

Thangaratinam, S., & Redman, C. (2005). The Delphi technique. *The Obstetrician & Gynaecologist, 7*, 120–125.

Vorgrimler, D., & Wübben, D. (2003). Die Delphi-Methode und ihre Eignung als Prognoseinstrument. *Wirtschaft und Statistik, 8*(2003), 763–774.

Woudenberg, F. (1991). An evaluation of Delphi. *Technological Forecasting and Social Change, 40*(2), 131–150.

Delphi Studies in the Health Sciences: Epistemic Potentials and Challenges

Saskia Jünger

Abstract

The aim of this chapter is to consider the epistemological potentials and challenges of the Delphi technique in the health sciences from the perspective of the sociology of knowledge. In particular, reference is made to the writings of Ludwik Fleck on the social construction of scientific facts, Berger and Luckmann on the social construction of reality, and Thomas Kuhn on the collaborative production of 'normal science' in terms of an accepted scientific paradigm. Against this background, different ways of looking at the Delphi method in terms of the production of knowledge in health research will be examined. Following this, different approaches will be discussed, which have been postulated in the literature as possible epistemological and scientific-theoretical/philosophical foundations of the Delphi technique – as well as their significance for the methodological design and practical implementation of Delphi studies. On the basis of these preliminary theoretical considerations, epistemological potentials and opportunities, as well as limitations and challenges regarding the use of Delphi studies in the health sciences will be discussed.

S. Jünger (✉)
Department of Community Health, University of Applied Health Sciences, Bochum, Germany
e-mail: saskia.juenger@hs-gesundheit.de

M. Niederberger, O. Renn (eds.), *Delphi Methods In The Social And Health Sciences*, https://doi.org/10.1007/978-3-658-38862-1_3

1 Introduction: The Strength and Power of the Delphi Technique for Creating Knowledge

Participation in various national and international Delphi processes in the field of palliative care allowed me to gain diverse insights into the power and effectiveness of this method for knowledge generation as well as for professional politics in a newly forming discipline. I witnessed discussions within research teams, debates in expert panels and negotiation processes between research teams and expert panels. In the wake of this, the influence of power and opinion leadership on the process of knowledge production in Delphi procedures was easy to observe – especially the transformation of first preliminary ideas into unanimously accepted consensus-supported statements and finally manifest recognised expertise. At the same time, I got a sense of the challenges and limitations of the process in striving for homogeneity and consensus across professional, national, and cultural boundaries. The question arose of how to frame international Delphi processes in a way that was respectful of linguistic and cultural diversity in relation to health issues - and that not only accommodated views at the 'centre' of discourse, but also valued divergent ideas and voices beyond the mainstream of knowledge production. This tension became the impetus for me to take a closer look at the role of Delphi procedures for knowledge production in the health sciences and to analyse them from a sociology of knowledge perspective.

2 The Role of the Delphi Technique in Health Research Using the Example of Palliative Care

The focus of current Delphi studies in the health sciences is primarily on bringing together expert perspectives on complex topic areas on which there is no consensus, and on facilitating collective reflection in order to promote a common understanding or to identify divergences between expert opinions (Guzys et al., 2015). Possible tasks and objectives of Delphi processes are, for example, the ranking of aspects according to their importance, the definition of a problem or a concept, the determination and classification of characteristics or the identification of 'best practice' with regard to a care question (Fletcher & Marchildon, 2014). Typical areas of application include (1) development of practice guidelines and professional standards; (2) criteria and curriculum content for education, training and professional development; (3) development and validation of assessment tools; (4) quality indicators; (5) criteria in the field of diagnosis, prognosis and classification

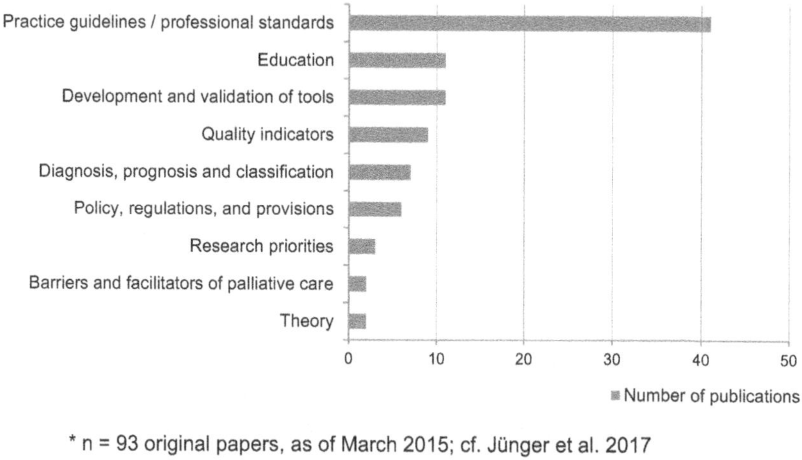

Fig. 1 Delphi studies in palliative care. (Own representation)

of symptoms and syndromes; (6) statements for policy, regulations or provisions; (7) identification and setting of research priorities; (8) identification of barriers and gaps in care; and (9) theory building. Figure 1 shows the use of the Delphi method for the aforementioned objectives in the field of palliative care as an example (result of a systematic literature search in PubMed, EMBASE, CINAHL, Web of Science and Academic Search Complete, as of March 2015; cf. Jünger et al., 2017).

2.1 Framework for Knowledge Acquisition in Medical Research

The dominant paradigm of knowledge generation in medical research since the 1990s has been evidence-based medicine (EBM). It has been defined as "the conscientious, explicit and judicious use of current best evidence in making decisions about the care of the individual patient. In this definition, the practice of evidence-based medicine means integrating individual clinical expertise a critical appraisal of the best available external clinical evidence from systematic research" (Sackett, 1997; p. 3). The randomised clinical trial, or better still, the systematic review of multiple randomised controlled trials, is seen as the highest-ranking foundation of clinical practice and has thus become the gold standard for evaluating medical interventions (Cochrane, 1972; Greenhalgh et al., 2014; Shah & Chung, 2009;

Sackett, 1997). Expert judgements, for example in the context of Delphi processes, on the other hand, represent the lowest level of knowledge generation according to EBM principles (Burns et al., 2011).

2.2 Context of Standardisation

Since the mid-1990s, standardisation, quality measurement and benchmarking in healthcare have increasingly become a priority (Donahue & van Ostenberg, 2000; Heidemann, 2000; van Niekerk et al., 2003; Segouin et al., 2005), accompanied by the development of standard operating procedures, quality indicators and measurement tools, audits and certification systems (Donahue & van Ostenberg, 2000; Heidemann, 2000; Segouin et al., 2005). Increasingly, there have been calls for unified strategies to meet the challenges of health care delivery in a globalised world (WHO, 2007). Against this background, the Delphi technique as a method of pooling expert assessments across geographical borders gained particular importance for the establishment of standards and for achieving homogeneity and standardisation.

2.3 Historical and (Health) Policy Context: Professionalisation and Differentiation

For the significance of the Delphi method as a group process, the historical and (health) political context also plays a role, as is shown here using the example of palliative care. Originating from the hospice movement, leading pioneers have continuously endeavoured constituting palliative care as a medical discipline over the past decades. Tension and hegemonic negotiation processes arose between the community-based civic engagement of the hospice movement and the desire for recognition in the medical community. In addition, with increasing professionalization, there was a desire to establish quality standards for care as well as political lobbying. Against this background, various instruments for benchmarking and standardisation were developed, as well as a series of White Papers by the European Association for Palliative Care (EAPC), in the preparation of which the Delphi method played a key role from the outset (Table 1).

The White Papers became a central tool for advocacy on funding and legislation, as well as for making the case to policymakers. The *White Paper for Global Palliative Care Advocacy* (Centeno et al., 2018), also based on a Delphi process, condenses this claim of the global reach of strategic recommendations. Delphi

Table 1 White Papers of the European Association for Palliative Care (EAPC). (Own representation)

EAPC recommended framework for the use of sedation in palliative care (Cherny et al., 2009)
EAPC White Paper on Standards and Norms for Hospice and Palliative Care in Europe (Radbruch et al., 2009, 2010)[a]
EAPC White Paper on improving support for family carers in palliative care (Payne and EAPC, 2010a, b)[a]
Core competencies in palliative care: an EAPC White Paper on palliative care education (Gamondi et al., 2013a, b)
White Paper on core competencies for education in paediatric palliative care (Downing et al., 2013)
White paper defining optimal palliative care in older people with dementia (van der Steen et al., 2014)[a]
Core competencies for palliative care social work in Europe: an EAPC White Paper (Hughes et al., 2014)
EAPC White Paper on Outcome Measurement in Palliative Care (Bausewein et al., 2016)
Defining volunteering in hospice and palliative care in Europe: an EAPC White Paper (Goossensen et al., 2016)[a]
White paper on euthanasia and physician assisted suicide (Radbruch et al., 2016)[a]
Defining consensus norms for palliative care of people with intellectual disabilities (Tuffrey-Wijne et al., 2016)[a]
Definition and recommendations for advance care planning: an international consensus (Rietjens et al., 2017)[a]

[a]The recommendations in the highlighted White Papers are based on Delphi studies

processes have thus become a fundamental methodological companion for those who are involved in the constitution of palliative care as an acknowledged medical discipline in professional, scientific and professional policy terms.

2.4 Methodological Framework of Knowledge Generation

The example of palliative care can also be used to show how the framework of knowledge generation affect the choice of methods and research designs. Against the background of the claim of evidence-based good clinical practice, research in the field of palliative care faces various challenges. Due to its specific objective, namely the maintenance or improvement of quality of life within a holistic approach to care, there are limits to obtaining 'high-level' evidence in the sense of EBM rules (Aoun & Nekolaichuk, 2014; Visser et al., 2015). In addition to ethical and methodological challenges, the question is how to operationalise clinical outcome parameters in a meaningful way (Addington-Hall, 2007; Aoun & Nekolaichuk, 2014; Visser et al., 2015). Traditional clinical outcomes such as survival rate or physical indicators of disease regression are by definition hardly applicable to the field of palliative care. It has therefore been questioned whether EBM sufficiently accounts for the complexity of severe advanced illness, particularly in older people with multiple chronic conditions (Upshur, 2005; Upshur & Tracy, 2008; Bonisteel, 2009). Delphi processes have thus become a significant alternative for establishing recognised expert knowledge and developing guidelines for clinical practice, education, training and quality control.

3 Consulting and Interpreting the Oracle: Projection Screen for Research Fantasies?

The etymological source of the method – the Delphic oracle – serves as an epistemological metaphor; the importance of the ritual for the institutionalisation of knowledge played a pivotal role in both the ancient oracle and the modern scientific process (Häder, 2014). However, for all its charm, the comparison also has its pitfalls, as especially the mystical, nebulous character of the Delphic oracle sometimes proved detrimental to the claim of scientificity of modern Delphi processes (Marchais-Roubelat & Roubelat, 2011; Dayé, 2018).

3.1 Epistemological Foundations of the Delphi Technique

The specific philosophical and epistemological basis of a scientific approach has implications for methodological practice and the nature of the insights gained (Mitroff & Turoff, 2002). In the literature, different considerations can be found regarding possible epistemological foundations of the Delphi technique (Mitroff & Turoff, 2002; Marchais-Roubelat & Roubelat, 2011; Fletcher & Marchildon, 2014; Guzys et al., 2015). Basically, the Delphi method can be considered as a heuristic technique that makes use of experts' opinions, experiences, intuition and tacit knowledge (Guzys et al., 2015). Dayé (2018) traces the historical lines of development of Delphi and describes its epistemological evolution in the first two decades of its genesis (1948–1968). While Delphi was originally conceived as a technique for aggregating expert opinions, efforts were later made to create an epistemological basis for the use of expert opinions, thus establishing Delphi as a scientific method. In the 1960s, the method underwent a stronger standardisation and institutionalisation, with an emphasis on convergence and a greater importance of numerical estimates – at the expense of the flexibility and openness that were still characteristic of the first studies. In a sense, Delphi was reconfigured as a tool that could be applied without specific prior scientific knowledge (Dayé, 2018). Against this background, it seems unsurprising that Delphi today turns out to be a collective term for heterogeneous approaches; the versatile shape of the method can be understood as a consequence of its multi-layered use, adaptation and 'socialisation' in different contexts and disciplines as well as for diverse objectives (Dayé, 2018). Mitroff and Turoff (2002), in a sense, make a virtue of necessity; they argue that there is no specific or 'best' philosophical basis for the Delphi method - but that the philosophy of science standpoint does play a role in the design of the procedure as well as the expectation of its outcomes. In this respect, a conscious reflection on one's own presuppositions as well as the presentation of a well-founded theoretical framework for the choice and design of the Delphi procedure are of importance for the epistemological consistency and rigour of the research process.

3.2 Dramaturgy of Delphi Procedures

In the methodological design of a Delphi procedure, the staging of the expert panel sets the tone with regard to the self-perception of the participants, their perception of the task set for them, and their expectations of the group and interaction dynamics (Scheele, 2002). The monitoring group thus has a significant responsibility here, as the experts' self-definition as part of a Delphi panel will influence the nature of their individual contributions as well as the quality of the interaction, and thus also the characteristics of the results. Dayé (2014) speaks here of the epistemic role attributed to participants in the study. This is characterised by normative expectations regarding their knowledge and skills (knowledge dimension), their behaviour and contribution to the knowledge process (task dimension), and their interaction with each other (interaction dimension). Scheele (2002) has shown a taxonomy of different types of group constellations, corresponding forms of interaction, and their consequences for the forms of reality produced (p. 55). Here it makes a difference, for example, whether the experts see themselves as part of a scientific group whose aim is to produce the most neutral, valid results possible – or whether they see themselves as the chosen representatives and advocates of a community who are to address a socially and/or politically explosive issue as convincingly as possible. In the former case, the exchange between the panel members will be more formal and the focus of the individual contribution will be on the accuracy and precision of the answers; in the latter case, however, the interaction may be more characterized by ideology and polemics and the individual contribution will be in the service of a specific socio-political interest.

3.3 Reopening the Methodological Spectrum

In the health sciences, the Delphi technique is often counted among consensus methods (Jones & Hunter, 1995; Murphy et al., 1998). However, this classification is based on a reductionist understanding of the Delphi technique as a consensus process, while other key objectives such as generation of ideas or future prediction are disregarded (Häder, 2014; Scheele, 2002; Mitroff & Turoff, 2002). This narrow focus on consensus-building as the motivation for using the method in healthcare has raised some issues, as will be discussed in more detail later.

In the health sciences, a distinction is often made between quantitative and qualitative research methods, each of which is rooted in a rather positivist or constructivist understanding of the world and science. In recent years, mixed-methods approaches in the sense of combining qualitative and quantitative research methods to answer questions have become increasingly popular, and the benefits of a plurality of methods for generating knowledge have come into focus (Kuckartz, 2014; Burzan, 2016; Zhang & Creswell, 2013). The Delphi technique cannot be classified exclusively under the positivist research paradigm, nor can it be counted purely among constructivist approaches. Delphi studies contain social constructivist elements in the sense of negotiation and co-construction of a shared reality within a group of people (Brady, 2015; Guzys et al., 2015). At the same time, they are characterised by strategies of standardisation and process control, which are typically features of positivist research, such as the rigour of formalisation and the anchoring of expert judgments in the best available evidence (Akins et al., 2005; Birko et al., 2015; Holey et al., 2007). In principle, then, Delphi studies can combine elements of different methodological approaches to data collection and analysis. The idea of a spectrum or typology therefore does more justice to the question of epistemological foundation as well as methodological design, rather than a dichotomous division into quantitative, positivist as well as qualitative, constructivist approaches (Hasson & Keeney, 2011). Indeed, the first Delphi study in 1951 was characterised by a combination of quantitative survey and qualitative interviews, in an effort to explicate the reasoning underlying the numerical estimates – and thus the experts' tacit knowledge (Dayé, 2018). Dayé speaks here of a 'flexible positivism' in the sense of seeking to legitimise the controlled use of intuitive expertise as a source of scientific knowledge (Dayé 2018).

Mitroff and Turoff (2002) analyse the importance of different theoretical and philosophical positions in science for the choice of the Delphi procedure and the methodological decisions in the process. Empirically anchored approaches with a stronger emphasis on data than on theory are, according to the authors, better suited for well-structured problems for which a solid consensual basis already exists. If this is not the case, Delphi studies with a focus on generating alternatives rather than achieving consensus are more suitable (Mitroff & Turoff, 2002). It is inherent in social or health-related issues in particular that there is no *one* answer or *one* best approach; they therefore require a more complex philosophy of science approach. However, given the strong focus on consensus building, the use of conflict as a methodological element in Delphi studies is strikingly underrepresented in the health sciences.

Another potential that has hardly been used so far is the integration of participatory approaches in Delphi research. This would open up new perspectives for the Delphi process, as experts would not only be considered as participants, but also as stakeholders in the design and implementation of the study. Thus, a self-reflexive element could be included in Delphi studies, as they would not only contribute to the generation of knowledge with regard to the topic of research as such, but equally to the acquisition of knowledge with regard to the participants themselves as well as the research field as a whole (Mitroff & Turoff, 2002). A pioneering example of the possibility of combining Delphi and participatory action research to involve participants more consciously in the design of the process is provided by the study by Fletcher and Marchildon (2014), which is described in more detail in Sect. 7.1.2.

Based on a literature review on the methodological foundations of Delphi methods in health research, Guzys et al. (2015) were able to show that only a minority of the identified publications provide information on the methodological-theoretical assumptions. At the same time, a variety of approaches were found; in terms of the overarching epistemology, reference was mostly made to qualitative research approaches and interpretivism (as an antithesis to positivism); individual studies referred in particular to grounded theory or phenomenology, among others. In addition, Delphi was described as a mixed methods approach or pragmatic research approach. Interestingly, no publications were found in the review that specifically referred to quantitative perspectives with a focus on, for example, mathematical modelling. Based on their findings, the authors discuss the cyclical process of hermeneutics as a purposeful methodological framework for Delphi research (Guzys et al., 2015). The hermeneutic circle visualizes the iterative process of concept formation between individuals and a collective, which finally results in a shared understanding, while divergent views can still remain represented.

3.4 Conclusion

A look at the current use of the Delphi technique suggests that a creative reopening of the epistemological discourse has taken place in the health sciences, in which scientists dare to rediscover the original flexibility of the method and adapt its implementation to the requirements of a complex research field. With regard to the epistemological foundations, it is not only the question of which philosophical approaches have already been discussed and used in relation to the Delphi technique that counts - but especially which ones have been largely neglected so far - because this is where possibly untapped potential lies in the sense of the further development of the Delphi technique (Mitroff & Turoff, 2002). This deserves special consideration against the background that up to now, mainly Western understandings of the world and of science have prevailed in the use of the Delphi method, as well as in research in the health sciences as a whole. In addition, the fit between the research question and the research interest as well as the choice and design of the Delphi procedure deserve particularly careful reflection; to say it with the words of Mitroff and Turoff (2002): *But then, believing in conflict as we do, we might have a good debate on the matter. If one were to design a Delphi to investigate the matter, which Delphi inquirer design do you think we (you) ought to use?* (Mitroff & Turoff, 2002, p. 34).

4 Excursus into the Sociology of Knowledge

> What realities have been or are being socially constructed – and what does this question mean for conducting Delphis? (Scheele, 2002, p. 41).

From the perspective of social constructivism and symbolic interactionism, science can be seen as an interactive negotiation process between individuals and within groups (Fleck, 2012; Bourdieu, 1984; Keller, 2011). Knowledge is thus created in a process of discursive co-construction (Keller, 2011). Unlike positivism or critical rationalism, scientific facts are not considered as detached, ahistorical objective goods. Scientific knowledge is understood as socially, culturally, and historically conditioned (Foucault, 1976; Fleck, 2012). Instead of natural phenomena to be uncovered only by means of the appropriate methods of empirical research, facts are constructed within particular scientific groups – so-called 'thought collectives' (Fleck, 2012); their 'styles of thinking' influence the generation of knowledge. This 'habitus mentalis' (Scheele, 2002) in the sense of the global reality of an era is characterized by a shared assumption about what valid knowledge is, how it can be generated or discovered, and how its acceptance or proof is constituted (epistemology), as well as by the ground rules elaborated and accepted on the part of the members of a community (Brown, 1995; Scheele, 2002). Here a reference can also be made to Kuhn's idea of a normal science – the scientific community accepts a paradigm on the basis of which it can conduct research and devote itself to the exploration of new questions (Kuhn, 1970).

The central interest of the sociology of knowledge is the social production, transformation and circulation of knowledge (Keller, 2011). A crucial criterion for evaluating knowledge is its fit in a context of meaning and not the abstract assessment as 'true' or 'false'. From this perspective, Delphi processes can be seen as a purposeful and effective method for the generation of collaboratively negotiated context-relevant knowledge.

5 Epistemological Opportunities and Potentials

From the perspective of the sociology of knowledge, Delphi procedures offer potential for knowledge generation in health research in three respects: for the creation of a common foundation on which science can be conducted; as a source of identity and cohesion; and for orientation in a complex professional terrain.

5.1 Habitualisation and Institutionalisation: Building a Scientific Foundation

Delphi procedures, from a philosophy of science perspective, can be seen as a resource for establishing foundational elements of scientific research and knowledge production; *"a type of foundational methodology upon which all other methodologies rest"* (Jorm, 2015, p. 888). Only consensus on fundamentals, such as what counts as knowledge or what is a legitimate research question, enables a state of "normal science" (Kuhn, 1970). The implicit styles of thinking, basic assumptions, metaphors and rules of argumentation guide and legitimise our scientific thinking and acting. It is on this ground that further differentiation of a discipline is possible, such as the study of more specific questions, the founding of professional societies, the publishing of journals, or the claim to a place value in the curriculum of academic training (Kuhn, 1970). Negotiation processes within the framework of Delphi procedures thus contribute to the formation and continuation of a paradigm, a common commitment and thus a progression of knowledge production.

5.2 Cohesion and Cohesiveness

Another function of Delphi procedures in health research is the creation and consolidation of cohesion between members of the scientific community. Participation in a collaborative process of gaining knowledge can foster identification with a thought collective and thought style (Fleck, 2012), as well as with the results of a Delphi procedure. In terms of normal science (Kuhn, 1970), the knowledge dynamic is characterized by scientists' efforts to create a collective normative framework and to defend it against external pressures. The co-construction of a common knowledge base and the suppression of latent differences of opinion in the context of Delphi procedures thus allow a higher common unified idea to be represented.

5.3 Orientation in a Complex and Uncertain Professional Terrain

Given the aforementioned challenges and limitations regarding the generation of scientific evidence through RCTs or observational studies for some fields and questions in health care, Delphi studies represent a relevant source of evidence and form the basis for clinical consultation, care planning and political decision-making (Biondo et al., 2008; Jünger et al., 2017). This can be particularly important in the case of existential or complex, difficult to solve issues. The example of the historical development of palliative care as a medical discipline shows how Delphi processes have been used to reach agreement on core values, definitions, theoretical concepts and standards for clinical practice, as well as rules for scientific practice. Leading authorities in health care refer to recommendations based on the results of Delphi studies, for example professional associations, scientific societies or the World Health Organization; they are cited and used as a resource for scientific argumentation and health policy decisions, reflecting the central relevance of Delphi processes for orientation and action in health issues.

6 Limitations and Challenges

Limitations and challenges with regard to the use of the Delphi technique in health research concern the question of the appropriateness of the method for certain questions in health care, the reproduction of power and hegemony in and through Delphi studies, as well as methodological challenges.

6.1 Limitations to the Appropriateness of the Delphi Technique to the Subject Matter

In order to answer value-laden, explosive questions in health research, for example with regard to recommendations and decisions in prenatal diagnostics or at the end of life, the use of the Delphi technique may be inappropriate - especially in view of the focus on the goal of consensus building, which is prominent in health research. The danger of consensus is that it can suppress conflict and debate precisely where it would be most needed. Particularly in quantitatively oriented Delphi studies with the goal of consensus building, it is important to note that the expert judgments that 'survive' the process are not necessarily the best, but represent a statistical compromise (Mitroff & Turoff, 2002; Dayé, 2018). As a consequence, these prevailing judgments may lack the significance and meaningfulness of extreme or conflicting positions.

6.2 Power and Hegemony In and Through Delphi Procedures

What knowledge is ultimately recognised and institutionalised as expertise and finds further dissemination depends on power relations as well as on the professional habitus (Fleck, 2012; Foucault, 1976; Bourdieu, 1984). Following this logic, hegemonic structures in academia imply a dominance of certain ideas as well as an underrepresentation of others (Bourdieu, 1984; Pellegrino, 1992; Pastrana et al., 2010). Accordingly, it can be assumed that the *habitus mentalis* of an era influences the design as well as the outcome of Delphi procedures – not only in the sense of what is sought, accepted and communicated as knowledge, but also in the way information is categorised and organised (Scheele, 2002; Dayé, 2018).

Power is present in Delphi processes on different levels. This concerns the composition of the monitoring team and the expert panel, the use of language, the design of the process as well as the basic attitudes and assumptions, which in turn influence the definition of the research question and the interpretation of the results. Research in medicine and health sciences is deeply rooted in 'Western' thinking (Pellegrino, 1992). Academic science is characterised by highly specialised forms of language and hierarchical power structures (Smith, 2012). The negotiation processes of knowledge production through Delphi processes tend to take place within this framework; however, in terms of outcomes, there is a claim of validity for a much wider community. This bears the risk of a bias in favour of the dominant positions of the experts involved, especially if the project lead or the monitoring team enjoy a high status in the scientific community and the results are thus widely recognised and disseminated.

6.3 Methodological Challenges

With the increasing popularity of Delphi studies in health research, a certain arbitrariness has also set in with regard to their use – both in terms of the objectives and the object of investigation, as well as in terms of the methodology of implementation. *"In their enthusiasm some analysts have urged Delphi for practically every use except cure of the common cold."* (Linstone & Turoff, 2002, p. 569). The original aspirations of the Delphi method were, in a sense, adapted to the realities of the epistemic marketplace in the course of its socialisation process (Dayé, 2018). In addition, there is the aforementioned problem that Delphi processes are sometimes used in health research as a methodological fig leaf for scientific consensus: "... *although the Delphi technique is widely regarded as a consensus development technique, our impression from reading Delphi publications was that achievement of consensus is often assumed to occur by virtue of performing a Delphi study.*" (Diamond et al., 2014, p. 402). While the flexibility of the Delphi process can be seen as a methodological strength, it also carries the risk of the method being used like an unreflective label for a collection of approaches with widely divergent methodological diligence (Green et al., 1999; Humphrey-Murto et al., 2017). Another challenge is the often lack of transparency regarding the procedure, including the methodological decisions made during the process (Fletcher & Marchildon, 2014). This relates, for example, to the processing of interim results to design the next Delphi round (Jünger et al., 2017; Fletcher & Marchildon, 2014). In particular, transforming data from an open, qualitative Delphi round into closed, quantitative questions, entails the dilemma of considerable loss of information and inappropriate reduction of meaning (Green et al., 1999).

7 Food for Thought for a Creative Vision of Delphi in the Health Sciences

In view of the described potentials and challenges in the use of the Delphi technique in the health sciences, some food for thought may be helpful in the sense of a careful use of the method. These concern the rationale for the choice of the procedure, the design of the process, the processing and analysis of the data, the interpretation of the results and their translation into a scientific finding. Based on recommendations for conducting and reporting Delphi studies (Jünger et al., 2017), the guiding questions described below can support these considerations. These are intended less as fixed rules regarding the 'correct' conduct, but rather as questions for reflection in terms of one's own research attitude as well as the appropriateness to the subject matter and transparency in the context of the study in question.

7.1 Reflections on the Research Attitude

The literature from the field of *'decolonising research methodologies'* (Ermine et al., 2004; Smith, 2012) offers helpful arguments and reflective approaches based on the principles of participation, consultation and inclusion of different stakeholders. As a prerequisite, researchers need to be aware of the historical dominance and hegemonic superiority of Western scientific approaches and worldviews. In order to avoid the reproduction of paternalistic structures, a continuous critical self-reflection with regard to one's own goals, ambitions and possible conflicts of interest is appropriate. To a certain extent, Delphi studies always involve negotiation processes with regard to power of definition and interpretative authority. Especially for researchers with reputation and authority in their scientific community it is therefore important to be aware of their own power in the production, dissemination and institutionalisation of health knowledge. This is the prerequisite for doing justice to different cultures, traditions and perspectives on health in the context of Delphi studies.

7.1.1 Diversity: Language, Culture, Theoretical Concepts and Health Practice

The use of language and definitions deserves special attention in Delphi processes, as these play a key role in the institutionalisation of knowledge. For example, international Delphi studies are usually conducted in English as the dominant language in science. Implicit concepts closely intertwined with language are thus adopted in consensus building and knowledge production. Therefore, when a Delphi study covers a wide geographical area with many different cultures, traditions and languages, translation and cross-cultural adaptation of the survey instruments should be considered. The selection of experts also deserves close attention. In order to enable context-sensitive knowledge production, researchers should ensure that worldviews and knowledge systems other than the dominant ones are represented. In Delphi processes in healthcare, it is therefore advisable to involve not only opinion leaders at the centre of knowledge production, but also representatives of the "periphery". Researchers can ask themselves the following questions: "Will my research question lead to surprising results?" Will my study design – including the composition of the research team and the selection of the expert panel – do justice to the scope of the contexts I want to address with the results of this Delphi procedure?" "Does the range of ideas and concepts covered in the study correspond to the reality of the contexts and practices involved – or does my design inappropriately exclude certain facets of reality?"

7.1.2 Delphi and Participatory Research Approaches

Epistemologically, participatory methods – such as participatory action research (PAR) – and Delphi methods can be seen as complementary approaches to collective knowledge production as well as to informing clinical practice and health policy decision-making. In PAR, participants are not solely in the role of being 'researched' but are actively involved in the study design, data collection and interpretation of results (Brazil, 2012; von Unger, 2012). They are seen as collaborative partners, equipped with the knowledge and agency to contribute to the understanding of the research process and the production of the results. In return, the participants are enabled to use the research results for their own goals and purposes. Thus, the focus is on opening up a dialogue and generating knowledge through interaction between researchers and participants. To date, the combination of the Delphi technique with PAR has hardly been discussed. Fletcher and Marchildon (2014) describe the integration of a two-stage Delphi process into a PAR approach research project on the role of healthcare leaders.

The authors cite central arguments for the choice of the Delphi method in the context of this PAR project. PAR focuses on the relevances and life-worlds of participants, gives authority to experience-based knowledge and thus opens up the space for non-academic persons and groups to contribute to knowledge production. The Delphi method defines actors and stakeholders of a field as experts on the respective research topic and thus allows attainment of action-oriented conclusions regarding unresolved health care issues grounded in the experience-based insights of the participants. In addition, the Delphi method facilitates transparency towards the participants in the course of processing, analysing and interpreting the (interim) results; this can be regarded as an extended form of communicative validation. Furthermore, Delphi is conducive to the PAR objective of action and change – the method can accompany change processes in real time and thus fulfil the function of a formative evaluation with the participation of the decision-makers involved. Finally, the study by Fletcher and Marchildon (2014) was able to show how a Delphi process can be used not only to achieve consensus, but also to openly reflect on the results. Participants are thus given the opportunity to assert their own interpretations, rather than solely ranking or guessing the items selected and formulated by the researchers. This can reveal disagreement, controversy and conflict.

7.2 Research Practice and Methodological Rigour

Due to its complexity and adaptability, the Delphi technique is reminiscent of a methodological chameleon – the procedure can be flexibly designed and modified depending on the theoretical presuppositions, epistemological interest and objective of a project. To ensure methodological quality, researchers are at the same time required to be able to draw on the knowledge and tools of a wide range of approaches and methods, e.g. the basics of statistics and questionnaire construction, the analysis of qualitative data, and the shaping of group dynamics. Criteria for assessing the quality of Delphi studies should also take into account the possible methodological diversity – instead of the classic quality criteria of quantitative research (objectivity, validity and reliability), the following criteria for the trustworthiness of Delphi studies were therefore proposed, following Lincoln and Guba (1985): confirmability, credibility, dependability and transferability (Day & Bobeva, 2005). Based on the results of a systematic literature review, a reporting standard for conducting and publishing Delphi studies (Recommendations for Conducting and REporting DElphi Studies CREDES) was developed (Jünger et al., 2017). This includes guiding questions for reflection on the methodological rationale for the choice of the Delphi technique, on planning and study design, on process quality and rigour in the conduct of the study, as well as on transparency and quality of reporting.

7.2.1 Appropriateness to the Subject Matter: Objective and Operationalisation

Central to the choice of a research design or method is the question of appropriateness to the subject matter. When choosing the Delphi technique to answer a particular research question in health research, it is important to consider the constructivist nature of the method (Birko et al., 2015; Guzys et al., 2015; Mitroff & Turoff, 2002; Scheele, 2002). The previously described focus on consensus-building Delphi studies in the health sciences can force an apparent consensus across groups, while the individual experts adhere to their differing positions (Birko et al., 2015; Hasson & Keeney, 2011). Scheele (2002) therefore suggests deliberately and intentionally introducing ambiguity or even irritation into Delphi studies to avoid undesirable convergence and agreement. Moreover, the importance of (non-)consensus should be reflected when interpreting the results; the value of stable disagreements in particular should not be underestimated, as these provide revealing insights findings and highlight differences in perspectives regarding complex issues (Mitroff & Turoff, 2002; Guzys et al., 2015).

7.2.2 Ensuring Credibility

It is the responsibility of the monitoring team to provide a space for the experts to reach valid and credible judgments. While the monitoring team needs to steer the process and make decisions even in unclear situations, care should be taken to include the voices of the different stakeholders affected by the outcomes of the process during all phases of the study. This includes defining the overall study goal, operationalising the research questions, generating items, the language and wording of statements and definitions, selecting response options, preparing data for the following round of data collection, and interpreting the results. Research projects are for the most part initiated due to the interest of leading scientists in their field, who as a rule represent a certain position on a certain topic. The monitoring team can take specific measures here to ensure that no direct or indirect influence is exerted on the judgements of the experts. First and foremost is the reflection on one's own interests. A balanced composition of the monitoring team and the opportunity for critical exchange within the team are also helpful. Another possibility is, for example, to delegate the methodological coordination of the study to an independent 'neutral' person. In addition, the draft results can be submitted to an external body or advisory board for critical review before publication.

7.2.3 Knowledge Production through Delphi Processes: Presentation, Publication and Dissemination

In the course of knowledge generation through Delphi processes, it is helpful for researchers to keep in mind the significance of the method for the dissemination and institutionalisation of health knowledge. In this context, researchers can ask themselves the following questions: "Are the terms used in the final publication stigmatising, too prescriptive, or too ambitious?" "Do definitions exclude options and choices, thereby unduly limiting the range of 'legitimate' ideas and practices?" Again, approaches based on participation and public deliberation can be a constructive way to ensure balanced conclusions.

When publishing, disseminating and implementing the results of Delphi studies, it serves transparency to make the methodological decisions during the Delphi process explicit, so that recipients can understand the respective steps, retrace the development of expert judgements and assess the results achieved (Diamond et al., 2014; Hasson et al., 2000). This encompasses a transparent description of the entire process, including the expert panel and the impact of possible methodological limitations on the interpretation of the findings and the resulting guidelines or recommendations for health care. With regard to the format of reporting, the publication of an additional methodological paper or study protocol can be considered – in addition to a quality standard or guidelines for good clinical practice – in order to provide transparent information on the details of the study process.

7.3 Outlook

In summary, the Delphi technique represents a valuable contribution to the production, transformation, circulation and institutionalisation of health knowledge. In this context, the premises of context sensitivity and scientific reason are of utmost relevance: Particularly in international Delphi processes, different normative, ethical and legal frameworks deserve consideration. Only in this way can researchers and health policy makers do justice to a globalised context of health care. This requires careful attention to the limitations and potential risks of (international) Delphi studies, including the disproportionate dominance of certain viewpoints, which in the process of knowledge production concomitantly implies the marginality of other perspectives. In view of existing controversies and continuing disagreements on some core issues of health care, it must be questioned whether consensus and convergence at any price are desirable and appropriate – they risk unduly narrowing the range of desirable and acceptable choices, attitudes and practices in health care, creating new taboos and preparing the ground for undesirable paternalism or even criminalisation. 'Normal science' (Kuhn, 1970) enables habitualisation and consolidation, but at the same time, especially in health care, continues to be characterised by complex existential questions and ambivalences. It therefore remains important to keep the dialogue alive. Ultimately, a conscientious use of the Delphi technique will contribute to a higher respect and recognition of expert judgements in scientific knowledge production. The study by Fletcher and Marchildon (2014) has demonstrated the potential of the Delphi methodology in the context of a qualitative participatory research project. This is where further research can begin: How can Delphi studies in the health sciences contribute to scientific mobility between the 'centre' and 'periphery' of knowledge production?

Literature

Addington-Hall, J. M. (2007). Introduction. In J. M. Addington-Hall, E. Bruera, I. J. Higginson, & S. Payne (Eds.), *Research methods in palliative care*. Oxford University Press.

Akins, R. B., Tolson, H., & Cole, B. R. (2005). Stability of response characteristics of a Delphi panel: Application of bootstrap data expansion. *BMC Medical Research Methodology, 5*(37), 1–12.

Aoun, S. M., & Nekolaichuk, C. (2014). Improving the evidence base in palliative care to inform practice and policy: Thinking outside the box. *Journal of Pain and Symptom Management, 48*(6), 1222–1235.

Bausewein, C., Daveson, B. A., Currow, D. C., Downing, J., Deliens, L., Radbruch, L., Defilippi, K., Lopes Ferreira, P., Costantini, M., Harding, R., & Higginson, I. J. (2016). EAPC white paper on outcome measurement in palliative care: Improving practice, attaining outcomes and delivering quality services – Recommendations from the European Association for Palliative Care (EAPC) task force on outcome measurement. *Palliative Medicine, 30*(1), 6–22.

Brady, S. R. (2015). Utilizing and adapting the Delphi method for use in qualitative research. *International Journal of Qualitative Methods, 14*(5), 1–6.

Brazil, K. (2012). Issues of diversity: Participatory action research with indigenous peoples. In J. Hockley, K. Froggatt, & K. Heimerl (Eds.), *Participatory research in palliative care: Actions and reflections*. Oxford University Press.

Biondo, P. D., Nekolaichuk, C. L., Stiles, C., Fainsinger, R., & Hagen, N. A. (2008). Applying the Delphi process to palliative care tool development: Lessons learned. *Supportive Care in Cancer, 16*, 935–942.

Birko, S., Dove, E. S., & Özdemir, V. (2015). Evaluation of nine consensus indices in Delphi foresight research and their dependency on Delphi survey characteristics: A simulation study and debate on Delphi design and interpretation. *PLoS One, 10*(8), e0135162.

Bonisteel, P. (2009). The tyranny of evidence-based medicine. *Canadian Family Physician, 55*, 979.

Bourdieu, P. (1984). *Homo academicus*. Stanford University Press.

Brown, H. R. (1995). Postmodern representation, postmodern affirmation. In H. R. Brown (Ed.), *Postmodern representations. Truth, power, and mimesis in the human sciences and public culture* (pp. 1–19). University of Illinois Press.

Burns, P. B., Rohrich, R. J., & Chung, K. C. (2011). The levels of evidence and their role in evidence-based medicine. *Plastic Reconstruction Surgery, 128*(1), 305–310.

Burzan, N. (2016). *Methodenplurale forschung. Chancen und methoden von mixed methods*. Beltz Juventa.

Centeno, C., Sitte, T., de Lima, L., Alsirafy, S., Bruera, E., Callaway, M., Foley, K., Luyirika, E., Mosoiu, D., Pettus, K., Puchalski, C., Rajagopal, M. R., Yong, J., Garralda, E., Rhee, J. Y., & Comoretto, N. (2018). White Paper for global palliative care advocacy: Recommendations from a PAL-LIFE Expert Advisory Group of the Pontifical Academy for Life, Vatican City. *Journal of Palliative Medicine* (Epub ahead of print).

Cherny, N. I., Radbruch, L., & The Board of the European Association for Palliative Care. (2009). European Association for Palliative Care (EAPC) recommended framework for the use of sedation in palliative care. *Palliative Medicine, 23*(7), 581–593.

Cochrane, A. L. (1972). *Effectiveness and efficiency. Random reflections on health services.* The Nuffield Provincial Hospitals Trust/The Royal Society of Medicine Press.

Day, J., & Bobeva, M. (2005). A generic toolkit for the successful management of Delphi studies. *Electronic Journal of Business Research Methods, 3*(2), 103–116.

Dayé, C. (2014). In fremden Territorien: Delphi, Political Gaming und die subkutane Bedeutung tribaler Wissenskulturen. *Österreichische Zeitschrift für Geschichtswissenschaften, 25*(3), 83–115.

Dayé, C. (2018). How to train your oracle: The Delphi method and its turbulent youth in operations research and the policy sciences. *Social Studies of Science, 48*(6), 846–868.

Diamond, I. R., Grant, R. C., Feldman, B. M., et al. (2014). Defining consensus: A systematic review recommends methodologic criteria for reporting of Delphi studies. *Journal of Clinical Epidemiology, 67*(4), 401–409.

Donahue, K. T., & van Ostenberg, P. (2000). Joint Commission International accreditation: Relationship to four models of evaluation. *International Journal for Quality in Health Care, 12*(3), 243–246.

Downing, J., Ling, J., Benini, F., Payne, S., & Papadatou, D. (2013). *Core competencies for education in paediatric palliative care. Report of the EAPC Children's palliative care education taskforce*. European Association for Palliative Care.

Ermine, W., Sinclair, R., & Jeffery, B. (2004). *The ethics of research involving indigenous peoples. Report of the indigenous People's Health Research Centre to the interagency advisory panel on research ethics*. Indigenous People's Health Research Centre.

Fleck, L. (2012). *Entstehung und Entwicklung einer wissenschaftlichen Tatsache* (9th ed.). Suhrkamp Taschenbuch Wissenschaft.

Fletcher, A. J., & Marchildon, G. P. (2014). Using the Delphi method for qualitative, participatory action research in health leadership. *International Journal of Qualitative Methods, 13*, 1–18.

Foucault, M. (1976). *The birth of the clinic. An archaeology of medical perception*. Tavistock.

Gamondi, C., Larkin, P., & Payne, S. (2013a). Core competencies in palliative care: An EAPC white paper on palliative care education – Part 1. *European Journal of Palliative Care, 20*(2), 86–91.

Gamondi, C., Larkin, P., & Payne, S. (2013b). Core competencies in palliative care: An EAPC white paper on palliative care education – Part 2. *European Journal of Palliative Care, 20*(3), 140–145.

Goossensen, A., Somsen, J., Scott, R., & Pelttari, I. (2016). Defining volunteering in hospice and palliative care in Europe: An EAPC white paper. *European Journal of Palliative Care, 23*(4), 184–191.

Green, B., Jones, M., Hughes, D., & Williams, A. (1999). Applying the Delphi technique in a study of GPs' information requirements. *Health and Social Care in the Community, 7*(3), 198–205.

Greenhalgh, T., Howick, J., Maskrey, N., & The Evidence Based Medicine Renaissance Group. (2014). Evidence based medicine: A movement in crisis? *British Medical Journal, 348*(3725), 1–7.

Guzys, D., Dickson-Swift, V., Kenny, A., & Threlkeld, G. (2015). Gadamerian philosophical hermeneutics as a useful framework for the Delphi technique. *International Journal of Qualitative Studies on Health and Wellbeing, 10*, 26291.

Häder, M. (2014). *Delphi-Befragungen: Ein Arbeitsbuch* (3rd ed.). Springer.

Hasson, F., & Keeney, S. (2011). Enhancing rigour in the Delphi technique research. *Technological Forecasting and Social Change, 78*, 1695–1704.

Hasson, F., Keeney, S., & McKenna, H. (2000). Research guidelines for the Delphi survey technique. *Journal of Advanced Nursing, 32*(4), 1008–1015.

Heidemann, E. M. (2000). Moving to global standards for accreditation processes: The ExPeRT Project in a larger context. *International Journal for Quality in Health Care, 12*(3), 227–230.

Holey, E. A., Feeley, J. L., Dixon, J., & Whittaker, V. J. (2007). An exploration of the use of simple statistics to measure consensus and stability in Delphi studies. *BMC Medical Research Methodology, 7*(52), 1–10.

Hughes, S., Firth, P., & Oliviere, D. (2014). Core competencies for palliative care social work in Europe: An EAPC white paper – Part 1. *European Journal of Palliative Care, 21*(6), 300–305.

Humphrey-Murto, S., Varpio, L., Wood, T. J., Gonsalves, C., Ufholz, L.-A., Mascioli, K., Wang, C., & Foth, T. (2017). The use of the Delphi and other consensus group methods in medical education research: A review. *Academic Medicine, 92*, 1491–1498.

Jones, J., & Hunter, D. (1995). Consensus methods for medical and health services research. *British Medical Journal, 311*, 376–380.

Jorm, A. J. (2015). Using the Delphi expert consensus method in mental health research. *Australian & New Zealand Journal of Psychiatry, 49*(10), 887–897.

Jünger, S., Payne, S. A., Brine, J., Radbruch, L., & Brearley, S. G. (2017). Guidance on Conducting and Reporting Delphi Studies (CREDES) in palliative care: Recommendations based on a methodological systematic review. *Palliative Medicine, 31*(8), 684–706.

Keller, R. (2011). The sociology of knowledge approach to discourse (SKAD). *Human Studies, 34*, 43–65.

Kuckartz, U. (2014). *Mixed methods. Methodologie, Forschungsdesigns und Analyseverfahren*. Springer.

Kuhn, T. S. (1970). *The structure of scientific revolutions* (2nd ed.). The University of Chicago Press.

Lincoln, Y. S., & Guba, E. G. (1985). *Naturalistic inquiry*. Sage.

Linstone, H. A., & Turoff, M. (Eds.). (2002). *The Delphi method: Techniques and applications*. Addison-Wesley.

Marchais-Roubelat, A., & Roubelat, F. (2011). The Delphi method as a ritual: Inquiring the Delphic Oracle. *Technological Forecasting and Social Change, 78*, 1491–1499.

Mitroff, I. I., & Turoff, M. (2002). Philosophical and methodological foundations of Delphi. In H. A. Linstone & M. Turoff (Eds.), *The Delphi method: Techniques and applications* (pp. 17–34). Addison-Wesley.

Murphy, M. K., Black, N. A., Lamping, D. L., et al. (1998). Consensus development methods, and their use in clinical guideline development. *Health Technology Assessment, 2*(3): i–iv, 1–88.

Pastrana, T., Vallath, N., Mastrojohn, J., Namukwaya, E., Kumar, S., Radbruch, L., & Clark, D. (2010). Disparities in the contribution of low and middle-income countries to palliative care research. *Journal of Pain and Symptom Management, 39*(1), 54–68.

Payne, S., & the EAPC Task Force on Family Carers. (2010a). White paper on improving support for family carers in palliative care: Part 1. *European Journal of Palliative Care, 17*(5), 238–245.

Payne, S., & the EAPC Task Force on Family Carers. (2010b). White paper on improving support for family carers in palliative care: Part 2. *European Journal of Palliative Care, 17*(6), 286–290.

Pellegrino, E. D. (1992). Intersections of western biomedical ethics and world culture: Problematic and possibility. *Cambridge Quarterly of Healthcare Ethics, 3*, 191–196.

Radbruch, L., Payne, S., & the Board of Directors of the European Association for Palliative Care (EAPC). (2009). White paper on standards and norms for hospice and palliative care in Europe: Part 1. *European Journal of Palliative Care, 16*(6), 278–289.

Radbruch, L., Payne, S., & the Board of Directors of the European Association for Palliative Care (EAPC). (2010). White paper on standards and norms for hospice and palliative care in Europe: Part 2. *European Journal of Palliative Care, 17*(1), 22–33.

Radbruch, L., Leget, C., Bahr, P., Müller-Busch, C., Ellershaw, J., de Conno, F., Vanden Berghe, P., & on behalf of the board members of the European Association for Palliative Care. (2016). Euthanasia and physician-assisted suicide: A white paper from the European Association for Palliative Care. *Palliative Medicine, 30*(2), 104–116.

Rietjens, J. A. C., Sudore, R. L., Connolly, M., van Delden, J. J., Drickamer, M. A., Droger, M., van der Heide, A., Heyland, D. K., Houttekier, D., Janssen, D. J. A., Orsi, L., Payne, S., Seymour, J., Jox, R. J., Korfage, I. J., & on behalf of the European Association for Palliative Care. (2017). Definition and recommendations for advance care planning: An international consensus supported by the European Association for Palliative Care. *Lancet Oncology, 18*(9), e543–e551.

Sackett, D. L. (1997). Evidence-based medicine. *Seminars in Perinatology, 21*(1), 3–5.

Scheele, D. S. (2002). Reality construction as a product of Delphi interaction. In H. A. Linstone & M. Turoff (Eds.), *The Delphi method: Techniques and applications* (pp. 35–67). Addison-Wesley.

Segouin, C., Hodges, B., & Brechat, P. H. (2005). Globalization in health care: Is international standardization of quality a step toward outsourcing? *International Journal for Quality in Health Care, 17*(4), 277–279.

Shah, H. M., & Chung, K. C. (2009). Archie Cochrane and his vision for evidence-based medicine. *Plastic Reconstruction Surgery, 124*(3), 982–988.

Smith, L. T. (2012). *Decolonizing methodologies: Research and indigenous peoples* (2nd ed.). Zed Books.

Tuffrey-Wijne, I., McLaughlin, D., Curfs, L., Dusart, A., Hoenger, C., McEnhill, L., Read, S., Ryan, K., Satgé, D., Straßer, B., Westergård, B.-E., & Oliver, D. (2016). Defining consensus norms for palliative care of people with intellectual disabilities in Europe, using Delphi methods: A white paper from the European Association of Palliative Care. *Palliative Medicine, 30*(5), 446–455.

Upshur, R. (2005). Looking for rules in a world of exceptions: Reflections on evidence-based practice. *Perspectives in Biology and Medicine, 48*(4), 477–489.

Upshur, R. E. G., & Tracy, S. (2008). Chronicity and complexity. Is what's good for the disease always good for the patients? *Canadian Family Physician, 54*, 1655–1658.

van der Steen, J. T., Radbruch, L., Hertogh, C. M. P. M., de Boer, M., Hughes, J. C., Larkin, P., Francke, A. L., Jünger, S., Gove, D., Firth, P., Koopmans, R. T. C. M., Volicer, L., & on behalf of the European Association for Palliative Care (EAPC). (2014). White paper defining optimal palliative care in older people with dementia: A Delphi study and recommendations from the European Association for Palliative Care. *Palliative Medicine, 28*(3), 197–209.

van Niekerk, J. P. D. V., Christensen, L., Karle, H., Lindgren, S., & Nystrup, J. (2003). WFME global standards in medical education: Status and perspectives following the 2003 WFME world conference. *Medical Education, 37*, 1050–1054.

Visser, C., Hadley, G., & Wee, B. (2015). Reality of evidence-based practice in palliative care. *Cancer Biology & Medicine, 12*, 193–200.

von Unger, H. (2012). Partizipative Gesundheitsforschung: Wer partizipiert woran? *Forum: Qualitative Sozialforschung, 13*(1) (Article 7).

World Health Organisation. (2007). *Towards health-equitable globalisation: Rights, regulation and redistribution. Final report to the commission on social determinants of health.* Institute of Population Health, Globalization and Health Equity.

Zhang, W., & Creswell, J. (2013). The use of "mixing" procedure of mixed methods in health services research. *Medical Care, 51*(8), e51–e57.

The Group Delphi Process in the Social and Health Sciences

Marlen Niederberger and Ortwin Renn

Abstract

The group Delphi method is a Delphi variant in which the anonymity of the experts is abandoned in favour of an open exchange among professinals. The experts are invited to a joint workshop and evaluate a standardized questionnaire in successive small groups with rotating composition. Through the open exchange, arguments for the evaluations are revealed and one can test (i) whether divergent judgements can be resolved argumentatively or semantically or (ii) whether there is an agreement about an unresolved dissent (consensus on dissent). At the end of the group Delphi workshop, there is usually a much clearer distribution of judgements and substantive justifications for each of the prevailing judgements. The group Delphi method thus facilitates a quantitative and qualitative improvement in knowledge. For the health sciences, the method is particularly suitable for inter- and transdisciplinary consensus-finding on the effectiveness of diagnostic or therapeutic advances, as an evaluation instrument for various strategies, and for the discursive investigation of social or transformation processes that are appropriate for specific settings. The application for a group Delphi relies clearly on a defined research question the answering of

M. Niederberger (✉)
University of Education Schwäbisch Gmünd, Schwäbisch Gmünd, Germany
e-mail: marlen.niederberger@ph-gmuend.de

O. Renn
Research Institute for Sustainability - Helmholtz Center Potsdam, Potsdam, Germany
e-mail: ortwin.renn@rifs-potsdam.de

M. Niederberger, O. Renn (eds.), *Delphi Methods In The Social And Health Sciences*, https://doi.org/10.1007/978-3-658-38862-1_4

which requires methodological expertise. However, compared to other Delphi variants, ithe group Delphi has been used rather rarely so far.

1 Introduction

When conducting a group Delphi, experts are invited to a joint workshop rather than addressing them individually per mail. The Delphi principle of repeated and iterated questioning with a feedback of the statistical outcome to all participants is compressed in such a way that it can be carried out in one or two days. A group Delphi provides the opportunity that through the personal exchange, substantive reasons of the experts can be recorded, debated and disclosed. At the same time, however, the anonymity of the experts is given up. In the following, the concept and the procedure of the group Delphi method will be presented. Subsequently, the specific opportunities and challenges for the health sciences will be discussed.

2 The Group Delphi: Concept and Definition

The group Delphi was developed in the 1980s as a variant of the Delphi method. The concern was to retain the characteristics of a classic Delphi while compensating for its negative aspects, especially the lack of substantive justifications (cf. Hill & Fowles, 1975; Renn & Kotte, 1984; Renn et al., 1985; Webler et al., 1991; Schulz & Renn, 2009; Niederberger & Renn, 2018). It is assumed that aspects such as discipline-specific perspectives, life-world experiences, or even semantic articuations influence the judgmental behavior of experts. For example, the distinction between whether someone rejects further research in a certain topic area because enough research has already been done or because further research is considered unimportant (cf. Goodman, 1987), makes a major difference for interpretation.

The aim of group Delphi is to identify a true consensus or a joint agreement about disagreement ("consensus on dissent") among experts. Consensus or consensus on dissent is reached in a group Delphi when further discussion does not lead to any significant change in judgement. Depending on how far apart the judgements are, a consensus or a consensus on dissent is reached. A mathematical precision of the formulation "how far" is not given, because this depends among other things on the choice of the response options or scale widths in the questionnaire used. It is therefore primarily a matter of determining stable distributions of the estimated values. The basic premise is that not all experts share the same opinion or assessment, but that there is a variability when choosing different degrees of approval or disapproval (cf. Williams & Webb, 1994). The aim of the group Delphi is to find out whether this variability is due to differences in the content of the assessments, to knowledge deficits, to measurement errors, to different semantic understandings of the questions or the scaling options, or to other artifacts (such as associations with certain numerical values). Ideally, consensus can evolve when all differences are based on misunderstanding rather than substantive disagreement. Frequently, however, a consensus can be reached that all agree on a dissent in assessing a specific topic or judgement. In the end, all experts involved share the common knowledge about why differences exist and why they cannot be resolved. Such information can be used by decision makers, for example, to derive further research needs, but also for making decisions under uncertainty.

A group Delphi is not exclusively about resolving differences on purely quantitative assessments, but also about integration of qualitative data. Although these are not usually systematically evaluated in the sense of numerical coding, they can reveal semantic ambiguities, provide clues for the interpretation and produce background information for interrpeting the statistical results. In this way, the group Delphi method shows conceptual parallels to an in-depth design, in which qualitative data are collected as a follow-up to the explanation or substantiation of quantitative findings (Creswell, 2008; Curry & Nunez-Smith, 2015).

While the classic Delphi method can primarily capture contextual and structural factors of a certain issue, the group Delphi additionally allows for interpretations of these factors with regard to possible individual or institutional relevance, backgrounds and meanings. Thus, the group Delphi represents a kind of "mixed methods instrument" for the integration of qualitative (free statements of the experts) and quantitative elements (standardized questionnaire). On the one hand, statistical estimations can characterize the scenarios or projections asked for in many Delphi procedures according to the degree of probability of their realization and quantified grades of approval or disapproval; on the other hand, content-related statements can contribute to understanding the variance in the experts' answers order to allow sufficient time for the experts' substantive explanations in the context of a workshop, the number of experts is limited to a maximin of 30 in a group setting (Niederberger & Renn, 2018).

3 The Main Characteristics of Group Delphi Procedures

The main difference between the classic Delphi and the group Delphi is that a group Delphi is not based on a written survey forwaded to the experts in advance, but on a face-to-face situation (real or virtual). A group Delphi is characterized by the following characteristics:

1. *Lack of anonymity:* The group Delphi method is the only modification of Delphi methods in which the anonymity of the experts is sacrificed in favour of personal exchange (Aengenheyster et al., 2017). However, the concrete list of participants can be made anonymous to the public.
2. *Joint answering of the questionnaire:* Instead of an individual questioning, the experts answer the questionnaire in small groups (2–5 members) during the workshop. They are encouraged to exchange arguments and views and to agree or disagree on a given questions
3. *Small group deliberation:* The group of experts is divided by random selection in small groups (3–5). These groups respond to the questionnaire and try to reach a consensus among them. If they cannot reach an agreement, majority and minority responses are recorded and later fed back to the plenary.
4. *Iterative small group discussions:* After each small group deliberation, the moderating team processes the numerical and narrative data from the questionnaires and provides a summary for the plenary discussion. The moderator selects those questions for the plenary debate that show the highest degree of vaiability (deviation from the mean or median value). Those group scores (or minority scores from each group) that deviate the most from the mean or median value are asked to present their arguments to the plenary. So all experts are exposed to the arguments on the both sides right or left from the mean value (for example on a scale from 1 to 10). All group scores that are selected because of the wide variability of assessments are then subject of an intensive discussion. Are the dissenting scores based on misunderstanding of the question's content, differences in the semantic attribution of meaning, lack of knowledge by one or the other side or true differences in judgment? Once this has been clarified, the deliberation process is continued in small grousp again, this time with systematic permutation of particpants. Ideally each new group should include one representative of the deviating parties. This process can be repeated several times until all groups feel comfortable with the resulting scores or time constrains do now allow for another round. In practice, three rounds of iteration are normally sufficient to reach a robust result.
5. *Consensus goal:* Group Delphi procedures pursue the goal of obtaining consensus or consensus on dissent. Consensus is established statistically and through arguments.

(a) Statistically, it involves the analysis of means and variances. In a ten-point scale, coefficients of variation[1] below 1 or below 0.5 are usually defined as consensus (Niederberger & Renn, 2018, p. 88).
(b) Argumentatively, it is a matter of the experts themselves establishing consensus or consensus on dissent during the workshop.

6. *Equality of expert judgements regardless of frequency:* If no consensus can be reached between the experts, minority votes can be recorded. They are included in the report on the results together with the substantive justifications. There is no distinction between majority or minority votes. If there is disagreement, *consensus on dissent* is recorded. In this case, the statistical discrepancy between the verdicts is irrelevant. The recording of minority votes summarizes the discussion during the workshop and the experts' adherence to certain judgements independent of the group numerical judgements.
7. *Real-time presentation of results:* The statistical results of the small group deliberations are not made available to the experts in written form as in the classic Delphi, but the results are evaluated during the workshop and fed back to the experts immediately. On the spot, the experts have the opportunity to explain and, if necessary, defend their judgements, but also to ask questions about the evaluation of all the other groups.

4 Procedure of a Group Pendulum

In the group Delphi, the experts are invited to a one to two-day workshop. A standardized questionnaire is handed out to them. The group is divided into rotating small groups of experts, who are asked to reach a consensus or a consensus on dissent (majority minority judgements). Once the small group members have reached their final judgments, they return to the plenary session where they are asked to defend their judgment if it deviates considerably from the means of all groups. The plenary discission are facilitated by a professional moderator.

In a group Delphi, the experts perfrom their deliberations in several successive small groups with rotating composition (based on systematic mutation) and discuss the answers as well as the reasons backing the answers together in the plenary. Thus, there is an alternation between the work in small groups and in the plenary.

[1] This puts the arithmetic mean and the variability in relation to each other and allows a comparison of the variability across all questions/items.

The experts can defend, modify or revise their opinions in both discussion forums or acknowledge the opinions of the others. Only the discussion in the plenary is moderated, in the small group setting, the experts remain among themselves and organize the deliberations without external assistance.

The procedure of such a group Delphi is similar to the classic procedure and is shown in Fig. 1.

The number of iterations of the small group deliberations depends on the judgements of the experts and on the time available. As a rule, three Delphi rounds (analogy to Delphi waves) are carried out, as in the classical Delphi method, in order to produce or determine relatively stable statistical findings (cf. Cuhls et al., 1998; Rowe & Wright, 1999). Thus, a duration of 2 days proves to be an ideal time window for conducting a group Delphi workshop. However, the preparation of such a workshop can take up to 6 months, also because it is important to contact the designated experts early on and to prepare them for their function during the Delphi process.

It is possible to combine the Group Delphi workshop with a written survey of the designated experts or even a larger group of experts before the group Delphi process takes place. In this case, the standardized questionnaire with the request for an individual response is sent out in advance of the workshop and subsequently processed by statistical means. The answers of the experts are treated anonymously

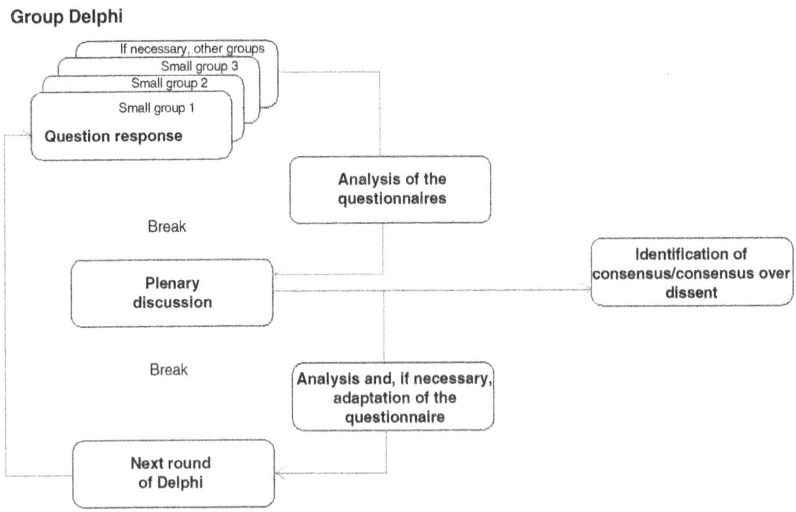

Fig. 1 Sequence of a group Delphi. (Own representation, Niederberger & Renn, 2018)

and statistically evaluated with regard to mean values and other distributional characteristics (such as variability, scope, extremes, variance etc.)

When conducting a preliminary survey, the research team receives a first impression of the experts' opinions and sensitivities and, based on the results, can focus the workshop on the particularly contentious and controversial aspects. In this case, items with hardly any deviations from the mean can be excluded for the workshop and consensus can be assumed. The experts also get a good insight about what their colleagues deem important and controversial before they meet in small groups. This gives them the opportunity to be beter prepared or, if necessary, to do further research. In this preliminary survey, a larger number of experts can be integrated in order to gain a more comprehensive representation of expert judgements. The extent to which this preliminary survey seems useful or necessary is a matter of balancing resources and the presumed gain in knowledge. On the one hand, it means a further expenditure of resources, but, on the other hand, both the research team and the experts can use this preliminary survey to prepare the workshop and to focus on those topics that seem to be most controversial or contested. A possible disadvantage can be that experts have made an inner commitment by answering the questions individually in advance, which may prevent them from taking up new aspects and rethinking their positions in the course of the group discussions. The group discussion thrives on mutual learning processes and is therefore inportant that participants are not already predetermined in their judgments and positions.

5 Selection of Experts

As in other Delphi methods, group Delphi methods usually involve experts and practitioners from different disciplines and institutional affiliations. The experts are usually identified and approached through a deliberate selection based on professional status and/or institutional affiliation. Due to the limited number of experts for the workshop, the concrete selection of the experts for a group Delphi is a particular challenge. The following aspects must be taken into account when identifying experts for a group Delphi:

- *Early planning of the workshop:* The challenge of a group Delphi is to bring together all the designated experts on a common workshop date. However, renowned experts, in particular, are often booked up for months. Therefore, the experts are usually invited several months before the workshop is scheduled (Niederberger & Renn, 2018).

- *Content range:* The invited experts should represent the entire range of relevant opinions and institutions. Experts with extreme, supposedly outsider positions need to be invited together with experts representing mainstream views. Through the open exchange during the workshop, the arguments and reasons for divergent votes are recorded. In addition, experts with extreme positions often sensitize the other participants to the relevance of often neglected or ignored observations or to the variability of interpretations associated with specific data or evidence.
- *Equal distribution of expertise:* As a rule, the aim for the designated experts is to represent the relevant institutions or opinion leaders roughly in proportion to the expert communities that they stand for. Usually, the experts come in roughly equal numbers from academia, politics and business and represent different disciplines (Niederberger & Renn, 2018). The integration of science and practice is associated with the claim to combine theoretical and real-world expertise. Thus, a group Delphi can be regarded as a formal method of transdisciplinary research (Bergmann et al., 2010; Pohl & Hirsch Hadorn, 2008).
- *Status and seniority:* For consensus building and the quality of the results, it is important that all experts participate equally in the discussion and express their opinions openly. In order to increase the opportunity for a free and non-coercive discourse, effects of group dynamics or group composition are crucial for the success of a group Delphi. Therefore, it is important that the experts have a similar status and seniority so that communication can take place on an equal footing (Niederberger & Renn, 2018). Therefore, in the field of science, for example, either professors or post-docs or doctoral students should be selected but not mixed.
- *Experts and practitioners are the requsted target groups:* In contrast to other Delphi methods, a group Delphi is based on a narrower understanding of the term expert. Civil society actors, interested citizens or interest groups (e.g. users, patients) are usually not included, unless they have a specific expertise that others do not possess. In this way, possible strategic reasoning can be reduced. Conceptually, this is based on the analytical separation of knowledge and interest. Those who argue on the basis of their own interest are less willing to engage in a learning and adaptive processes based on knowledge-related argumentation.

In principle, there is a risk in every group Delphi workshop that the experts deliberately manipulate the results, position themselves as spokespersons of particular intersts or do not contribute sufficiently beause they cannot deal appropriately with the experience of dissent. These risks are conceptually countered by the alternation between small group and plenary discussion, the permutation of the expert composition in the small groups and the neutral moderation in the plenary. In addition, the questionnaire serves as an anchor and reminder to stick to the tasks and not to digress. Thus, the focus of the discussion in the small groups as well as in the plenary is directed towards concrete issues. Discussions of principles or "window dressing speeches" can be largely avoided. However, it is not possible to exclude deliberate manipulation by experts.

6 Moderation

The tasks of every moderator of a group discussion are, first, to ensure a neutral and impartial facilitation of the plenary deliberations and, second, to provide equal opportunities for each participant to voice his or her judgement and to critique those of others (Hartmann et al., 2009). A moderator is, on the one hand, the "sovereign" of the entire discussion process, who wants to reach closure on each discussion point, and, on the other hand, the person who supports a group in fulfilling its task (Hartmann et al., 2009). The course of the discussion and thus the success of the entire exercise depend crucially on the moderator's competencies. Compared to other discussion settings, the moderation of a group Delphi is particularly demanding in terms of the following aspects:

1. *Experts are a demanding target group:* Experts sometimes react indignantly if they have the feeling that their time and expertise are not sufficiently taken into account or that their fellow professionals are not sufficiently prepared. Therefore, a certain sensitivity is necessary when dealing with different communication styles of experts. While some experts answer extensively with many technical details, others react rather anecdotally or authoritatively. Still others remain rather stuck on the abstract level in their explanations (Martens & Brüggemann, 2006).
2. *Challenging topics:* The topics or questions of a group Delphi require a minimum of expertise in the suject area. In addition, a certain inter- and transdisciplinary competence is necessary, because the topics often touch on different domains and areas of expertise.
3. *Different schools of thought:* The experts come from different disciplines and represent different academic traditions, i.e. they are bearers of diverse manifestations of knowledge and culture (Fleck, 2011; Sabisch, 2017). In the health sciences, for example, different disciplines (e.g. medicine, psychology, sociology and nutritional science) come together which are bound to different methodological paradigms. Taking this into account and supporting a common language is a challenge and requires the research and facilitation team to be

familiar with the terminology and language styles of each of the respective external parties involved.
4. *Political subtexts:* The attributed or actual knowledge of experts is the basis for their judgments. This knowledge is not only based on theoretical and discipline-specific foundations, it also includes functional, operational and experiential knowledge (Dreiack & Niederberger, 2018; Meuser & Nagel, 1997). These bodies of knowledge can be laden with personal values and political convictions (Niederberger & Dreiack, 2018; Molitor, 2009). On the one hand, experts can use this contextual knowledge specifically to influence and manipulate outcomes and instrumentalize the discourse. On the other hand, discussion and disclosure can reveal the background for divergent votes and, if necessary, contribute to consensus-building.
5. *Risk of heated controversies:* The experts in a group Delphi are deliberately selected because they hold different opinions, which can lead to heated discussions. An experienced moderator can mitigate conflict situations through strategies such as objectification, confrontation or concretisation (Niederberger & Renn, 2018).

The moderator of a group discussion ultimately needs expertise in leading the discussion, experience in dealing with controversies and a basic knowledge of the topic. There is the possibility to involve co-moderators. In this case, one person can take over the task of facilitating the discussion and the other is a specialist for responding to content-related issues. Simultaneous recording on a flipchart or with the help of presentation software has also proven successful in many cases.

7 Statistical Evaluation in Real Time

One of the biggest challenges in a group Delphi is the processing of statistical data during the workshop. The stastistical results are the basis for the plenary discussions and must therefore be available immediately after the small group discussions. For this purpose, the experts are sent into a 15 min break and the research team processes the data from the questionnaires. Different variants are possible here: either the small groups enter their answers directly into a digital response device and the results are compiled and evaluated automatically or the experts fill out the questionnaire in paper form. Inthis case, the research team feeds the data into the computer system and processes them with a statistical program (e.g. Excel, SPSS). It is important that this evaluation is done quickly. Therefore, a group Delphi questionnaire is mostly based on rating scales (Niederberger & Renn,

2018). This allows mean values and distributional charcateristics to be calculated expeditiously. Moreover, the results can be ordered according to the degree of variability. This gives the moderator/facilitator the opportunity to start with the most contentious points during the plenary discussion. Elaborated statistical calculations are not possible due to the small time frame during the workshop, and are usually not necessary.

8 Result of a Group Delphi

The results of a group Delphi are usually presented in the form of a report. This report does not record the discussion process itself but summarises the final results of the workshop. Descriptive frequency tables and statistical data are provided together with arguments when dissenting views are recorded. Dissenting judgements are listed without identifiying the individuals that represent each of the dissenting views and also without specifiying the number of experts that support each of the final positions.

The report can be sent to the designated experts with a request for possible corrections before publication or handover to the commissioning party of the group's report. This gives the experts a final opportunity to check whether their opinion is sufficiently reflected in the results. However, this reflection may jeopardise potential consensus or re-frame the entire task.

The results of a group Delphi can be used, for example, to derive recommendations for action or for further processing in a research process.

9 Research and Application Area of Group Delphi Procedures in Health Sciences

The group Delphi process has proven useful in various research and application areas for developing consensus or consensus on dissent.[2] In principle, it is suitable for:

- *Knowledge integration:* This is particularly useful for summarizing the state of knowledge beyond the boundaries of one's own discipline. Triggers for group Delphi processes can be political debates, social transformation processes or specific knowledge gaps. For example, the current state of knowledge can be

[2] For concrete project examples, cf. Niederberger and Renn (2018).

assessed for initiating organisational, technical or social innovations. The focus is on evidence-based findings and on the experts' assessment of the feasibility, acceptance and chances of implementation of possible interventions in all domains of human action, in particular individual behavioral routines. Concrete examples would be the traffic light labelling of food, the introduction of deterrent images on cigarette packets or the promotion of physical activity in cities and municipalities.
- *Knowledge transfer:* This area is primarily concerned with discussing, evaluating and prioritising scientific research results together with the relevant experts from practice. Bringing the two groups together enhances the opportunity for policies to be effective and efficient.
- *Evaluation:* Evaluations often involve having experts assess the progress or effects of projects, campaigns or interventions (Niederberger & Kuhn, 2013). The group Delphi method has proven itself as na appropriate evaluation instrument for evaluating educational programmes (Niederberger & Kuhn, 2013). In this case, the experts have been instructores for education or training.Their invovlement in a group Delphi led to an early identification of potential problems and contributed to a participatory development of effective solution strategies. In addition, the Delphi process increased the rate of acceptance among the instructors and enhanced their readiness to implement the results.

In principle, a group Delphi is suitable for integrating expert judgements, for deriving recommendations for common action, for resolving dissenting or controversial expert judgements and for identifying and evaluating interventions or measures. Prerequisites for the application are:

- the trans- or multidisciplinary topic must be clearly defined,
- the answers to the questions require solid expertise and professional judgement,
- the participating experts cover a large range of opinions and positions, and
- are willing to contribute.

The group Delphi method is mainly used in the fields of innovation, sustainability and environmental research (Niederberger & Renn, 2018). In the health sciences, group Delphi methods have rarely been used to date, when compared to other Delphi variants (Jünger et al., 2017). Nevertheless, initial experiences from the health sciences confirm the potential and feasibility of group Delphi. Particularly in the case of divergent expert judgements and at the interface between research, practice and policy, they have proven their worth. The group Delphi appears relevant when different scientific findings about the effects of interventions compete with each other, different disciplines are involved, and both real-life and theoretical expertise are equally relevant. Concrete examples could include the identification of competence profiles of health managers or the identification of suitable measures for the reduction of particulate matter in large cities.

10 Opportunities and Challenges of Group Delphi Procedures in the Health Sciences

A group Delphi is associated with a number of opportunities, but also challenges, when applied to the health sciences (Table 1).

The resilience and quality of the results of a group Delphi process depend significantly on the selection and willingness of the designated experts to participate. If it is possible to represent a wide range of opinions and to establish a culture of discussion on a equal footing. Different levels of knowledge and judgements can be reconciled and integrated. A group Delphi helps to discern whether there is real dissent or whether there are divergent understandings of the questions, semantic ambiguities or merely gaps in knowledge.

In the group Delphi workshop, the anonymity of the experts is abandoned in favour of a personal, direct exchange. The workshop situation allows the experts to

Table 1 Opportunities and challenges of group Delphi processes, own presentation

Opportunities	Challenges
Recording of majority and minority votes	Coverage of the whole range of opinions by the limited number of experts
Identification of areas of consensus or dissent in the case of divergent expert judgements	Selection and focus on a few, central topics/ questions
Direct exchange between experts from different disciplines and institutional affiliations (inter- and transdisciplinary)	Willingness of relevant experts to participate
Reduction of uncertainty within the expert group	No "representativeness" of the results
Clarification of reasons for dissent (e.g. factual or semantic reasons)	Opinion leaders and window-dressing (special moderation skills required)
Relatively fast procedure (especially compared to the classical Delphi procedure)	Risk of instrumentalisation of the procedure, especially in the case of politically and socially contested issues
High connectivity in the research process	Limited scope of forecasts due to uncertain possible futures

exchange arguments and to justify, confirm, modify or revise judgements. This is accompanied by the risk that group dynamics may play a undue role. Some participnats may dominate the discussion and try to influence the others with the help of convincing rhetoric. However, this is countered by the fact that minority votes are given special weight. They are not lost in the "statistical noise", as in other Delphi methods, but are integral part of the results. However, the relative importance of anonymity as a major feature of classic Delphi versus direct interaction as a major property of group Delphi is still contested and it may depend on the context to decide which of the two criteria is more valuable.

A major advantage of group Delphi process is clearly the possibility to have a full representation of majority and minority judgements together with the reasons to back up each position. This is particularly relevant for policymaking when looking at the full range of positions, including minority judgements.

- Minority votes can take on a kind of "early warning function" for politics and society. This is because minority votes can anticipate major changes that are about to come. Minority opinions can develop into majority opinions over time (Xie et al., 2011). At the same time, it is possible that individual experts have new or previously unnoticed information that turns out to be particularly relevant for the policy context in which the question is raised.
- Minority votes influence the group discussion processes at a workshop. Social psychological research shows that consistently and persistently held minority opinions can also unsettle a majority and influence latent judgment processes, which may lead to substantial changes in opinion and judgment (Erb & Bohner, 2010). However, if too rigid, a minority opinion can also have a repellent effect (Nemeth et al., 1974). Experience shows that in group Delphis, it is precisely the minority votes that are discussed and reflected on in detail; however, if there is genuine dissent, this cannot be resolved in the course of a two-day workshop, but is recorded as a consensus on the dissent.

Whether a group Delphi actually succeeds in capturing the minority votes is debatable. It is known from impact research that people often follow the current majority opinion (Schubert, 2000). The dominant motive is fear of isolation, i.e. the representatives are afraid of falling into social isolation or disgrace by their peers. It is possible that in a group Delphi workshop experts are more likely to withhold minority opinions than people with the supposed majority opinion because of the open and direct exchange. However, from previous experience with group Delphis, this behaviour of conformity pressure have been rare and not lasting over the entire 2 day period.

In principle, the group-delphi method can be applied to complex research processes. It can be used at the beginning to identify research gaps or at the end to check the plausibility and evaluate research results. As a procedure, it can be carried out relatively quickly and inexpensively. However, as with other methods of expert involvement, there is a risk of instrumentalization and manipulation of results (Dreiack & Niederberger, 2018). In addition, the results of a group pendulum are snapshots of often complex and highly topical issues. It may be necessary to conduct a series of group Delphis on the same topic over a longer time period. The procedure is well suited for regularly revisiting the topic at fixed intervals with the same or different experts.

11 Conclusion

The group Delphi is a suitable procedure for involving experts in assessment and judgemental processes. It is particularly suitable when different expert judgements exist, the knowledge of different disciplines (inter- and transdisciplinary) needs to be integrated and projects or interventions with unclear consequences should be assessed. The procedure can be carried out with a limited managerial effort and promises above all a better calibration of diverse judgements. Differences in the assessment or in the evaluation of data and the meaning of research results can be due to diverging knowledge assumptions, different evaluation criteria, weighting differences between criteria, uncertainties or ambiguities of the data base. A group Delphi is particularly well suited for identifying true consensus or true dissent. It helps to trace differences in the evaluation of statements back to the underlying causes. These differences cannot always be resolved during the limited time period of a Delphi workshop. But at least there is a plausible explanation for these differences and a basis of argumentation for the position taken by the respective representatives of each camp. This is as valuable for academic discussions as it is for political discourse and collectively binding decision-making.

For the health sciences, it has potential above all for finding potential areas of consensus and dissent and, as an evaluation instrument for different diagnostic or therapeutic options. Overall, it may be well suited to be an integral part of transdisciplinary research designs. However, compared to other Delphi variants, there is still a lack of experience and empirical evaluations to come up with a robust assessment of the strengths and weaknesses associated with group Delphi processes.

Literature

Aengenheyster, S., Cuhls, K., Gerhold, L., Heiskanen-Schüttler, M., Huck, J., & Muszynska, M. (2017). Real-time Delphi in practice – A comparative analysis of existing soft-ware-based tools. *Technological Forecasting and Social Change, 118*, 15–27.

Bergmann, M., Jahn, T., Knobloch, T., Krohn, W., Pohl, C., & Schramm, E. (2010). *Methoden transdisziplinärer Forschung: Ein Überblick mit Anwendungsbeispielen*. Campus.

Creswell, J. (2008). *Research design: Qualitative, quantitative and mixed methods approaches*. Sage.

Cuhls, K., Blind, K., & Grupp, H. (1998). *Delphi '98: Studie zur globalen Entwicklung von Wissenschaft und Technik.* Fraunhofer-Institut für Systemtechnik und Innovationsforschung.

Curry, L., & Nunez-Smith, M. (2015). *Mixed methods in health sciences research: A practical primer*. Sage.

Dreiack, S., & Niederberger, M. (2018). Qualitative Experteninterviews in internationalen Organisationen. *Politische Vierteljahresschrift, 59*(2), 293–318.

Erb, H.-P., & Bohner, G. (2010). Consensus as a key: Towards parsimony in explaining minority and majority influence. In R. Martin & M. Hewstone (Eds.), *Minority influence and innovation: Antecedents, processes and consequences* (pp. 79–103). Psychology Press.

Fleck, L. (2011). Das Problem der wissenschaftlichen Beobachtung. In S. Werner & C. Zittel (Eds.), *Denkstile und Tatsachen: Gesammelte Schriften und Zeugnisse* (pp. 534–537). Suhrkamp. (First published 1948).

Goodman, C. (1987). The Delphi technique: A critique. *Journal of Advanced Nursing, 12*, 729–734.

Hartmann, M., Besser, R., Maleh, C., Frank, H.-J., Rieger, M., & Funk, R. (2009). Ergebnisorientiert moderieren: Besprechungen, Versammlungen und Großgruppen. In I. Sachsenmeier (Ed.), *Mit Kommunikation zum Erfolg* Vol. 5. Beltz.

Hill, K. Q., & Fowles, J. (1975). The methodological worth of the Delphi forecasting technique. *Technological Forecasting and Social Change, 7*, 179–192.

Jünger, S., Payne, S. A., Brine, J., Radbruch, L., & Brearley, S. G. (2017). Guidance on conducting and reporting Delphi studies (CREDES) in palliative care: Recommendations based on a methodological systematic review. *Palliative Medicine, 31*(8), 684–706. https://doi.org/10.1177/0269216317690685

Martens, K., & Brüggemann, M. (2006). *Kein Experte ist wie der andere: Vom Umgang mit Missionaren und Geschichtenerzählern* (TransState working papers, 39).

Meuser, M., & Nagel, U. (1997). Das ExpertInneninterview – Wissenssoziologische Voraussetzungen und methodische Durchführung. In B. Friebertshäuser & A. Prengel (Eds.), *Handbuch qualitative Forschungsmethoden in der Erziehungswissenschaft* (pp. 481–491). Juventa.

Molitor, M. (2009). *Bildungskompetenzen im Fokus des aktuellen ethischen Diskurses: Explorative Studien zu inhaltlichen Parametern verantwortlichen pädagogischen Handelns*. Utz.

Nemeth, C., Swedlung, M., & Kanki, B. (1974). Patterning of the minority's responses and their influence on the majority. *European Journal of Social Psychology, 4*, 53–64.

Niederberger, M., & Dreiack, S. (2018). Wissensarten und deren politischer Gehalt bei Expert_inneninterviews in internationalen Organisationen. *Zeitschrift für Internationale Beziehungen, 25*(1), 189–198. https://doi.org/10.5771/0946-7165-2018-1-3.

Niederberger, M., & Kuhn, R. (2013). Das Gruppendelphi als Evaluationsinstrument. *Zeitschrift für Evaluation, 1*, 53–77.

Niederberger, M., & Renn, O. (2018). *Das Gruppendelphi: Vom Konzept zur Anwendung*. Springer.

Pohl, C., & Hirsch Hadorn, G. (2008). Methodenentwicklung in der transdisziplinären Forschung. In M. Bergmann & E. Schramm (Eds.), *Transdisziplinäre Forschung: Integrative Forschungsprozesse verstehen und bewerten* (pp. 69–92). Campus.

Renn, O., & Kotte, U. (1984). Umfassende Bewertung der vier Pfade der Enquete-Kommission auf der Basis eines Indikatorkatalogs. In G. Albrecht & H. U. Stegelmann (Eds.), *Energie im Brennpunkt: Zwischenbilanz der Energiedebatte* (pp. 190–232). High Tech Verlag.

Renn, O., Albrecht, R., Kotte, U., Peters, H. P., & Stegelmann, U. (1985). *Sozialverträgliche Energiepolitik: Ein Gutachten für die Bundesregierung*. High Tech Verlag.

Rowe, G., & Wright, G. (1999). The Delphi technique as a forecasting tool: Issues and analysis. *International Journal of Forecasting, 15*, 353–375.

Sabisch, K. (2017). Die Denkstilanalyse nach Ludwik Fleck als Methode der qualitativen Sozialforschung – Theorie und Anwendung [34 Absätze]. *Forum Qualitative Sozialforschung/Forum: Qualitative Social Research, 18*(2), Art. 5. http://nbn-resolving.de/urn:nbn:de:0114-fqs170258.

Schubert, B. (2000). *Shell in der Krise: Zum Verhältnis von Journalismus und PR in Deutschland. Dargestellt am Beispiel der "Brent Spar"*. LIT.

Schulz, M., & Renn, O. (Eds.). (2009). *Gruppen-Delphi: Konzept und Fragebogenkonstruktion*. VS Verlag.

Webler, T., Levine, D., Rakel, H., & Renn, O. (1991). The group Delphi: A novel attempt at reducing uncertainty. *Technological Forecasting and Social Change, 39*, 253–263.

Williams, P. L., & Webb, C. (1994). The Delphi technique: A methological discussion. *Journal of Advanced Nursing, 19*, 180–186.

Xie, J., Sreenivasan, S., Korniss, G., Zhang, W., Lim, C., & Szymanski, B. K. (2011). Social consensus through the influence of committed minorities. *Physical Review E, 84*, 011130.

Real-Time Delphi

Lars Gerhold

Abstract
In the classic Delphi method, results are processed only after the conclusion of a round, and the numerical and qualitative information is reported back to the experts. This article describes a "real-time Delphi" approach, which eliminates the conventional "round logic" in favor of intermediate result feedback. The article describes the requirements of this efficiency-centered approach and discusses the biases and problems as well as the specifics of the survey procedure. In addition, the paper presents providers of software tools and identifies current developments regarding real-time Delphis.

1 Introduction

Real-time Delphi[1] is a methodological extension of the classical Delphi approach (see Cuhls & Steinmüller in this volume) that leads to more discussion and reflection of expert judgments. Like classic Delphi, real-time Delphi is an expert survey

[1] Different notations are common in the literature, including RT Delphi (Gordon & Pease, 2006) and real-time Delphi (Geist, 2010; Gnatzy et al., 2011; Gordon, 2009).

L. Gerhold (✉)
Institute of Psychology, Psychology of Sociotechnical Systems, Technische Universität Braunschweig, Berlin, Germany
e-mail: lars.gerhold@tu-braunschweig.de

M. Niederberger, O. Renn (eds.), *Delphi Methods In The Social And Health Sciences*, https://doi.org/10.1007/978-3-658-38862-1_5

that, depending on type, can serve to aggregate ideas, determine a future state of affairs, ascertain expert opinions on future developments, or reach a consensus (Häder, 2009, p. 30 ff.). The central difference between real-time and classic Delphi is that the former relies on the immediate feedback of intermediate results. In classic Delphi, results are processed only after the conclusion of a round, and the numerical and qualitative information is reported back to the experts. Participants gain a comprehensive understanding of the first-round results before checking and prevising their statements. Real-time Delphis, by contrast, jettison the classic "round logic" so that participants have immediate access to the interim results after responding. This enables them to re-evaluate their assessments on the fly. It replaces the sequential elicitation and feedback process of the classic approach with a continuous process.

The initial spark for the establishment of the method was the paper "RT Delphi: An efficient, 'round-less' almost real time Delphi method" by Gordon and Pease (2006). There, Gordon and Pease present the real-time Delphi method as the result of a study commissioned by the US Defense Advanced Research Projects Agency (DARPA) (Gordon & Pease, 2006). In commissioning the study, DARPA was seeking to accelerate coordination between decision-IN ORDER to enable "rapid decisions in tactical situations" (Gordon & Pease, 2006, p. 322). Gordon and Pease's solution was to have several experts simultaneously and synchronously or asynchronously make their judgments about the value of alternative solutions or statistical estimates of future developments. Originally requested by DARPA for a small number of experts (10–15), the real-time method is capable of handling a higher number of participants.

The central function of the real-time Delphi for DARPA was to enable efficient and fast consensus-building among experts. The focus was on the improvement of group communication and the collection of group opinions. But Häder (2009, p. 19) identifies a second essential form of Delphi studies: solving particular problems. Problem-solving aims to assess future states of affairs that are uncertain or contingent (Neuhaus & Steinmüller, 2015). Based on previous Delphi studies, Häder (2009) developed four types of Delphi methods (type 1: idea aggregation; type 2: determination of a future issue; type 3: determination of expert opinions; type 4: consensus building). Häder's types also serve as a framework for conducting real-time Delphis.[2]

[2] The typification helps Delphi developers be clear about objectives, enables a methodological framing (e.g. design of the questions depending on the objective), and shows the possibilities that Delphi surveys offer (Häder, 2009, p. 31).

2 How Real-Time Delphi Works

This section presents the foundations and functions of real-time Delphi. The point is to provide a basic understanding of the method and explain the added benefits of the real-time approach, which are not always obvious to those who conduct real-time Delphi studies or those who participate in the surveys.

According to Gordon and Pease, a real-time Delphi is based on an existing survey in electronic form and on numerical information. The following information is displayed for all participants (adapted from Gordon & Pease, 2006, p. 323):

1. The arithmetic mean or median as the average of all previous responses to a question.
2. The number of responses so far.
3. The qualitative rationale for the numerical data.
4. A button for numerical responses to the respective question.
5. A button for qualitative rationales in addition to numerical estimations.

In a real-time Delphi, participants can repeat responses to individual questions or even the entire survey multiple times. This means that they can also change their assessment multiple times. This may result in a change of the average value of the group answer to a question. The interim results can thus evolve depending on when and how often a person participates in an ongoing real-time Delphi study. At the same time, the ratio (i.e. the difference) between one's own response and the group response can change. If the differences in values between the individual answers of the experts decrease, the dispersion of the values around the mean value also decreases. A low dispersion indicates a high consensus between the respondents' answers.

The layout of a real-time Delphi with technical support is more comprehensive than in classic surveys. Figure 1 shows the layout of an early Delphi (Gordon, 2007). Here, the time occurrence of different events (1.01–1.04) has to be estimated with regard to future developments in the field of energy supply (e.g. "business as usual," "environmental backlash"). It also supplies the average values and the number of previous responses. Clicking on the "Comments" button opens an additional window in which all previous comments are displayed.

By comparison, Fig. 2 shows a more modern layout, based on the real-time software programmed by Wes Boyer for the Millennium Project, which is embedded in the Global Futures Information System (GFIS). On the left side, a question is phrased regarding an uncertain future state of affairs. Here the future state is

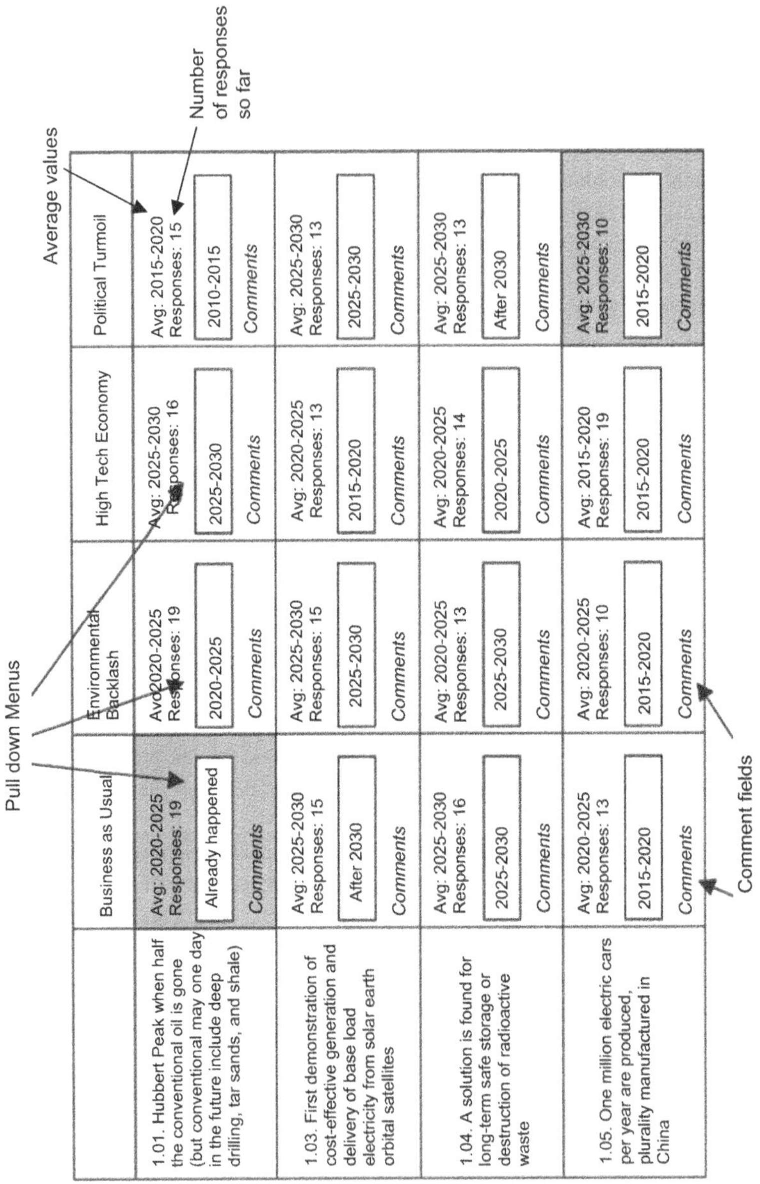

Fig. 1 Layout of an early online real-time Delphi questionnaire. (Gordon, 2007)

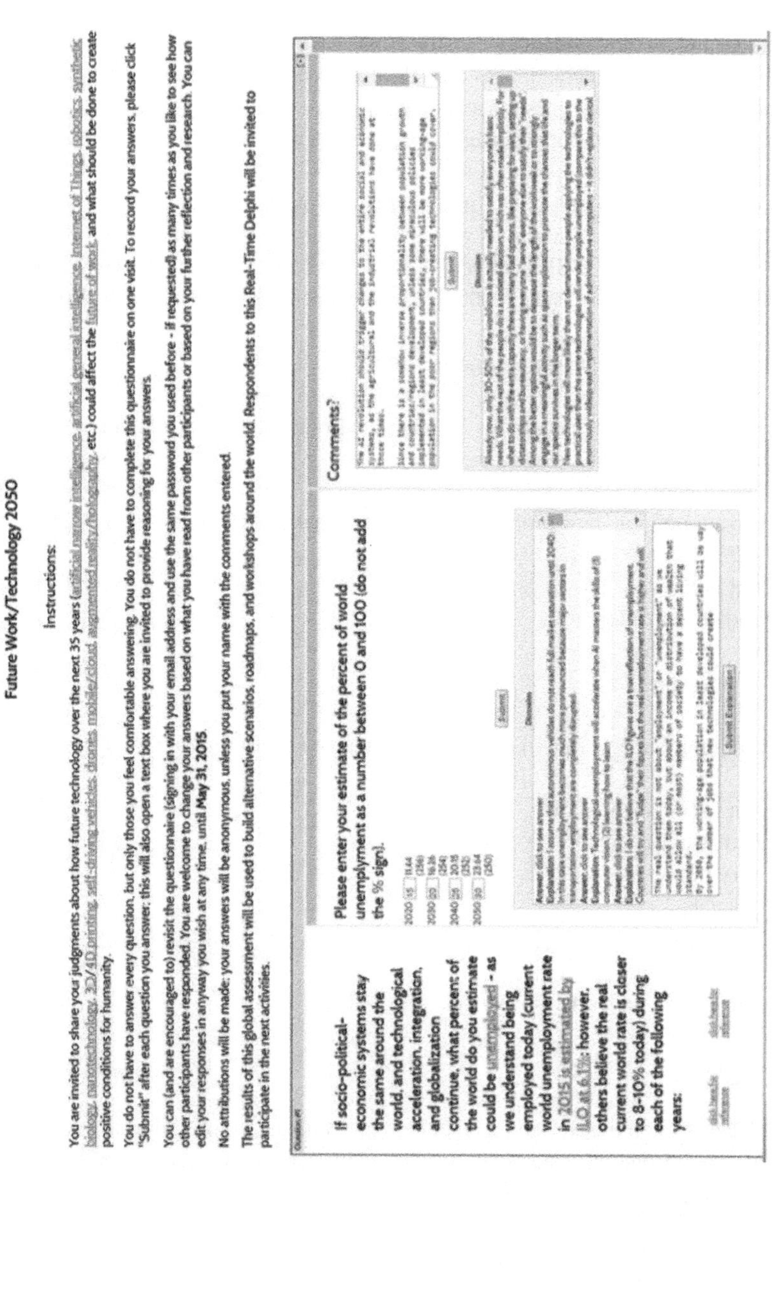

Fig. 2 Layout of a real-time Delphi of the Millenium Project/GFIS. (Screenshot provided by authors Glenn & Florescu, 2015)

"global unemployment." In the middle panel, respondents have the option of providing numerical information on future trends over various time periods. The "discussion" below shows qualitative justifications for the numerical statements, which also enables group interaction, as does the comment field on the right-hand side.

The use of different question and item formats does not differ between classical and real-time Delphi. Both open and closed items can be used, which are presented as questions, statements, or mini-scenarios.

With regard to item scaling, time intervals or expected occurrence periods are just as conceivable as questions regarding desirability, probability, and expected EFFECTS. Several OTHER studies ALSO deal with item determination (Linstone & Turoff, 1975, 2011; Häder, 2009; Häder & Häder, 2000; Cuhls, 2009, 2012).

Example: Item and questions (Aguirre-Bastos et al., 2009):

Item: Climate change causes extreme environmental conditions in some EU countries (incl. Storms, floods, draughts).

Questions:

In your opinion, how probable is it that this change will unfold until 2025?

- Not probable
- Rather probable
- Very probable
- Almost sure

In your opinion, how important will this change be for European security by then?

- Not important at all
- Rather important
- Very important
- Crucial

Example: Item and scales (Wagner et al., 2016, p. 437 f.):

Item:

- Because of an increase in social interconnection due to social media, citizens of all socioeconomic categories receive additional qualification to become involved in participation processes

Scales:

- probability of occurrence (0–100%)
- the potential impact on politicians (5-point Likert-type scale)
- desirability of occurrence (5-point Likert-type scale)

Example: Scenario and scales (Sonk n.V.)

The dream of many employees has come true in 2050: The standard work week has been reduced from 40 to 20 h. The cause is straightforward: Various productive innovations mean lower demand for human labor. The populace is now using the extra free time not only to cultivate their well-being, but also to perform charitable activities, such as beautifying the urban landscape.

Scales:

- Please rate the probability this scenario will occur (in %; or do not specify) (0–100%).
- Please also rate the desirability of this scenario (5-point scale ranging from "very desirable" to "very undesirable")

With increasing item complexity or when using scenarios or ideas about the future, the following challenges also arise:

- It is unclear how respondents rate the individual components of the item, or whether individual items are overrated.
- If individual components of the mini-scenario contradict each other, no clear answer is possible. This can be avoided by carrying out homogeneity checks (e.g. consistency analyses) and pre-tests.
- Individual components of the scenario are so extreme that respondents can evaluate the majority of the scenario, but the extreme aspect dominates the evaluation.

Since an ideal description of an item is impossible, Rowe and Wright (1999) recommend the following:

- Items should be meaningfully phrased, which means that they "relate to the domain of knowledge of the specific panelist" (Rowe & Wright, 1999, p. 368).
- Oversimplification can lead to unclear questions or results (Rowe & Wright, 1999).

Furthermore, a subjective estimation of the experts competencies with regard to the topic area is useful for filtering the data afterwards.

Sample questions regarding subjective competence include:

- How competent do you feel regarding the research subject?
- How confident are you in your judgment?
- How familiar are you with the subject area?
- How long have you been working in your field?

3 Real-Time Delphi and Classical Delphi: Similarities and Differences

As the discussion of the questionnaire items make clear, real-time Delphis are based on the Delphi method. Both rely on a survey method, use (online) questionnaires, guarantee the anonymity of the participants, identify group responses and elicit feedback (Häder, 2009). In addition, the assessment of both Delphis and real-time Delphis as to whether they can be assigned to a qualitative or quantitative research logic varies across different authors. While Steinmüller (1997) and Glenn and Gordon (2009) ascribe a qualitative and explorative character to the Delphi approach because it generates opinions on questions for which no hard data are available, Popper (2009) describes the method as semi-quantitative because it applies "mathematical principles to quantify subjectivity, rational judgments and viewpoints of experts and commentators." Schüll (2009), by contrast, argues that the Delphi method can encompass both qualitative and quantitative elements. However, this assessment requires more specificity. One must namely distinguish between three levels: research conception, data collection and data analysis (Gerhold, 2012).

In terms of research conception, each Delphi study needs to be located within a theoretical framework that does justice to the subject matter of research and its understanding. At the level of data collection, a Delphi study oriented towards the numerical estimation of occurrence probabilities leads to different statements about the future from that of a qualitative assessment. (See, for instance, Niederberger & Renn, in this volume.) Last, the relation between quantitative and qualitative data needs to be determined. For example, it must be determined whether open comments are understood as complementary information to numerical averages, or whether they are seen to have a validating function (leading to divergence or convergence). This is crucial for further processing the data.

The logic of a real-time Delphi also results in obvious differences to the classic Delphi method. It eliminates the classic "round logic" and does not require that all expert judgments are available before interim results can be reported back as mean values (see Fig. 3):

This results in a significant increase in efficiency and time savings, which can be valuable for decision-makers. Furthermore, a significant difference is that experts can always return to the interview to change their previous judgments. As a rule, they are shown both their original judgment and the relation of their judgment to that of the other participants. This is done by displaying the deviation of their own numerical indication from the group response, which may also be highlighted in different shadings (see Fig. 4).

The real-time Delphi places the learning effects of conventional Delphi studies in a different setting. Learning and reflection must begin more immediately. With the classic approach, the assumption is that the initial judgments are first made on the basis of expert knowledge, obvious sources, intentions to answer, and mental models. In the Delphi approach, this would mean that experts first evaluate the questions posed to them on the basis of the expert knowledge explicitly available to them, which may be supported by evidence-based sources. The evaluation is accompanied by intentional action: the experts answer in a way that is coherent with their personal expert assessment (i.e. their mental model) of the problem. These models – and the initial judgments derived from them – then undergo a review based on external anchors (i.e. the judgments of the other participants) and if necessary a subsequent readjustment based on learned information (Häder, 2009, p. 40 f.). But the aforementioned learning process is based on the assumption that the initial assessment is made independent of group opinion and put up for discussion only after statements from other participants emerge. In a real-time Delphi, however, the group judgment is usually displayed directly after the submission of an individual assessment (see Fig. 3). This means that the group assessment of the first question can have an effect on responses to later questions, as the next section discusses.

Table 1 summarizes the similarities and differences between classic and real-time Delphis:

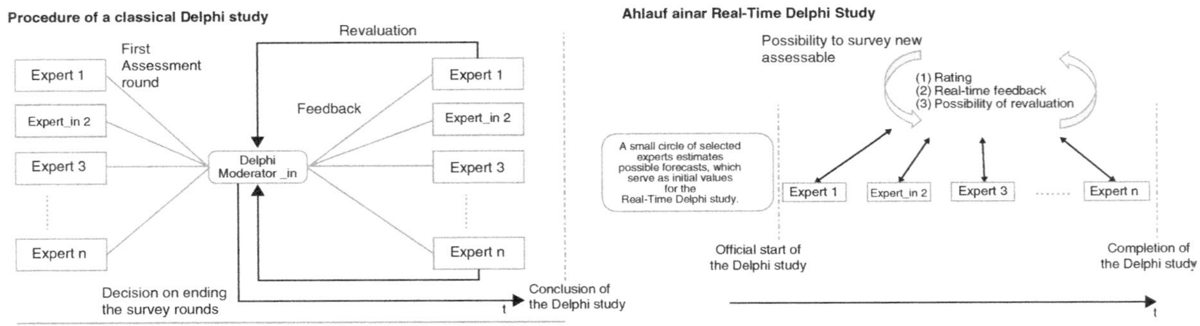

Fig. 3 Sequence of classic and a real-time Delphis. (Gnatzy et al., 2011, p. 1686)

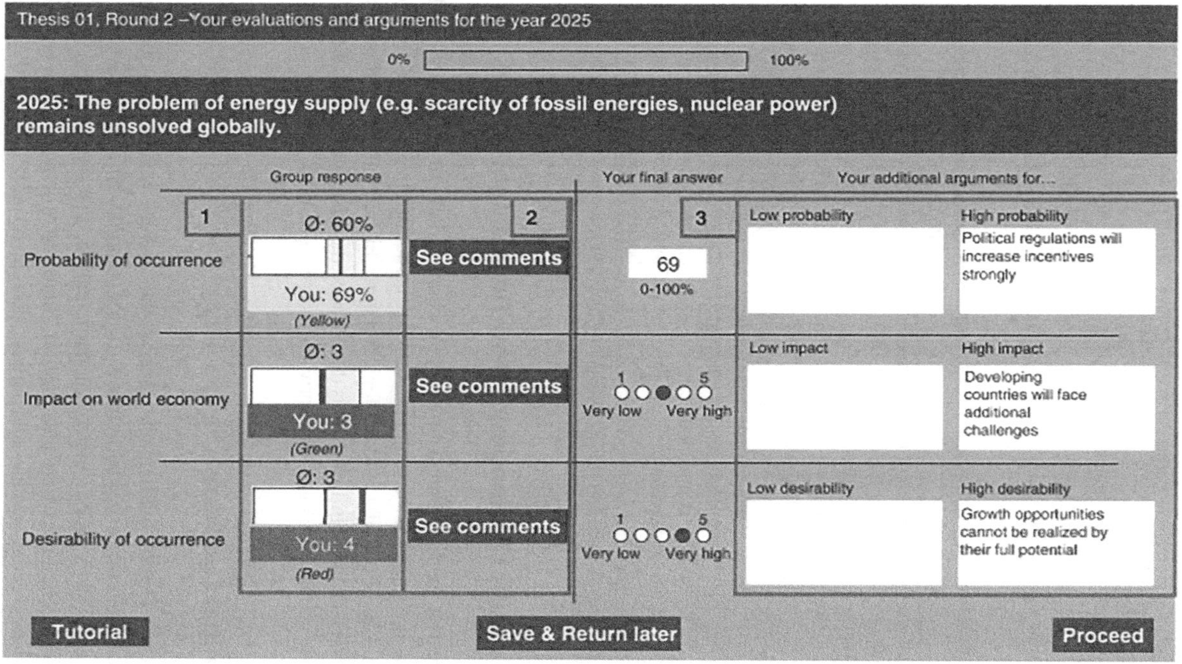

Fig. 4 Feedback screen of a real-time Delphi study. (Gnatzy et al., 2011, p. 1684, The software shown here is not publicly available. The color scheme used was available, however (Gnatzy et al., 2011, p. 1685))

Table 1 Characteristics of classic and real-time Delphis

Characteristic	Classic Delphi	Real-Time Delphi
Common ground		
Survey instrument	Questionnaire	Questionnaire
Sample	Expert panel	Expert panel
Anonymity of responses	Given	Given
Differences		
Number of rounds	Two or more	No rounds, but immediate feedback
Basis of feedback on judgments of other participants	Feedback of the arithmetic mean or the median of all expert assessments	Feedback of the arithmetic mean or the median of all previous expert assessments
Scope of qualitative feedback	Summary or complete presentation of all justifications given by participating experts for their numerical assessments	Complete presentation of all previous justifications given by the participating experts for their numerical assessments
Revision of participant assessment	No further changes possible after completion of the questionnaire	Changes are possible after completion of the questionnaire until the entire survey phase has been completed by a moderator

Adapted from Linstone and Turoff (1975), Häder (2009), Gordon and Pease (2006)

4 Specific Challenges of Real-Time Delphi Studies

As described at the beginning, an essential characteristic of a real-time Delphi study is that it eliminates the round logic from classical Delphis. This gives rise to two essential questions of a methodological nature: First, what is the initial condition (Sect. 4.1), i.e. what information is disclosed to the first participants of a study? Second, how should certain types of errors (Sect. 4.2) be dealt with?

4.1 Initial Condition

In a real-time Delphi, participants receive the average values and qualitative responses of previous survey participants. If, for example, 20 experts have already answered a question before their own participation, the average values of the answers are reported back for each question. Since the arithmetic mean is susceptible to statistical extreme values and outliers, this can be problematic if the number of cases is small, providing a distorted picture to those completing the questionnaire. The higher the number of cases (n) of survey participants, the smaller the effect of the problem.[3] Accordingly, the possible bias due to the initial condition is particularly evident at the beginning of real-time Delphi studies, since there must always be experts who are the first to fill out the questionnaire. Their judgement could have a particular influence on the responses of subsequent participants. This is true for both numerical values and for qualitative data because a framing effect (Sect. 4.2) for subsequent questions could arise from the latter.

Several options are possible for meeting the challenge of the initial condition:

- Activate the feedback function of group responses and qualitative information only when a critical mass of information has been achieved. Gordon (2009, p. 8), citing Finnish studies, suggests 5–10 "key experts" whose judgment should be taken as a starting point. However, this number is also more or less arbitrary and could be set higher if the subject demands it. Gnatzy et al. (2011) used a sample study in the field of energy to investigate the extent to which this variant would lead to a significant change vis-a-vis the classic Delphi and were unable to identify any significant differences. However, the methodological approach and the thematic focus mean that the significance of the study is also limited.
- Enter average values into the study before it is released to the experts. It is best to use beta tests or other plausible data collected in studies on similar questions (Gordon & Pease, 2006, p. 326). Particularly in the case of uncertain and/or complex research questions, it makes sense to conduct a "0-th round." In this case, a heterogeneous selection of experts evaluate the questions or statements of the Delphi and, if necessary, revise them or develop new ones. The experts can evaluate initial values together or independently.

4.2 Biases in Delphi Studies

While there are very few empirical studies on the initial condition effect, Winkler and Moser (2016) have investigated framing, anchoring, and bandwagon effects and have identified a number of methodological challenges that arise from them. These biases also apply in principle to real-time Delphi studies, but they have yet

[3] It should be noted, however, that a large sample size is not necessarily the objective. "In a statistically based study, Gordon observes, "such as a public opinion poll, participants are assumed to be representative of a larger population; in Delphi, non-representative, knowledgeable persons are needed" (Gordon, 2009, p. 5).

to be examined in this context. Based on the work of Winkler and Moser, these biases will be displayed with regard to their relevance for real-time Delphis in the following:

- *Framing effects* are especially likely to occur with homogeneous groups and extreme formulations. Depending on how an issue is presented in the scenario/question, it can influence the recipients' evaluation (e.g. their sense of its probability or desirability). In real-time Delphis, this applies not only to the formulation of the question, but also to the qualitative reasoning of the participants. Framing may prevent rational evaluations and thus limit the variability of responses.
- *Anchor effects* arise from the dependence of assessment and estimation on pre-existing anchor values (e.g. empirical values, the judgments of others). The problem arises when participants excessively weight a particular anchor value. If the anchor value is extreme because, say, the number of small number of cases is low and the arithmetic mean is used, the effect is amplified. Anchor effects are relevant in real-time Delphis to the extent that not all questions are initially answered independently of the average values of the other survey participants, as in the classic Delphi. Rather, one's own response is immediately presented in relation to the group response.
- Since Delphis usually deal with questions that involve a high degree of uncertainty, *bandwagon effects* are also salient here. Participants adapt their responses to that of the group because they feel pressure to conform, they want to avoid a controversial discussion, or they do not want to question weak arguments. Moreover, a group response reduces individual uncertainty regarding questions. The group, in turn, can be influenced by the first extreme arguments in the qualitative reasoning of other experts.

To reduce the effect of these biases, the following basic rules should be observed when creating a questionnaire, selecting experts, and designing feedback (see Winkler & Moser, 2016, and my own additional comments):

Creating a questionnaire

- Conduct a pretest to check whether the items or questions are formulated in a way that the experts can understand.
- Randomize questions so that responses are not influenced by particular previous questions (sequence effects).

Selecting experts

- Avoid snowballing (e.g. experts recommending other experts), as this may affect the heterogeneity of the sample composition.
- Pick participants with the highest possible level of expertise to keep anchoring effects to a minimum.
- Assemble a group that is as heterogenous as possible in case there are several "competing" anchor values.

Designing feedback

- Use high-quality, argumentative feedback rather than statistical averages. This allows a breadth of perspectives on a particular item/scenario.
- Edit feedback by deleting duplicate or particularly extreme arguments.
- Put different arguments, especially counter-arguments, at the top of the intermediate results in order to challenge participants who only "browse" through the rationales of others.

5 Technical Innovations and Real-Time Delphi Tools

The market for real-time Delphi is growing steadily, though the success and scope of products vary greatly. Some producers embed the real-time software in a methodological or futures research platform to offer a broader portfolio of methods (Global Futures Intelligence System, Foresight Cockpit, RAHS or FACT). Others concentrate exclusively or primarily on explicit real-time Delphi software (e.g. eDelphi, Surveylet).

Gordon and Pease developed the first attempts at a real-time Delphi under the name "Delphi Blue." Its code was adapted by Gordon and used under the name Real-Time Delphi in the Millenium Project, which was run jointly with Glenn. Meanwhile, new software was developed as part of the Millenium Project, resulting in the Global Futures Intelligence System (GFIS, www.themp.org), which is still available today. The real-time Delphi tool available from GFIS is available for all to purchase (from individual annual licenses for $99 to corporate annual licenses for $2100). These licenses include not only the use of the real-time Delphi tool, but also allow access to numerous method descriptions (e.g. cross-impact analysis, text mining, environmental scanning) as well as various reports and information on future global challenges.

The not yet (October 2021) available version of the Future Analysis Cooperation Tool (FACT) procured by the Bundeswehr is based on the prototype Risk

Assessment and Horizon Scanning (RAHS). RAHS is an Internet-based platform containing future analysis methods for security policy. Its 43 methods allow analysts to carry out computer-assisted collaborative research projects with other experts. The real-time Delphi survey is one of the most popular methods. Use by individuals outside the Bundeswehr is only possible on request.

Among the pure real-time Delphi tools are eDelphi and Surveylet. The Finnish eDelphi (formerly eDelfoi) offers a free basic version, but it does not allow data export. Various services and others options can be purchased. The tool includes all common question types described here as well as a comprehensive management area for the organization of the survey and the panel. Surveylet is an another professional tool. It offers different variants of Delphis (real-time, classic, and "RTD-2," which includes multiple repetitions of real-time Delphis). The costs here are essentially based on the intensity of use, i.e. the more answers that are generated, the higher the costs are for using the software.

In addition to these software solutions, which have already been used for several scientific studies, there are other offerings on the market or currently being developed. Expertsight is geared to the corporate environment and must be contacted directly to develop a study. The same applies to the toolbox "Foresight Cockpit", developed by the company 4strat, that includes a real-time Delphi software solution.

The aforementioned software solutions were mainly developed to pursue economic interests. Accordingly, various questions and challenges should be considered before their use. A systematic analysis exists only for the first four providers listed in Table 2. Aengenheyster et al. (2017) have assessed these tools on the basis

Table 2 A list of Delphi tools and providers. In some cases, the software is offered as part of larger method platforms, which are marked accordingly

Platform/software	Provider/Website
Global futures intelligence system (GFIS) (platform); Realtime Delphi (software)	www.themp.org
eDelphi (software)	www.edelphi.org
Risk assessment and horizon scanning (RAHS)/future analysis cooperation tool (FACT) (platform), real-time Delphi (software)	www.rahs-bundeswehr.de
Surveylet (software)	www.calibrum.com
Expertsight (company/software)	www.expertsight.com
Foresight cockpit (platform/software)	www.foresight-cockpit.de

The spelling of "real-time Delphi" follows that used by the providers

of 20 categories with regard to their features (e.g. layout of the survey instruments, question types, pretest functions, etc.), data output (e.g. data generated, compatibility with other programs, visual output, and options for qualitative analysis), user-friendliness (e.g. ease of use, functions, stability), and administration (quality of participant management, intuitiveness of the software). The authors conclude that all the tools they examine are basically comparable with the basic principles of the real-time Delphi method. Each have different advantages and disadvantages and all have room for improvement. But the authors point out a more fundamental flaw: in the real-time Delphi studies documented so far, few reflect seriously on the survey tools in use, even though each tool has limitations. For example, some tools may not offer every question option or response scale provided for in the original research design. It may not be possible to moderate open-ended responses to the extent necessary in light of the anticipated biases. The objective of the tools is to offer users the simplest possible implementation of real-time Delphis. This is particularly evident in the automated result displays. Most allow users to call up an automatic result report that presents the results in a clear layout. However, the basic rules of empirical work are sometimes disregarded, such as when arithmetic mean values are presented with a very small number of cases (n), or when group differences are represented on the basis of mean values without addressing the limitations of interpretation. In addition, no data cleaning takes place before the automated evaluation, even though such cleaning is indispensible. It is advisable, therefore, to export the collected data, to clean the data sets, and then to submit them to further processing with appropriate tools such as SPSS, R, Stata, and others for quantitative data and MAXQDA, Atlas.ti, and others. The decisive factor for conducting a real-time Delphi study is not that all tools have limitations, but, rather, that they are disclosed in the research process and reflected on with regard to the consequences so as to avoid system-inherent errors.

6 Discussion and Outlook

The above considerations point out the potential of the real-time Delphi method while identifying its limitations and challenges. "The greatest weakness of RT Delphi is that only a proof of concept prototype exists," Gordon and Pease note, adding that "more development is required to place it into full scale operation, particularly the asynchronous application" (2006, p. 332). This assessment is no longer true today, because real-time Delphis now come in many different forms, as described in the present study. Innovations revolve around individual technical components such as question formats, the display of results, panel management, layout, and adaptation to new technical standards, e.g. the optimization of the display for mobile devices such as smartphones or tablets (responsive design). Moreover, researchers have expanded the real-time idea: For instance, the real-time Delphi of Di Zio et al. (2017) uses geoinformation systems to enable spatially based decisions by expert groups. Another conceptual proposal is the "social real-time Delphi (sRTD)" by Kloker et al. (2018). The authors aim to improve group interactions with qualitative data by assigning random and anonymous usernames. The idea is to enable participants to refer to each other directly, making discussions on single questions/items more fruitful. Furthermore, they propose adding a function whereby participants can rate qualitative statements with tags such as "helpful" or "like."

There is no doubt that real-time Delphi represents a time-efficient solution for addressing future-related questions. The available tools are easily accessible and usually intuitive. Nevertheless, the technical possibilities of real-time Delphi tools are not yet of the same standard as those offered by providers of classic surveys such as Unipark, SurveyMonkey, LimeSurvey, etc. For example, real-time Delphi users cannot adapt the questionnaire layout and variability for handling data through automatically created codebooks or different data export formats. The fact that such options are limited in real-time Delphis is due, among other things, to the restricted circle of users and the significantly smaller market segment of Delphi software applications. Nevertheless, this is not the actual challenge in the implementation of real-time Delphi studies. Rather, the challenge lies in its critical methodological reflection. The number of studies that address methodological questions for real-time Delphis is limited; many studies on real-time Delphis omit a comprehensive description of methodology and its objectives. Going forward, studies must at least describe

- the typification of the real-time Delphi based on Häder's classification (2009, p. 36);
- the item and scale development (theoretical basis, procedure, pretest);
- the technical limitations in the programming of the survey instrument as well as problems in the survey phase;
- the reasons for expert selection;
- the process of data cleaning and data preparation (qualitative as well as quantitative); and
- the compliance with standards for the presentation of results (scaling, percentages, etc.; see Döring & Bortz, 2016).[4]

[4] The handbook *Standards of Futures Research. Guidelines for Practice and Evaluation* (Gerhold et al., 2021) provides guidelines for futures research.

Literature

Aengenheyster, S., Cuhls, K., Gerhold, L., & Muszynska, M. (2017). Real-time Delphi in practice – A comparative analysis of existing software-based tools. *Technological Forecasting and Social Change, 118*, 15–27. https://doi.org/10.1016/j.techfore.2017.01.023

Aguirre-Bastos, C., Giesecke, S., Wasserbacher, D., & Weber, M. (2009). FORESEC Deliverable D 4.3 1st Delphi Report 30 April 2009. No longer available online.

Cuhls, K. (2009). Delphi-Befragungen in der Zukunftsforschung. In R. Popp & E. Schüll (Eds.), *Zukunftsforschung und Zukunftsgestaltung: Beiträge aus Wissenschaft und Praxis* (pp. 207–221). Springer.

Cuhls, K. (2012). Zu den Unterschieden zwischen Delphi-Befragungen und "einfachen" Zukunftsbefragungen. In R. Popp & E. Schüll (Eds.), *Zukunft und Wissenschaft. Wege und Irrwege der Zukunftsforschung* (pp. 139–158). Springer (Zukunft und Forschung, 2).

Di Zio, S., Rosas, J. D. C., & Lamelza, L. (2017). Real time spatial Delphi: Fast convergence of experts' opinions on the territory. *Technological Forecasting and Social Change, 115*, 143–154.

Döring, N., & Bortz, J. (2016). *Forschungsmethoden und Evaluation in den Sozial- und Humanwissenschaften*. Springer.

Geist, M. (2010). Using the Delphi method to engage stakeholders: A comparison of two studies. *Evaluation and Program Planning, 33*(2), 147–154. https://doi.org/10.1016/j.evalprogplan.2009.06.006

Gerhold, L. (2012). Methodenkombination in der sozialwissenschaftlichen Zukunftsforschung. In R. Popp (Ed.), *Zukunft und Wissenschaft* (pp. 159–183). Springer. https://doi.org/10.1007/978-3-642-28954-5_8

Gerhold, L., Holtmannspötter, D., Neumann, C., Schüll, E., Schulz-Montag, B., Steinmüller, K., & Zweck, A. (2021). *Standards of futures research. Guidelines for practice and evaluation*. Springer.

Glenn, J. C., & Florescu, E. (2015). *State of the future*. The Millennium Project. http://www.millennium-project.org/publications-2-3/#sof2015-16

Glenn, J. C., & Gordon, T. J. (2009). Integration, comparisons, and frontiers of futures research methods. In J. C. Glenn & T. J. Gordon (Eds.), *Futures research methodology version 3.0, the millennium project* (pp. 1–34). American Council for the United Nations University.

Gnatzy, T., Warth, J., von der Gracht, H., & Darkow, I.-L. (2011). Validating an innovative real-time Delphi approach – A methodological comparison between real-time and conventional Delphi studies. *Technological Forecasting and Social Change, 78*(9), 1681–1694. https://doi.org/10.1016/j.techfore.2011.04.006

Gordon, T. J. (2007). Energy forecasts using a "Roundless" approach to running a Delphi study. *Foresight, 9*(2), 27–35. https://doi.org/10.1108/14636680710737731

Gordon, T. J. (2009). The real-time Delphi method. In J. C. Glenn & T. J. Gordon (Eds.), *Futures research methodology version 3.0, the millennium project*. American Council for the United Nations University.

Gordon, T., & Pease, A. (2006). RT Delphi: An efficient, "round-less" almost real time Delphi method. *Technological Forecasting and Social Change, 73*(4), 321–333. https://doi.org/10.1016/j.techfore.2005.09.005

Häder, M. (2009). *Delphi Befragungen. Ein Arbeitsbuch* (2nd ed.). Springer. https://doi.org/10.1007/978-3-658-01928-0

Häder, M., & Häder, S. (Eds.). (2000). *Die Delphi-Technik in den Sozialwissenschaften. Methodische Forschungen und innovative Anwendungen*. Springer.

Kloker, S., Straub, T., Morana, S. & Weinhardt, C. (2018). *The effect of social reputation on retention: Designing a social real-time Delphi platform* (Research papers. 46). https://aisel.aisnet.org/ecis2018_rp/46

Linstone, H. A., & Turoff, M. (1975). Introduction. In H. A. Linestone & M. Turoff (Eds.), *The Delphi method. Techniques and applications*. Addison-Wesley Educational Publishers.

Linstone, H. A., & Turoff, M. (2011). Delphi: A brief look backward and forward. Technological forecasting and social change on ScienceDirect *Technological Forecasting and Social Change, 78*(9), 1712–1719. https://www.sciencedirect.com/science/journal/00401625. https://www.sciencedirect.com/science/journal/00401625/78/9

Neuhaus, C., & Steinmüller, K. (2015). Grundlagen der Standards Gruppe 1. In L. Gerhold, D. Holtmannspötter, C. Neuhaus, E. Schüll, B. Schulz-Montag, K. Steinmüller, & A. Zweck (Eds.), *Standards und Gütekriterien der Zukunftsforschung* (pp. 17–20). Springer. https://doi.org/10.1007/978-3-658-07363-3_2

Popper, R. (2009). *Mapping foresight. Revealing how Europe and other world regions navigate into the future*. European Foresight Monitoring Network. https://doi.org/10.2777/47203

Rowe, G., & Wright, G. (1999). The Delphi technique as a forecasting tool: Issues and analysis. *International Journal of Forecasting, 15*, 353–375.

Schüll, E. (2009). Zur Forschungslogik explorativer und normativer Zukunftsforschung. In R. Popp & E. Schüll (Eds.), *Zukunftsforschung und Zukunftsgestaltung. Beiträge aus Wissenschaft und Praxis* (pp. 223–234). Springer. https://doi.org/10.1007/978-3-540-78564-4

Steinmüller, K. (1997). *Grundlagen und Methoden der Zukunftsforschung. Szenarien. Delphi. Technikvorausschau*. Werkstattbericht 21. Gelsenkirchen.

Wagner, S., Vogt, S., & Kabst, R. (2016). How IT and social change facilitates public participation: A stakeholder-oriented approach. *Government Information Quarterly, 33*, 435–443.

Winkler, J., & Moser, R. (2016). Biases in future-oriented Delphi studies: A cognitive perspective. *Technological Forecasting and Social Change, 105*(2016), 63–76. https://doi.org/10.1016/j.techfore.2016.01.021

Delphi Markets

Simon Kloker, Tim Straub, Tobias T. Kranz,
and Christof Weinhardt

Abstract

Delphi markets refer to approaches and implementations of integrating prediction markets and Delphi studies (Real-time Delphi). The combination of the two methods for producing forecasts can potentially compensate for each other's weaknesses. For example, prediction markets can be used to select participants with expertise and also motivate long-term participation through their gamified approach and incentive mechanisms. In this paper, two potentials for prediction markets and four potentials for Delphi studies, which are made possible by integration, are derived theoretically. Subsequently, three different integration approaches are presented, on the basis of which the integration on user, market and Delphi question-level is exemplified and it is shown that, depending on the approach, not all potentials can be achieved. At the end, recommendations for the use of Delphi markets are derived, existing limitations for Delphi markets as well as future developments are pointed out.

S. Kloker (✉) · T. T. Kranz · C. Weinhardt
Institute for Information Management and Marketing, Karlsruhe Institute of Technology, Karlsruhe, Germany
e-mail: simon.kloker@kit.edu; weinhardt@kit.edu

T. Straub
FZI Research Center for Information Technology, Karlsruhe, Germany
e-mail: straub@fzi.de

M. Niederberger, O. Renn (eds.), *Delphi Methods In The Social And Health Sciences*, https://doi.org/10.1007/978-3-658-38862-1_6

1 Forecasts by Means of Markets

> In these democratic days, any investigation into the trustworthiness and peculiarities of popular judgments is of interest. The material about to be discussed refers to a small matter, but is much to the point[1] (Galton, 1907).

Long before Surowiecki officially launched an entire field of research on the aggregation and use of distributed information and expertise with his well-known book "The wisdom of crowds" in 2005, the relevance of the question of the reliability of decisions by a large number of people was already undisputedly topical. Galton (1907) dealt with this question and introduced one of today's most famous parables for the wisdom of crowds. At an exhibition of fattening cattle and poultry in Plymouth, England, in 1906, a contest was called for an ox. For a negligible amount of money, lots could be purchased that entitled the owner to give an estimate of the weight of the ox. The prize for the best guess was to be the ox itself. While many individual estimates missed the mark to a greater or lesser extent, Galton was particularly stunned by the result of the mean: an error of only 0.08% (Shrier et al., 2016). To Galton, the comparison seemed apt that the average participants in his contest knew about as little about oxen as average voters knew about politics. The parable is just one of many pieces of evidence since then that predictions by a group or set of estimators are often even better than the opinions of individual experts (Shrier et al., 2016; Green et al., 2007). In the 1950s, the Delphi method was introduced as an anonymous, round-based feedback process by the military-funded RAND Corporation, specifically to aggregate expertise regardless of hierarchy, status, or reputation (Linstone & Turoff, 2002). This has been continuously developed and successfully used in many application contexts (Linstone & Turoff, 2002). However, other ideas for aggregating many individual opinions also made their way before and since. Prediction markets have been used to forecast political events since the mid-nineteenth century (Rhode & Strumpf, 2004). The theoretical basis was provided by Hayek in 1945 with his view of the market price as a (weighted) information carrier of all public as well as private information, and later by Fama (1970): the information efficiency of markets.

[1] German: "In these democratic days any investigation of the trustworthiness and peculiarities of popular judgments is of interest. The material to be discussed relates to a small matter, but is very pertinent."

1.1 Information Efficiency

In 1984, economists studied the relationship between futures on the orange price (bets on the price of oranges) in the US and weather forecast errors in the corresponding growing regions (Shrier et al., 2016). They found that the day's closing futures price (around 2:45 p.m.) predicted the error regarding the minimum temperature of the weather report that evening. The economists explained this by the fact that the market price reflects all publicly available information (e.g. weather report), but additionally all private information. This is all the information that only local market participants have, who know the area, can watch the sky and know that fresh oranges do not survive at low temperatures. So if the local market participants see a cold weather front coming up, they will adjust the market price upwards by buying, assuming a falling supply and rising prices, and thus are likely to realize a profit. The fact that all available information is priced in by forming the market price through this mechanism is called the "market efficiency hypothesis" (Fama, 1970).[2] Our stock exchanges today are also based on this principle. Therefore, stock prices or stock indices such as the DAX-30 are also interpreted as indicators of economic or corporate growth, i.e. as projections of the future. Prediction markets are also based on the principle of market efficiency. The prerequisite for this, however, is that trading is profitable for the individual participants, as is the case, for example, on a stock exchange or stock markets.

1.2 Prediction Markets

Prediction markets can be thought of as a kind of gambling stock market. In such a market, one can define contracts (shares) that are paid out depending on the realization of a defined event. Prediction markets are thus markets in which contracts are traded that are paid out based on future events (Graefe et al., 2010). The prices on such markets can be interpreted both as the current most likely value or directly as the probability of the future event occurring (Wolfers & Zitzewitz, 2006).

A simple example: Suppose a stock defined as follows: "If A wins the next mayoral election, each share of this stock pays out 100 monetary units (MU), otherwise 0 MU." Now, if a person has an estimate at the current time that A has a 20% probability of winning, then each share of this stock is worth 20 MU to him, since he

[2] The market efficiency hypothesis is further differentiated into "strong", "medium-strong" and "weak" market efficiency on the basis of assumptions about the information contained in the price.

receives 100 MU at 20% chance and 0 MU at 80% (0.2 × 100 MU + 0.8 × 0 MU = 20 MU). If the current market price is 10 MU, it is worthwhile for this person to buy shares because a profit of 10 MU can be expected for each share purchased (the person pays 10 MU for a share that is worth 20 MU in the person's opinion). However, this person's assessment can change at any time as a result of receiving new information. For example, if this person receives information that before the election A's involvement in a corruption scandal will come to light, this may immediately change the estimate to a 0% probability of winning. The person now believes that this news will destroy politician A's chances of winning the election. According to this new assessment, it is therefore worthwhile for the person to sell all his shares of this stock at any market price offered, so as not to end up empty-handed if, according to his assumption, it is paid out at 0 MU.

If all participants proceed according to this principle of maximising their expected profit on the basis of their expectations and information, a market price will settle that reflects all these expectations and information – and thus also reflects back to everyone what the others think. In theory, a number (the market price) that reflects all available information and expectations at a point in time (Fama, 1970) can be interpreted as the best forecast for the event at that point in time (market prediction).

Prediction markets are used in a wide variety of fields, such as politics, sports, entertainment, economic development (including business cycles), project management, idea management, and risk assessment (Luckner et al., 2005; Graefe, 2017; Teschner et al., 2011; Bothos et al., 2009; Cowgill et al., 2009; Prokesch et al., 2015; Cipriano & Gruca, 2014). Underlying this are also the many advantages of prediction markets, such as a fast response time to new information (Graefe et al., 2010), continuous forecasting (Graefe et al., 2010), ease of incentive creation and good implementability of incentive compatibility[3] (Luckner & Weinhardt, 2007), motivation through gamification (Buckley & Doyle, 2017), implicit long-term weighting of good and bad predictors (Arrow et al., 2008), and robustness (at least theoretically) to out-of-balance sampling (Kranz et al., 2014a). Various disadvantages of prediction markets, as well as the advantages, are mentioned again in Table 1 and will be explained in more detail directly afterwards in Sect. 2.1. The design of a prediction market is relatively open. The market mechanism can vary from a continuous double auction (similar to real stock exchanges) to hidden markets (Teschner & Weinhardt, 2012), which can be based on a market scoring

---

[3] Incentive compatibility exists if each individual participant maximizes his expected benefits exactly thenwhen he acts in accordance with his true assessment or attitude, i.e. when he acts in accordance with or states his true expectation.

Table 1 Selected strengths and weaknesses of prediction markets and Delphi studies compared. (Own representation)

	Prediction markets	Delphi studies/Real-time Delphi
Strengths	Playfulness (Buckley & Doyle, 2017) Implicit long-term weighting of individual participants and participants (Arrow et al., 2008) Fast reaction time to new information (Graefe et al., 2010) Tendency to always challenge current forecast (Green et al., 2007) Very high number of participants possible (Green et al., 2007) Continuous prediction (Graefe et al., 2010) Direct feedback on own assessment (Kranz et al., 2014b) Robustness to out-of-balance samples (Kranz et al., 2014a)	Acquisition of quantitative information, backgrounds and correlations Hypothetical questions and questions with a long time horizon possible (Linstone & Turoff, 2002) More than one question can be asked The questions can be adapted to new findings
Weaknesses	No qualitative information No background information (correlations) Not every question/issue can be defined as a share (causalities, hypothetical questions) (Wolfers & Zitzewitz, 2006) Observable events are a prerequisite (Slamka et al., 2012) Low visibility of alternative viewpoints Complexity (Green et al., 2007)	Incentive design, little incentive compatibility (Green et al., 2007) Long-term motivation to participate is difficult to maintain (Mullen, 2003) Tendency to conformity (Woudenberg, 1991) (Only) medium to high number of participants possible (Vernon, 2009; Linstone & Turoff, 2002)

rule[4] and are practically indistinguishable from simple surveys (Laskey et al., 2015). At least in the background, however, the aggregation of individual assessments about a market, i.e. contracts, money holdings and deposits, is always aggregated.

[4] A (market) scoring rule defines a set of rules in which all assessments made are assigned a utility depending on the realization of the underlying event, so that one can/could calculate an expected utility according to his assessment. A "proper scoring rule" meets several criteria, including incentive compatibility.

2 Commonalities and Potentials for Integration

Both Delphi studies[5] and prediction markets pursue similar goals in some respects. Both procedures aggregate many individual opinions (Green et al., 2007) and can be described as feedback procedures (Sprenger et al., 2007). This means that both procedures reflect the (aggregated) opinion of the group back to all participants in order to give them the opportunity to correct their own assessment. Moreover, both procedures work anonymously (or quasi-anonymously, Kochtanek & Hein, 1999), so that identification of the other participants is not possible, or only with difficulty. Prediction markets are usually designed as online platforms, which makes the integration with the Real-time Delphi method as an adaptation of the Delphi method particularly interesting. The Real-time Delphi concept,[6] initially introduced by Gordon and Pease in 2006, is an online adaptation of the classical Delphi method to reduce the duration of surveys. It is particularly characterized by an asynchronous feedback cycle (Kloker et al., 2016). The concept of Real-time Delphi, which adapts the rigid round-based character of the Delphi method to an asynchronous individualized process, can be compared and connected well with participation in markets. A comparison "across" the fields in Table 1 quickly and clearly shows that the two methods could potentially complement each other in many respects and that some advantages or the compensation of various weaknesses could be derived.

2.1 Potential for Prediction Markets

In prediction markets, all information is exchanged via price/quantity bundles. Therefore, prediction markets do not allow qualitatively differentiated statements of individual opinions, e.g. on the basis of which information and against which backgrounds the participants in the market act and change the market forecast.

By integrating the prediction market and the Delphi study, participants can be given the opportunity to qualitatively support their assessment or to share information. In principle, there is no incentive to share new information in prediction markets, since profit can be realized from it. However, this potential is usually quickly exhausted for a single participant, so participants are willing to disclose it in exchange for other information (Kloker et al., 2017). In many Real-time Delphi

[5] Whenever Delphi studies or surveys are mentioned in the following, the implementation as Real-Time Delphi is implicitly meant. In all other cases it is explicitly referred to.

[6] For detailed information, the reader is referred to another chapter in this anthology that deals explicitly with the Real-Time Delphi method.

applications, participants cannot view arguments until they participate in the survey themselves. In the spirit of reciprocity, but also due to self-presentation and prestige (reputation), this encourages information sharing (Kloker et al., 2016). While in classic prediction markets all participants have to acquire information independently of each other, participants in Delphi studies learn directly from the other participants. This is also a better way to communicate new ideas or scenarios than through market prices. According to Green et al. (2007), this exchange of information leads to greater efficiency in the search for information and also to fewer information cascades. The latter especially because participants know the background of a price movement and do not have to evaluate it without background and infer important information they do not know. A first potential is therefore the improved qualitative information flow and exchange.

Due to the one-dimensional representation as a share, the abstraction load of the participants increases in the case of complex predictions. Even simple markets are a hurdle for many participants who have little background knowledge of stock trading, as they lack the necessary knowledge of how expectations are translated into market prices (Green et al., 2007). This can lead both to participants dropping out (with all the resulting problems such as biased samples) and to trading that does not actually match the assessment. The hidden market approach (Teschner & Weinhardt, 2012) solves this problem at least to some extent. Moreover, interrelationships and causalities are difficult to represent in contracts, though they can be interrogated well in Delphi studies. A second potential of the integration with Delphi studies is therefore the more flexible design of the forecast object.

Depending on the implementation, further downstream potentials are a lower necessary number of participants (Abramowicz, 2004), a higher resistance to manipulation (Green et al., 2007), a better visibility of alternative viewpoints and a higher acceptance of the results by the individual participants (Graefe & Armstrong, 2011).

2.2 Potentials for Real-Time Delphi

In Delphi studies, the selection of participants (with expertise) is the critical factor for the quality of the results and therefore still a potential weak point (Gordon, 2007; Welty, 1972; Ammon, 2009). In the case of participants without (enough) background knowledge or if all participants draw from the same pool of information, the use of the Delphi method is not advisable or purposeful (Green et al., 2007; Sniezek, 1990). In many Delphi studies, participants have been selected on the basis of their reputation, which does not necessarily reflect their individual predictive ability (Hill & Fowles, 1975), and often at relatively high cost (acquisition, salary/compensation) for participants with high reputations (Welty, 1972). Thus, as a third potential, integrated approaches can use markets to select participants with expertise and potential information and very high predictive accuracy. Procedures for this are described in Kloker et al., (2017) and Sect. 3.1.

Another problem of Delphi studies is the decreasing motivation of the participants in the course of the implementation (Cuhls, 2003; Kloker et al., 2018c), as the traditional Delphi process is often very rigid and lengthy for the participants. The problem of high dropout rates arises, which can only be addressed to a limited extent in traditional Delphi studies (Okoli & Pawlowski, 2004; Reid, 1988). Prediction markets offer the possibility of intrinsic as well as extrinsic incentives and motivate participants to take part in the long term, as this is the way to achieve the greatest gains (Green et al., 2007). Thus, sustained and active participation in the Delphi study can benefit from an integration of these methods (fourth potential).

Winkler and Moser (2016) deal with cognitive heuristics that lead to systematic errors in predictions, including in Delphi studies. The persistence of such errors, such as the anchor heuristic, is also pointed out by de Wilde et al. (2018). Winkler and Moser (2016) and de Wilde et al. (2018) recommend the targeted creation of proper incentives as a countermeasure. These can be financial, given in the form of reputation (Winkler & Moser, 2016), or designed as accountability of the predictors so that they thus have to bear the consequences (de Wilde et al., 2018). In line with the literal meaning of the proverb "put your money where your mouth is", participants in prediction markets thus also have to prove the credibility of their argument with an "investment" or "bet", which may well encourage reconsideration (Levin et al., 1988). Depending on the underlying market mechanism, this can create a performance-compatible or even an incentive-compatible environment (Chen & Pennock, 2010; Luckner & Weinhardt, 2007; Jurca & Faltings, 2008). Besides the fact that the estimation has to be given by the trade, if this is coupled with the giving of an argument,[7] this can provide participants with further information regarding the credibility and confidence behind a single argument. As a fifth potential, Delphi studies benefit from a prediction market through better incentive creation, reduction of cognitive biases, and possibly information enrichment of arguments.

A final characteristic of Delphi studies, which is problematic depending on the context, is that they are designed in principle to find a consensus and thus implicitly suppress disagreement (Green et al., 2007). This leads to the fact that only opinions

[7] See later the integration approach in Sect. 3.2.

that lie outside the currently existing consensus are questioned, while an opinion within the consensus is simply accepted. In prediction markets, profits can only be realized from a good forecast if one's opinion differs from that of the "crowd", i.e. the current market price (Green et al., 2007).[8] This means that every opinion must be questioned and challenged. Nevertheless, Delphi studies may result in the formation of two or more clusters of opinion (Gnatzy et al., 2011). As a sixth potential, prediction markets offer the advantage that a consensus, the price, is (must be) found even for questions where different world views and values clash and/or opinion clusters are formed.

Another downstream potential, depending on implementation and market mechanism, is existing incentive compatibility[9] (Chen & Pennock, 2010).

3 Integration Approaches

The term Delphi markets, as a designation for approaches to the integration of the Delphi method with prediction markets, does not, however, make any concrete statement about the many possible ways of designing this integration. Not all potentials mentioned in Sect. 2 can be realized in every approach to integration. In the following, three approaches to integration are presented in order to give an impression of the breadth and possible deployment scenarios. A distinction is made between integration at user-, market- and question-level.

3.1 Integration at User-Level

In user-level integration, a prediction market and a Real-time Delphi platform are operated in parallel. The two platforms are connected via a common user base. This possibility also underlies the work of Kloker et al. (2017) and the prediction market "FAZ.NET Oracle"[10] and is conceptually illustrated in Fig. 1.

[8] Manipulation and uninformed trading strategies aside.

[9] At least the forecast. Does not apply to the delivery of truthful arguments.

[10] http://orakel.faz.net. The FAZ.NET Oracle is a cooperation between the Frankfurter Allgemeine Zeitung and the Institute for Information Science and Marketing (IISM) at the Karlsruher Institut für Technologie (KIT) and is accessible to the readership of FAZ.NET. The FAZ.NET Oracle is mainly used for forecasting election events and economic indicators, as well as individual questions on current topics.

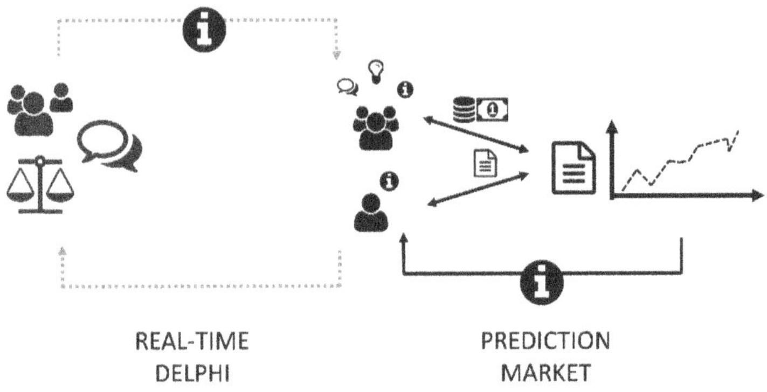

Fig. 1 Integration at the user-level. The prediction market and Real-time Delphi run in parallel. Users can be active on both platforms and, if necessary, transfer information from one to the other. (Own illustration)

The focus is on a panel of prediction market participants. This panel has several characteristics: (1) It includes both informed and uninformed market participants (Gruca & Berg, 2007). (2) All market participants bring some interest in the topic (Servan-Schreiber et al., 2004). (3) Panel participants possess both public and private information (Gruca & Berg, 2007). Participants act according to their expectation in the prediction market and also face the expectations of other participants. With user-level integration, a Real-time Delphi survey can now make use of the participants in this panel. In addition to the option of inviting all participants from thematically related markets to the Delphi survey, which would only partially solve the problem of selecting participants with expertise for the Delphi round mentioned in Sect. 2.2, there are three interesting alternatives for selecting participants (Kloker et al., 2017):

- "The Topscorer": In prediction markets, participants are usually ranked based on their trading success, which according to Hayek (1945) can only be achieved in the long run by participants with true (and private) information. Participants who are ranked higher are more likely to possess important and correct information and thus qualify for the Delphi study as participants with expertise.
- "The Potential": One problem with "The Topcscorer" method is that a truly meaningful ranking for a market can only be created after it has been paid out. For Delphi surveys for which no topic-related market exists yet, participants with expertise cannot be selected based on their past trading success. The selection procedure "The Potential" therefore selects participants based on their trad-

ing behaviour. It can be shown that certain features of trading behavior in prediction markets are correlated with a higher probability of success (Kloker et al., 2018a). Attributes of such behavior can be learned on historical data and can then be used to select participants with expertise.

- "The Bohemian": This selection procedure also selects the participants for the Delphi survey on the basis of current trading behavior. The central difference to the selection procedure "The Potential" is that not only participants with a high probability of success are selected, but also those with trading behavior that shows significant deviation from the "average" trading behaviour in the market. Participants who are more likely to buy shares may have different information or viewpoints than participants who are more likely to sell shares. Against this background, it seems reasonable to consider both opinions in the Delphi survey and to invite them as participants. In particular, these participants, whose trading behaviour obviously represents different opinions than the "mainstream" of other market participants, potentially have new, interesting, or at least previously unnoticed information and viewpoints that may be of interest for the Delphi survey. This selection procedure thus leads to high heterogeneity.

In addition to the above-mentioned selection procedures, a random selection would also be possible, since a general level of knowledge on the topic can already be assumed through participation in the market. Also, conceivable would be a self-selection strategy, according to which the participants themselves decide whether they want to take part in the Delphi survey. According to Green et al. (2007), only those participants take part in the market anyway who think that their private information is not yet included in the previous forecast.

Actions in the Delphi market thus have no direct (rule-based) influence on the prediction market, or the market forecast. Nevertheless, information can be exchanged between methods through the participants. In markets, market participants usually realize profits from available information very quickly, which is why this information loses its value for the individual market participant within a short time (cf. Fama, 1970, market efficiency). In order to be able to make further profits from future price developments, market participants are constantly dependent on finding new information. This can happen, among other things, in the exchange with other participants in the Delphi survey, which encourages the participants to participate actively and in the long term in the Delphi survey.

Another advantage of this integration approach is that the design of the market and Real-time Delphi can be adapted to the specific requirements of the respective context completely independently of each other. This also applies to the way in which participants are invited from the market to the Real-time Delphi platform.

Kranz et al. (2014b) recommends a more integrated solution that allows individual questions to be answered directly from the Delphi study.

Thus, user-level integration leverages the first and third potential and should be used when technical integration is not desired or possible, when Delphi survey implementation should be decoupled from profit-seeking incentives and trading strategies, or when participants are recruited from multiple pools of individuals, some of whom, however, have no understanding of markets. In particular, Delphi studies also benefit from this integration approach when the objective selection of participants is of great importance for the outcome or is not possible (for example, due to a lack of historical data on potential participants).

3.2 Integration at Market-Level

In the case of integration at market-level, basically a Real-time Delphi is operated within the context of a prediction market. This approach is also based on the "Delphi markets"[11] platform and is shown conceptually in Fig. 2.

The focus here is on the market with the market question (forecast target of the market). This is also the first limitation of this approach. Since a market can only answer one question at a time, the Delphi survey also consists of only one single question. The market acts directly as an aggregation mechanism for the individual

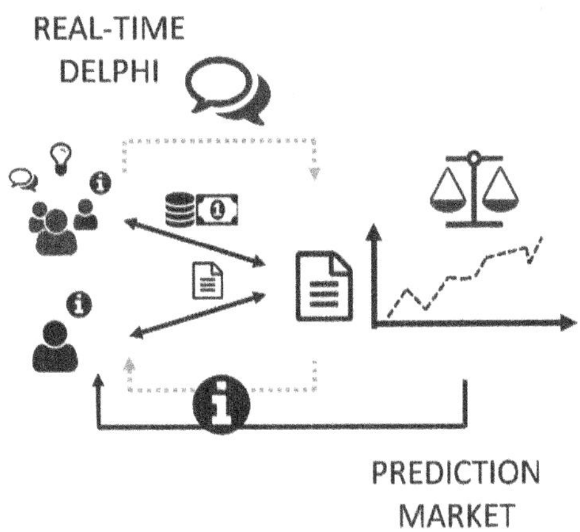

Fig. 2 Integration at the market-level. Real-time Delphi is conducted in the context of the prediction market. Participation in Real-time Delphi is not possible without participation in the prediction market. (Own representation)

[11] https://delphimarkets.net. Delphimarkets.net is a privately operated site that uses open and closed Delphi markets to forecast issues from various subject areas (including risk management).

opinions of all participants. Participants in the prediction market have the option to provide the underlying information and background each time they submit a trade order. Therefore, each comment must also be assigned to a price-increasing or price-decreasing effect and thus, in theory, to a positive or negative effect on the variable or probability being predicted. Ensuring the "optionality" of this argument output is crucial, as otherwise many market-calming and liquidity-providing trading strategies that seek small profits would be prevented. These arguments can then be sorted visually, for example, as in "Delphi markets", on the sides of the market according to pro and con. If participants disagree with an argument and wish to write a counter-argument to it, this must automatically be accompanied by the submission of a trade order. The advantages of this approach are explained in the fifth potential.

This approach has some advantages and disadvantages that need to be weighed depending on the use case. Depending on the market mechanism, integration at the market-level creates a performance and/or incentive compatible environment for forecasting the market question, therefore participants can be expected to forecast truthfully and with less cognitive heuristics. Moreover, this approach allows participants to be motivated both intrinsically, via the opportunity to share their knowledge (contribute), or extrinsically, via a leaderboard, via prizes, or even via trading real money, in the long run. This encourages active and long-term participation in the market and in the Delphi survey as well as continuous research of information (Gangur, 2016). The question of game or real money is secondary for the forecasting quality (Servan-Schreiber, 2017).[12] Another advantage is the user-friendly design of the interaction. Market-level integration theoretically allows all relevant elements to be displayed on one screen, eliminating the need to switch between different platforms or views. The final advantage of this approach, as mentioned in Sect. 2.2, is that a market always finds a price, even when different values and opinions are in opposition. According to Linstone and Turoff (2002), the Delphi method is also used especially for such issues where values and goals are in conflict. A market to find a consensus price and an argumentation in the style of the Delphi method to exchange points of view can complement each other very well here.

A disadvantage of this approach is that while incentive compatibility is achievable for forecasting, this does not necessarily hold for arguments. In some circumstances, the opposite effect can even be expected. Participants could use arguments

[12] According to Servan-Schreiber (2017), the choice between gambling and real money has an influence primarily on the self-selection of participants and thus only indirectly on the prediction (quality), whereby prediction markets are per se robust to unbalanced samples.

to lure other participants onto a false track and profit from the resulting trading orders in the market. Manipulation is a relevant aspect in prediction markets when making decisions regarding mechanism and design (Kloker & Kranz, 2017; Kloker et al., 2018b). Another drawback arises from the fact that prediction markets can actually only be used for issues for which there is also a realization in the foreseeable future (Green et al., 2007). Since in the other case the incentives for truthful assessments would no longer be guaranteed, the market price could possibly become the plaything of pure speculation and signalling[13] strategies.[14] Irrespective of the time horizon, however, there may be other difficulties (complexity or interrelationships between events) that make it very difficult or impossible to formulate an issue into a tradable contract as a market issue (Green et al., 2007; Wolfers & Zitzewitz, 2006). In this context, "combinatorial prediction markets" (Laskey et al., 2015) offer an interesting option. They allow the modelling of dependencies between individual markets and would thus address the problem of formulating complex questions as contracts, as well as that only one market question is possible so far. So far, however, no implementation or discussion of an integration of a combinatorial market with the Delphi method is known. Finally, the increased complexity of a market is an obstacle for participants who do not fully understand the market or do not want to deal with it, but would nevertheless participate in the Delphi study.

Integration at the market-level thus highlights the first, fourth, fifth and sixth potential and should be used when the question can be presented relatively easily in a market. In this case, the market will benefit from the arguments, while the Real-time Delphi study will be motivated by the market. However, many Delphi studies will not be able to be broken down to a market question, so the advantages for the prediction market clearly outweigh the disadvantages for this approach.

At this point, the question legitimately arises as to how this approach differs from a simple (or combinatorial) prediction market with a "forum" or "comment box" for each market question. These are mainly two points: (1) Each comment (or argument) is associated with a price movement, so it is not possible to simply comment without participating in trading at the same time. In addition, arguments in a Delphi market are more likely to refer to a specific piece of information, rather than

[13] When insiders trade new information, the price moves. This small price movement can be interpreted by other participants as a signal for new information(s) acting in a certain direction and possibly be assessed as credible. This then often leads to further price movements in the same direction. However, this effect can also be used to feign insider information and then take profits from the resulting price movements.

[14] Signalling refers to a receiver-related disclosure of information.

simply commenting generally on the question or engaging in side discussions (e.g., fun comments, flaming, etc.). (2) As is common in many implementations of Real-time Delphi, the comments of other participants are not visible until an own assessment has been made. In principle, this would also be possible with the trading price (depending on the underlying market mechanism).

3.3 Integration on Delphi Question-Level

The integration on Delphi question-level basically uses a classic Real-time Delphi. Only the aggregation of the individual answers to each question takes place on the basis of markets. The integration is schematically shown in Fig. 3.

The focus here is on the Real-time Delphi survey as such and also follows its process. For each individual question, a prediction market is used on which the participants can trade the expectations regarding this question. However, there are two problems with this approach: (1) Integration at the Delphi question-level can quickly become complex and time-consuming for participants due to the large number of markets. (2) In addition, the questions in Delphi surveys are usually thematically related and conditional. This also leads to the fact that the markets condition each other and this in turn promotes arbitrage opportunities[15] and signalling strategies with the potentially negative consequences (truthful answering is no longer the dominant strategy).

Hidden markets with scoring rules and combinatorial markets can address these two problems, but only at the cost of tradeoffs. The use of hidden markets can remedy the complexity and time intensity. Depending on the market mechanism

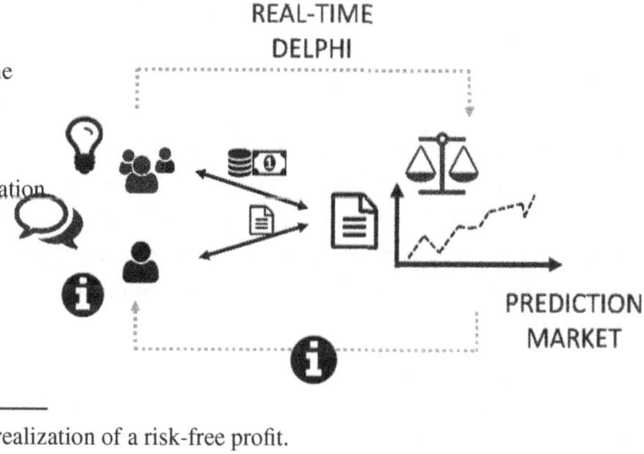

Fig. 3 Integration at the market-level. Real-time Delphi is conducted in the context of the prediction market. Participation in Real-time Delphi is not possible without participation in the prediction market. (Own representation)

[15] Arbitrage refers to the realization of a risk-free profit.

used, the Delphi survey with an integrated market is indistinguishable from other Delphi surveys (Teschner & Weinhardt, 2012; Laskey et al., 2015). If proper scoring rules are used (and communicated to participants), incentive compatibility can be maintained. Several proper scoring rules are known, probably the most widely implemented is the Logarithmic Market Scoring Rule (Hanson, 2002). Scoring rules also have the advantage that there are no liquidity requirements and many low-information trading strategies cannot be used. However, the survey loses some of its playful nature that promotes long-term motivation, as well as the money metaphor that might induce deeper thinking (Levin et al., 1988). However, other benefits remain. In particular, this is the long-term implicit weighting of participants depending on their past forecast goodness. Participants with good forecasts increase their portfolio value and hence their market influence. Participants with poor long-term forecasts, on the other hand, decrease their portfolio value and thus lose their forecast influence. Combinatorial markets can prevent arbitrage and signalling strategies because they can map conditions between individual markets. However, this in turn places various limits on the designability of the individual markets[16] and thus restricts the types of questions that can be asked. Moreover, combinatorial markets are so far known only on the basis of market scoring rules and no other market mechanisms.

An open question that needs to be assessed on a case-by-case basis is whether and how the individual markets (for the individual questions) can be fairly combined into an overall ranking without in turn encouraging arbitrage opportunities and signalling strategies. Also, a selection of participants with expertise by the market is no longer a given.

Thus, integration at the Delphi question-level raises the first and second potential, provided one sees the application from the perspective of prediction markets. But more importantly in this case, the approach to Delphi studies holds the fourth, the fifth and the sixth potential. Delphi studies benefit from the long-term motivation of participants, the additional information that underpins each argument, the potential incentive compatibility, the long-term stronger weighting of the better participants, and that consensus must be found.

This approach is therefore recommended for very complex questions where it can also be assumed that the participants have trading experience. The variant with hidden markets is recommended if only the former, but not the latter, applies, although this does weaken the long-term motivation somewhat.

[16] Combinatorial markets are only possible between market issues whose summed probabilities across all options add up to 100%. Index or spread contracts are not possible.

In 2015, Prokesch et al. presented an approach to integrate Delphi studies with prediction markets, which can basically be considered as a Delphi question-level integration with hidden markets. However, a scoring rule was used as the market mechanism, which no longer leads to any trading, making the term "Delphi market" no longer entirely appropriate and the advantage of classical markets of implicit long-term weighting and the money metaphor no longer present. As in a classical Delphi study, Prokesch et al. (2015) explicitly selected the participants beforehand. Nevertheless, this approach was also able to beat the relevant benchmarks (Prokesch et al., 2015) and shows that Delphi markets, applied correctly and in the right place, can compensate for the mutual weaknesses of the individual approaches.

4 Conclusion and Future Developments

The previous sections have shown three different approaches to give an impression of possible implementations. The integration on user-level has especially highlighted the potentials regarding the selection of participants with expertise for the Delphi study by the market. The integration on market-level shows how a prediction market can benefit from the advantages of Delphi studies (qualitative information). The integration on Delphi question-level has picked up the potentials for Delphi studies that arise through the market.

However, an integration of the methods can also take other forms. In general, in the vast majority of cases, a combination is only expedient if the realisation of the forecast event can also be observed in the "foreseeable" future, as otherwise the prediction market cannot be paid out and is therefore not incentive-compatible. Although there are individual approaches to the application of prediction markets for the prediction of events that may not be observable or for which no generally accepted objective payoff value can be determined (Slamka et al., 2012), these always entail losses in terms of accuracy and susceptibility to manipulation (Kloker & Kranz, 2017).

Delphi markets are currently still relatively little used and researched (Prokesch et al., 2015). However, some well-known studies report encouraging results. A significant obstacle and permanent limitation for the use of Delphi markets is certainly the increased complexity and the also greater implementation effort, which do not meet every application field and case. The still outstanding formalization and validation of Delphi markets as a research method also hinders their application in science - if this is possible at all given the breadth of design possibilities.

Nevertheless, a stronger research focus is recommended here. In particular, integration at user-level allows the "crowd" to be involved in the prediction process and can thus also be understood as a participatory approach (Niemeyer et al., 2016). In the thematic area of "health", too, Delphi markets can therefore both support the results of public discussions and increase their acceptance. While a panel of experts discusses the future design of health insurance contributions, a market integrated at user-level can serve to forecast relevant key figures (e.g. development of contributions and contributors, development of costs, ...). The market can then also be used, as described above, to allow individual prominent participants to have their say in the discussion.

Future research will have to focus in particular on quantifying the theoretically derived potentials, such as the objective selection of participants with expertise (third potential), or the positive effects of market structure on the aggregation of expectations for each individual question, as well as the increased (long-term) motivation in Delphi studies. The potentials are great, the possibilities all the greater. Delphi markets will almost certainly be used again and again and - if the results remain encouraging - will be recommended for use more often.

Literature

Abramowicz, M. (2004). Information markets, administrative Decisionmaking, and predictive cost-benefit analysis. *The University of Chicago Law Review, 71*(3), 933–1020. http://www.jstor.org/stable/1600601

Ammon, U. (2009). Delphi-Befragung. In S. Kühl, P. Strodtholz, & A. Taffertshofer (Hrsg.), *Handbuch Methoden der Organisationsforschung: Quantitative und Qualitative Methoden* (S. 458–476). VS Verlag. https://doi.org/10.1007/978-3-531-91570-8_22.

Arrow, K. J., Forsythe, R., Gorham, M., Hahn, R., Hanson, R., Ledyard, J. O., et al. (2008). The promise of prediction markets. *Science, 320*(5878), 877–878. https://doi.org/10.1126/science.1157679

Bothos, E., Apostolou, D., & Mentzas, G. (2009). IDEM: A prediction market for idea management. In C. Weinhardt, S. Luckner, & J. Stößer (Hrsg.), *WEB2008: Designing E-Business systems markets services and networks* (S. 1–13). Springer.

Buckley, P., & Doyle, E. (2017). Individualising gamification: An investigation of the impact of learning styles and personality traits on the efficacy of gamification using a prediction market. *Computers & Education, 106*, 43–55. https://doi.org/10.1016/j.compedu.2016.11.009

Chen, Y., & Pennock, D. M. (2010). Designing markets for prediction. *AI Magazine, 31*(4), 42–52.

Cipriano, M. C., & Gruca, T. S. (2014). The power of priors: How confirmation bias impacts market prices. *Journal of Prediction Markets, 8*(3), 34–56.

Cowgill, B., Wolfers, J., & Zitzewitz, E. (2009). Using prediction markets to track information flows: Evidence from Google. In S. Das, M. Ostrovsky, D. Pennock, & B. Szymanksi (Hrsg.), *1st International conference on auctions, market mechanisms and their applications 2009* (S. 3). Springer. https://doi.org/10.1007/978-3-642-03821-1_2
Cuhls, K. (2003). From forecasting to foresight processes – New participative foresight activities in Germany. *Journal of Forecasting, 22*(2–3), 93–111. https://doi.org/10.1002/for.848
de Wilde, T. R. W., Ten Velden, F. S., & De Dreu, C. K. W. (2018). The anchoring-bias in groups. *Journal of Experimental Social Psychology, 76*, 116–126. https://doi.org/10.1016/j.jesp.2018.02.001
Fama, E. F. (1970). Efficient capital markets: A review of theory and empirical work. *The Journal of Finance, 25*(2), 383–417. https://doi.org/10.2307/2325486
Galton, F. (1907). Vox populi (the wisdom of crowds). *Nature, 75*(7), 450–451.
Gangur, M. (2016). *Motivation system on prediction market*. In N. T. Nguyen, L. Iliadis, Y. Manolopoulos, & B. Trawiński (Hrsg.), Proceedings of the 8th International Conference on Computational Collective Intelligence, ICCCI 2016, Halkidiki, Greece, September 28–30, 2016, Part II (S. 354–363). Springer. https://doi.org/10.1007/978-3-319-45246-3_34.
Gnatzy, T., Warth, J., von der Gracht, H. A., & Darkow, I.-L. (2011). Validating an innovative real-time Delphi approach – A methodological comparison between real-time and conventional Delphi studies. *Technological Forecasting and Social Change, 78*(9), 1681–1694. https://doi.org/10.1016/j.techfore.2011.04.006
Gordon, T. J. (2007). Energy forecasts using a "Roundless" approach to running a Delphi study. *Foresight, 9*(2), 27–35. https://doi.org/10.1108/14636680710737731
Gordon, T. J., & Pease, A. (2006). RT Delphi: An efficient, "round-less" almost real time Delphi method. *Technological Forecasting and Social Change, 73*(4), 321–333. https://doi.org/10.1016/j.techfore.2005.09.005
Graefe, A. (2017). Prediction market performance in the 2016 U.S. presidential election. *Foresight: The International Journal of Applied Forecasting, 1*(45), 38–42. http://econpapers.repec.org/RePEc:for:ijafaa:y:2017:i:45:p:38-42
Graefe, A., & Armstrong, J. S. (2011). Comparing face-to-face meetings, nominal groups, Delphi and prediction markets on an estimation task. *International Journal of Forecasting, 27*(1), 183–195. https://doi.org/10.1016/j.ijforecast.2010.05.004
Graefe, A., Luckner, S., & Weinhardt, C. (2010). Prediction markets for foresight. *Futures, 42*(4), 394–404. https://doi.org/10.1016/j.futures.2009.11.024
Green, K. C., Armstrong, J. S., & Graefe, A. (2007). Methods to elicit forecasts from groups: Delphi and prediction markets compared. *The International Journal of Applied Forecasting, 8*, 17–20.
Gruca, T. S., & Berg, J. E. (2007). Public information bias and prediction market accuracy. *The Journal of Prediction Markets, 1*(3), 219–231. https://doi.org/10.5750/jpm.v1i3.430
Hanson, R. (2002). Logarithmic market scoring rules for modular combinatorial information aggregation. *Journal of Prediction Markets, 1*(1), 3–15. http://www.ubplj.org/index.php/jpm/article/view/417
Hayek, F. A. (1945). The use of knowledge in society. *American Economic Review, 35*(4), 519–530.

Hill, K. Q., & Fowles, J. (1975). The methodological worth of the Delphi forecasting technique. *Technological Forecasting and Social Change, 7*(2), 179–192. https://doi.org/10.1016/0040-1625(75)90057-8

Jurca, R., & Faltings, B. (2008). *Incentives for expressing opinions in online polls*. In Proceedings of the 9th ACM conference on electronic commerce (S. 119–128). ACM. https://doi.org/10.1145/1386790.1386812

Kloker, S., & Kranz, T. T. (2017). *Manipulation in prediction markets – Chasing the fraudsters*. In Proceedings of the 25th European conference of information systems, June 5th–10th 2017, Guimarães, Portugal.

Kloker, S., Kranz, T. T., Straub, T., & Weinhardt, C. (2016). *Shouldn't collaboration be social? – Proposal of a social real-time Delphi*. In Proceedings of the second Karlsruhe service summit research workshop. http://service-summit.ksri.kit.edu/downloads/Session_3B2_KSS_2016_paper_19.pdf

Kloker, S., Straub, T., & Weinhardt, C. (2017). Designing a crowd forecasting tool to combine prediction markets and real-time Delphi. In A. Maedche, J. vom Brocke, & A. Hevner (Hrsg.), *Designing the digital transformation. DESRIST 2017. Lecture notes in computer science* (10243rd Hrsg., S. 468–473). Springer. https://doi.org/10.1007/978-3-319-59144-5_33

Kloker, S., Klatt, F., Hoeffer, J., & Weinhardt, C. (2018a). Analyzing prediction market trading behavior to select Delphi-experts. *Foresight*. https://doi.org/10.1108/FS-01-2018-0009

Kloker, S., Straub, T., Morana, S., & Weinhardt, C. (2018b). *Fraud and manipulation prevention in prediction markets*. In Proceedings of the 13th international conference, DESRIST 2018, Chennai, India, June 3–6, 2018 (S. 1–6).

Kloker, S., Straub, T., Morana, S., & Weinhardt, C. (2018c). *The effect of social reputation on retention: Designing a social real-time Delphi platform*. In Proceedings of the 26th European conference on information systems (ECIS2018), Portsmouth, UK, 2018.

Kochtanek, T. R., & Hein, K. K. (1999). Delphi study of digital libraries. *Information Processing and Management, 35*(3), 245–254. https://doi.org/10.1016/S0306-4573(98)00060-0

Kranz, T. T., Teschner, F., Roüast, P., & Weinhardt, C. (2014a). *Identifying individual party preferences in political stock markets*. In Proceedings of the IADIS international conference on E-Society. (Madrid, Spain) (S. 162–169).

Kranz, T. T., Teschner, F., & Weinhardt, C. (2014b). *Combining prediction markets and surveys: An experimental study*. In Proceedings of the European conference on information systems (ECIS) 2014, Tel Aviv, Israel, June 9–11, 2014.

Laskey, K. B., Hanson, R., & Twardy, C. (2015). *Combinatorial prediction markets for fusing information from distributed experts and models*. In Proceedings of the 18th international conference on information fusion (Fusion) (S. 1892–1898).

Levin, I. P., Chapman, D. P., & Johnson, R. D. (1988). Confidence in judgments based on incomplete information: An investigation using both hypothetical and real gambles. *Journal of Behavioral Decision Making, 1*(1), 29–41. https://doi.org/10.1002/bdm.3960010105

Linstone, H. A., & Turoff, M. (2002). *The Delphi method: Techniques and applications*. Addison-Wesley.

Luckner, S., & Weinhardt, C. (2007). How to pay traders in information markets: Results from a field experiment. *Journal of Prediction Markets, 1*(2), 147–156. http://econpapers.repec.org/RePEc:buc:jpredm:v:1:y:2007:i:2:p:147-156

Luckner, S., Kratzer, F., & Weinhardt, C. (2005). *STOCCER-A forecasting market for the FIFA World Cup 2006*. In 4th Workshop on e-Business (WeB 2005), Las Vegas, USA.

Mullen, P. M. (2003). Delphi: Myths and reality. *Journal of Health Organization and Management, 17*(1), 37–52. https://doi.org/10.1108/14777260310469319

Niemeyer, C., Wagenknecht, T., Teubner, T., & Weinhardt, C. (2016). *Participatory crowdfunding: An approach towards engaging employees and citizens in institutional budgeting decisions*. In Proceedings of the annual Hawaii international conference on system sciences (S. 2800–2808). https://doi.org/10.1109/HICSS.2016.351.

Okoli, C., & Pawlowski, S. D. (2004). The Delphi method as a research tool: An example, design considerations and applications. *Information & Management, 42*(1), 15–29. https://doi.org/10.1016/j.im.2003.11.002

Prokesch, T., von der Gracht, H. A., & Wohlenberg, H. (2015). Integrating prediction market and Delphi methodology into a foresight support system – Insights from an online game. *Technological Forecasting and Social Change, 97*, 47–64. https://doi.org/10.1016/j.techfore.2014.02.021

Reid, N. (1988). The Delphi technique: Its contribution to the evaluation of professional practice. In R. Ellis (Hrsg.), *Professional competence and quality assurance in the caring professions* (S. 230–254). Chapman & Hall. https://doi.org/10.1016/0020-7489(90)90106-S.

Rhode, P. W., & Strumpf, K. S. (2004). Historical presidential betting markets. *Journal of Economic Perspectives, 18*(2), 127–141. http://www.aeaweb.org/articles?id=10.1257/0895330041371277

Servan-Schreiber, E. (2017). *Debunking three myths about crowd – Based forecasting*. In Collective intelligence conference, Brooklyn, New York, USA.

Servan-Schreiber, E., Wolfers, J., Pennock, D. M., & Galebach, B. (2004). Prediction markets: Does money matter? *Electronic Markets, 14*(3), 243–251. https://doi.org/10.1080/1019678042000245254

Shrier, D., Adjodah, D., Wu, W., & Pentland, A. (2016). *Prediction markets*. http://cdn.resources.getsmarter.ac/wp-content/uploads/2016/08/mit_prediction_markets_report.pdf

Slamka, C., Jank, W., & Skiera, B. (2012). Second-generation prediction markets for information aggregation: A comparison of payoff mechanisms. *Journal of Forecasting, 31*, 469–489. https://doi.org/10.1002/for.1225

Sniezek, J. A. (1990). A comparison of techniques for judgmental forecasting by groups with common information. *Group & Organization Studies, 15*(1), 5–19. https://doi.org/10.1177/105960119001500102

Sprenger, T., Bolster, P., & Venkateswaran, A. (2007). Conditional prediction markets as corporate decision support systems – An experimental comparison with group deliberation. *Journal of Prediction Markets, 1*(3), 189–208. https://doi.org/10.5750/jpm.v1i3.428

Surowiecki, J. (2005). *The wisdom of crowds*. Anchor.

Teschner, F., & Weinhardt, C. (2012). Evaluating hidden market design. In P. Coles, S. Das, S. Lahaie, & B. Szymanski (Hrsg.), *Auctions, market mechanisms, and their applications* (Bd. 80, S. 5–17). Springer. https://doi.org/10.1007/978-3-642-30913-7_3

Teschner, F., Stathel, S., & Weinhardt, C. (2011). *A prediction market for macro-economic variables*. In Proceedings of the Annual Hawaii international conference on system sciences (S. 1–9). https://doi.org/10.1109/HICSS.2011.23

Vernon, W. (2009). The Delphi technique: A review. *International Journal of Therapy and Rehabilitation, 16*(2), 69–76. https://doi.org/10.12968/ijtr.2009.16.2.38892

Welty, G. (1972). Problems of selecting experts for Delphi exercises. *Academy of Management Journal, 15*(1), 121–124.

Winkler, J., & Moser, R. (2016). Biases in future-oriented Delphi studies: A cognitive perspective. *Technological Forecasting and Social Change, 105*, 63–76. https://doi.org/10.1016/j.techfore.2016.01.021

Wolfers, J., & Zitzewitz, E. (2006). *Interpreting prediction market prices as probabilities* (Working paper series). http://www.nber.org/papers/w12200.

Woudenberg, F. (1991). An evaluation of Delphi. *Technological Forecasting and Social Change, 40*(2), 131–150.

Part II

Case Studies for Delphi Methods

New Qualification Requirements in the Health Care Sector

Methodology and Summary of Results of a Delphi Survey in the Field of Public Private Health

Johannes Leinert, Alexander Rommel, and Helmut Schröder

Abstract

The study "Public Private Health" was designed to answer the question of what consequences demographic, social, technical and economic change will have for the future qualification requirements of employees in training occupations in the health care sector and related areas from the perspective of experts. This question was investigated using a mix of methods from qualitative and quantitative approaches. The core element of the study was a multi-stage Delphi survey in which around 1500 experts were asked for their assessments. For this purpose,

J. Leinert (✉)
infas Institute for Applied Social Sciences GmbH, Bonn, Germany

Bertelsmann Stiftung, Gütersloh, Germany
e-mail: johannes.leinert@bertelsmann-stiftung.de

A. Rommel
Robert Koch Institute, Former Scientific Institute of Doctors in Germany (WIAD), Berlin, Germany
e-mail: RommelA@rki.de

H. Schröder
infas Institute for Applied Social Sciences GmbH, Bonn, Germany
e-mail: helmut-schroeder@unitybox.de

M. Niederberger, O. Renn (eds.), *Delphi Methods In The Social And Health Sciences*, https://doi.org/10.1007/978-3-658-38862-1_7

a differentiated sampling plan was developed. On this basis, a stratified sample of 19 main strata and 75 substrata was drawn. In the non-standardised, first Delphi round, experts' opinions on qualification-relevant developments in the German health care system were collected, which were evaluated in the second, standardised Delphi round with regard to their probability of occurrence and effects on qualification requirements. The third survey round, which is usual in Delphi methods, was replaced by three expert workshops. This paper primarily describes the methodological approach of the study. The focus is on the explanation of the study design, the selection of experts and the operationalization of the research question. Furthermore, the most important results of the study are summarised.

1 Introduction

This paper describes the methodological approach of the study "Public Private Health" (PPH). It is the revised, English-language version of the article by Leinert et al. (2019). The PPH study was conducted by the infas Institute for Applied Social Sciences (infas), which was the lead partner, and the Scientific Institute of Doctors in Germany (WIAD) in 2011. The study was commissioned by the Federal Ministry of Education and Research (BMBF). In Germany, the BMBF is responsible for the development and regulation of professions at the intermediate qualification level, i.e. apprenticed occupations, but not academic professions.

Accordingly, the study focused on the consequences of demographic, social, technical and economic change for the vocational training of employees in the health care sector and related areas (e.g., nursing, care for the elderly, wellness). The focus was on employees at the "middle" level (apprenticed occupations), such as medical assistants, nursing staff, social workers, nutritionists and non-physician or non-academic therapists.

This research question was investigated within the framework of the PPH study with a mix of methods from qualitative and quantitative approaches. The core element of the study was a multi-stage Delphi survey, which was designed to obtain expert assessments of qualification-relevant developments and future qualification needs.

The following explanations describe in more detail how this was done. Based on the research question, the study design is established and it is described how the special requirements that arose in the PPH study were dealt with. This applies in particular to the sample generation and the operationalisation of the research question, were dealt with.

In Section 2, the research question and the objectives of the study are described before the research object is delimited. In Section 3, the study design and method are presented, in Section 4 the selection of the experts is described. In Section 5, the operationalisation of the research question is explained. In Section 6, the field course of the Delphi rounds is summarised. In Section 7, some central results of the PPH study are presented.

The following explanations must be limited to a summary presentation. For a detailed description of the study, please refer to the comprehensive final report of the PPH study by Klaes et al. (2011), which largely forms the basis for the present explanations. The report includes a detailed presentation of the substantive study results and documentation of the survey materials. The study and its results are also described in Klaes et al. (2013); a summary focusing specifically on the nursing sector can be found in Schüler et al. (2013).

Since the PPH study is now more than 10 years old, new developments such as the pandemic situation could not yet be taken into account. However, this is not relevant for the present article, as it focuses on the study design. The methodology of the PPH study is time-independent. Even today, it is still impressive how the study findings were obtained by condensing the assessment of more than 240 experts from a carefully constructed sample.

2 Background

2.1 Research Question and Objective of the Study

The PPH study was funded within the framework of the BMBF initiative "Early recognition of qualification requirements in the network (FreQueNz)". This initiative was intended to act as an "early warning system", to identify at an early stage when the requirements for professional qualifications at the intermediate qualification level change. One of the aims of the PPH study was to obtain expert assessments on "how significant technological, organisational and social developments will affect the activities and qualification requirements of employees in the healthcare system (Klaes et al., 2011, p. 26)." The focus was on employees at the "middle" qualification level (training occupations).[1] Against this background, the PPH study investigated the following question:

> What are the qualification requirements in the medium term (5–10 years) for the middle level (training occupations) in the health care sector and related areas?

The aim of the study was to provide an empirically sound information base on emerging developments in the world of work and needs for adapting qualifications. On this basis the BMBF could both define further research needs and examine whether occupational regulations should be adapted or new occupational profiles should be developed.

In order to meet this requirement, a study design for obtaining expert opinions had to be developed that was suitable for collecting facts on future developments that naturally elude observation. The survey should also be open to the entire range of possible and presumably dissonant assessments. Conducting a survey of actors in the strongly hierarchically organised health care system, care had to be taken that the assessments and positions of certain professional groups did not dominate the results of the survey as a whole. In addition, innovative developments were to be detected even if they were still largely unknown in public and only seemed worth mentioning to a small number of experts. Therefore, it was important to include as many existing positions as possible in the sense of a screening approach.

2.2 Delimitation of the Research Object

The starting point for the delimitation of the research object outlined below (Klaes et al., 2011, pp. 29–30) was the assumption that a complex structure of demographic, socio-structural, technical and economic change acts as a driver for developments in the health care system and its related areas. This results in changed requirements for the performance of very specific activities that are carried out in one or more service areas (e.g. nursing) in one or more institutions (e.g. old people's homes) by one or more occupational groups (e.g. geriatric nurses).

It stands to reason that changing work requirements in the service areas will lead to work organisation being restructured. This may lead to a change in the division of labour between existing institutions or to the emergence of new institutions

[1] This meant "skilled workers with degrees in a recognised training occupation (according to BBiG/HwO), in one of the federally regulated non-medical health professions (according to Sect. 74 (1) No. 19 GG) or in one of the school-based training courses regulated by Land law, as well as graduates with advanced training degrees." (Klaes et al., 2011, p. 3).

and/or to a shift of activities between existing occupations and/or to the need for new occupations. As a consequence, it can be assumed that entirely new qualifications are created or that existing qualifications are transferred to occupational groups that did not need them before. In this context, shifts from one field of activity to another are conceivable both on a horizontal level at the same hierarchical level and on a vertical level between the occupational or professional levels.

It follows from these considerations that the changed qualification requirements arise in a three-dimensional space which is spanned by the dimensions described:

- *Service areas*
  e.g. prevention, diagnostics, curation, rehabilitation, care, pallation, etc.
- *Professions or occupational fields*
  nursing professions, non-physician health care professions, social care professions, technical professions, etc.
- *Organizations*
  e.g. hospitals, medical practices, medical care centres, outpatient services, etc.

This model was a good basis both for the development of the sampling plan for selecting the experts to be interviewed and for the development of the analysis schemes for evaluating the qualitative study elements. However, survey instruments based on such a three-dimensional model would have been too complex for the respondents. Therefore, the three-dimensional model was transformed into a sequential model for this purpose (see Fig. 1).

3 Study Design and Method

The following sections begin with a theoretical classification. First, we will explain why a Delphi method was used as the core element of the study. Then, we will discuss which type of Delphi method the study belongs to and what implications this has for the study design. Eventually, we will present the study design of the PPH.

3.1 Theoretical Classification

The aim of the study was to obtain expert assessments of the lines of development that can be expected in the health care system and its related areas in the future, and which changes in qualification requirements at the middle level are associated with

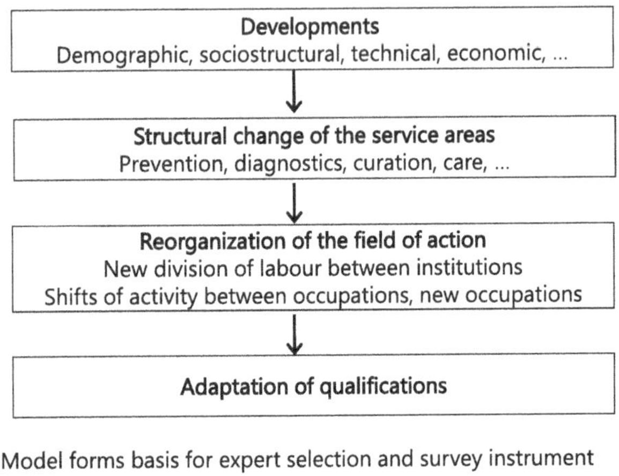

Fig. 1 Operationalization of the research object. (Source: own representation according to Klaes et al., 2011, p. 30)

Table 1 Types of expert interviews in comparison

Criterion	Group discussion	Expert survey	Delphi survey
Anonymity	No	Yes	Yes
Possibly influence by opinion leaders	Yes	No	No
Possibly influence through conformity pressure	Yes	No	Only limited
Possibility of high case numbers	No	Yes	Yes
Possibility of feedback	Yes	No	Yes
Possibility of specifically triggering cognitive processes	Yes	No	Yes
Time required	Low	Low	High

Source: own representation based on Häder (2014, p. 66)

this. In order to obtain expert assessments, different survey variants can be considered, such as group discussions, simple expert interviews and Delphi surveys. Each of these is associated with specific advantages and disadvantages. In the following Table 1, the characteristics of these three survey types are summarised based on Häder (2014, p. 66).

A group discussion to answer the research question was ruled out. On the one hand, the anonymity of the survey was necessary to avoid that mainly hierarchically higher placed professional groups or opinion leaders influence the results. On the other hand, a high number of cases was necessary to detect innovative, still largely unknown developments. Since the assessments of all experts on future developments were to be fed back and evaluated in a further survey round, a "simple" expert survey was also out of the question. Rather, a Delphi method was required to answer the question.

The basic idea of Delphi methods "is to use expert opinions in several waves to solve problems and to make use of anonymous feedback" (Häder, 2014, p. 22). There is a broad consensus in the literature that "classic" Delphi methods are characterised by the following steps (Häder, 2014, p. 24 f.):

- Operationalization of the general problem in order to derive concrete criteria that can be presented to the experts for evaluation in the standardised survey.
- Development of the survey instrument for the standardised expert survey.
- Processing of results and anonymous feedback.
- Repetition of the questioning.

Even though the Delphi method was developed as early as in the 1950s, there is still no uniform definition of the term today (Niederberger & Renn, 2018, p. 7). Rather, it has been further developed in a large number of studies and adapted to specific studies, so that numerous variants exist. Different approaches contribute to the richness of variants of the Delphi method, especially with regard to the following design features: Selection and number of experts interviewed, number of survey rounds, design of feedback to the experts, query of the respondents' self-assessment of their expertise, termination or consensus criteria, tasks to be worked on, and use of workshops to collect and discuss the data (Häder, 2014, p. 25). With a typology of Delphi methods, Häder (2014, pp. 30–36) makes an attempt to structure this diversity (see Table 2). In this typology, the PPH study corresponds to type 3, since the focus was on determining expert opinions.

3.2 Implementation of the Study-Specific Requirements

With the objective of the Delphi study (determination of expert opinions), central requirements for the design of the study were already defined according to the Delphi typology: It was crucial to operationalise the question to be answered as precisely as possible – a requirement that could be fulfilled in the first, non-standardised, qualitatively oriented Delphi round. On this basis, a standardised survey instrument with predominantly closed questions was to be developed (see Section 5).

Table 2 Types of Delphi methods according to Häder (2014)

Criterion	Type 1: idea aggregation	Type 2: stipulation	Type 3: determination of expert opinions	Type 4: consensus building
Objective	Brainstorming	Improvement in the determination of issues (predictions)	Identification and qualification of expert opinions	High level of agreement among participants
Criterion for the selection of experts	Expertise	Hypotheses necessary, rules cannot be formalised	Complete survey or deliberate selection	Possible by means of determinable frame
Operationalization	Hardly necessary	Operationalization of the question to be addressed as precisely as possible		Strongly differentiated operationalization
Qualitative Delphi rounds	Exclusively qualitative	Can be used for operationalization		Can be omitted, will be taken over by the monitoring team
Question type	Open questions	Mainly closed questions		Closed questions only

Source: Own representation based on Häder (2014, p. 37)

In addition, criteria for the deliberate selection of the experts to be interviewed had to be developed, since a full survey was not possible considering the size of the population - defined as persons with expertise in the health care system and related fields. In order to include the expertise of all groups of actors relevant to the research question, a differentiated sample was necessary. It was stratified according to several criteria with sufficient case numbers in all subgroups. With regard to the expected non-response, a gross sample of $n = 1500$ was specified (see Section 4).

In the sense of a screening approach, the PPH study was to detect developments that were previously largely unknown and to evaluate them by all participants. According to the project team's assessment, this could only be partially achieved with the literature research and qualitative expert interviews planned in advance of the Delphi study. Therefore, it was deliberately decided not to conduct the first qualitative Delphi round with a small sub-sample, but to interview the *entire* gross sample already at this stage. This was the only way to ensure that the experts in the standardised second Delphi round could be presented with as many qualification-relevant developments as possible for evaluation.

These two Delphi rounds already demanded a very high degree of motivation and willingness to participate from the experts. In order to keep the burden on the respondents within limits and to secure their participation in both survey rounds, a further standardised feedback and renewed evaluation by the expert sample was dispensed with, which classical Delphi methods usually still provide for. Instead of a third survey round, three expert workshops were held. These allowed an in-depth discussion and evaluation of the survey results and a discussion of the consequences that result from the assessments of the future development trends for the qualification of healthcare workers (Klaes et al., 2011, p. 69).

3.3 Overview of the Study Design

The study design consisted of a mixture of standardised and non-standardised survey instruments, which were designed in several stages (see Fig. 2). The first two study modules served to determine the current state of the discussion and the different positions and argumentations with regard to changes in qualification requirements and to derive experience-saturated hypotheses from this. To this end, a literature review and analysis was conducted. Subsequently, structured qualitative interviews were conducted with experts in key positions from central institutions of the health care system and related fields (Klaes et al., 2011, p. 56).

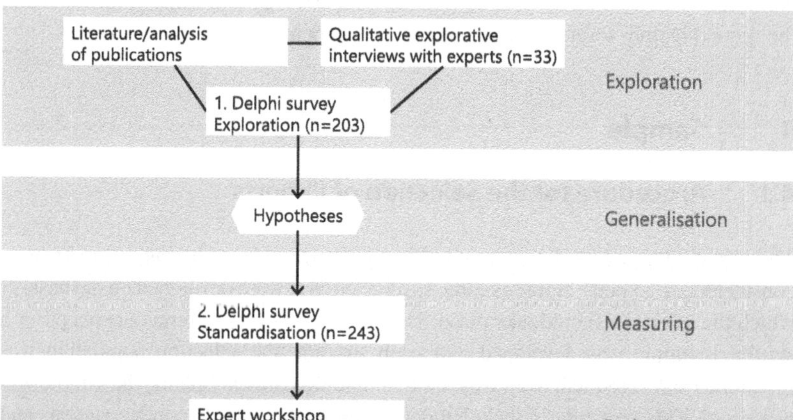

Fig. 2 Overview of the study design. (Source: Klaes et al., 2011, p. 57)

The core element of the PPH study was a subsequent three-stage Delphi process, which consisted of a qualitative and quantitative survey of a gross sample of about 1500 experts as well as three concluding expert workshops. In the first Delphi round, the experts' perceptions of future developments in the health care system and the associated qualification requirements for employees at the middle level were collected in a questionnaire with open questions (Klaes et al., 2011, p. 56).

The standardised questionnaire for the second Delphi round was created on the basis of a content-analytical evaluation of the first Delphi round and was also sent to the gross sample of the first Delphi round. The statements contained in the standardised questionnaire were to be evaluated by the respondents in terms of how probable and how relevant to action they considered the occurrence of the developments named in the first Delphi round and their impact on the qualification requirements (Klaes et al., 2011, p. 56).

The standardised questionnaire for the second Delphi round was developed on the basis of the results of the first Delphi round. For this purpose – after a content-analytical processing and hypothesis generation – the answers of the first round were condensed into a standardised questionnaire, which was sent to the gross sample of the first round. Thus, all respondents obtained knowledge about the developments and their consequences for the qualification requirements that had been mentioned by the other experts in the first round. Through the standardised survey in the second round, all participants now answered the same questions against their specific background of experience. This resulted in a quasi standardised, written group discussion (Klaes et al., 2011, p. 66). Finally, the results of the second Delphi round were discussed and deepened at three workshops.

4 Sample

4.1 Procedure for the Selection of Experts

The expert sample was drawn in a multi-stage process. First, it was defined who is considered an "expert". Subsequently, specific criteria were developed on the basis of which the selection should take place. Then, based on these criteria, a concept for a stratified sample was developed. For each stratum, the selection population was researched and classified, from which the sample was drawn. Finally, the sample was processed. This particularly included determining the concrete contact persons and their address data as well as a final adjustment of the sample for any duplications.

Persons with expert status were understood to be "actors in the system who have developed expertise for the research questions due to their activities in associations, organisations or as practitioners" (Klaes et al., 2011, p. 57). For the selection of the group of experts defined in this way, two criteria were determined in accordance with the model of the three-dimensional space of qualification requirements as described in Sect. 2.2; First, experts from all service areas, organisations and professional fields should be represented in the sample and second, actors from the normative, strategic and operational levels should be included. The definition of the selection criteria was based on two considerations.

> Due to their tasks in health care, in associations, supervisory bodies or in science and education, experts have a closer view on entire service areas of the health care system, on individual professions or professional fields or on work organisations. Thus, for example, the focus of representatives of a medical profession could presumably be directed more towards this professional field and the labour market, while the view of medical or nursing teachers could presumably be directed more towards the service areas and that of decision-makers presumably more towards the organisation of work.
>
> Depending on their institutional setting and function, the experts are more likely to be active in an operational, strategic or normative function. It is to be expected that the representatives of professional and other associations, who are professionally more involved with the processes of change, whether they analyse them scientifically, drive forward technical developments or create economic control instruments, belong predominantly to the normative and strategic level of the health and care system. To put it bluntly, they are more likely to have a dispositional attitude with regard to the service sector, with the intention of controlling change as far as possible. In contrast, it is to be expected that experts who are primarily professionally close to practical service provision are more likely to adopt a reorganising perspective, in that they react to pressure to change and attempt to adapt the consequences of change to the changed conditions by restructuring tasks or organisation (Klaes et al., 2011, p. 58).

On this basis, a sampling concept was developed that contained a total of 18 sampling strata plus a residual category as well as 75 subgroups (see following chapter). This detailed breakdown was intended to define the expertise to be included as transparently and completely as possible. In addition, the tabular overview enabled the sample composition to be verified intersubjectively without having to disclose names and institutions, which would have violated the promised confidentiality and data protection (Klaes et al., 2011, p. 58). For each sampling stratum or its subgroups, research then began on the selection population from which the sample was drawn. The starting point for the research was usually the institution in which the experts were located and the function they performed within this institution.

Ideally, complete lists of the population of interest existed at the level of the institutions, so that the sample population was identical to the population. This was the case, for example, for health insurance funds, medical associations, pharmacist's associations, or associations of statutory health insurance physiciens. As a rule, however, such lists did not exist. Then, if possible, lists covering at least a large part of the population were used as a basis for selection. These were, for example, lists of members of associations in which a large part of the population is organised (e.g. Federal Association of Pharmaceutical Manufacturers, Association of Medical Professions, German Network for Health Services Research) or accreditation lists of actors in the health care system (e.g. medical laboratories). If such lists were not available or were considered to be too incomplete, an additional search option was an internet search for keywords (e.g. chairs for "health services research"). It was important to keep in mind that the sample population included relevant organizations as collective actors in the health care system and related areas. Who within that organization was the expert to be interviewed was often best decided by the organization itself. In these cases, the organization as such was to be contacted.

Once the sample population had been researched for each subgroup, the sample – stratified by subgroups – was drawn from it. In the case of very small subgroups, all institutions or persons researched were included in the sample. In a large number of cases, however, until this stage it was only known which function the expert to be interviewed held in which institution; but the specific person behind a particular function (e.g. nursing director of a particular hospital) was not known. Which specific target person was to be interviewed (e.g. holders of the chair of health services research at a particular university) was only known from the outset in a few cases. Therefore, the address and contact data of a target person at the institution of interest were first researched – usually via Internet research. In a subsequent telephone search, it was determined which person in the respective institution performs the function of interest and should thus be included in the sample as an expert. In most cases, it was possible to research this person by name. If this was not possible, the Delphi survey questionnaire was sent to a specific function within the institution, which had been identified on the basis of organisation charts or internet directories (Klaes et al., 2011, p. 64). Finally, the experts known by name were cleared of duplicates.

4.2 Result of the Expert Selection: Gross Sample by Main Groups and Subgroups

The creation of the gross sample as described in the previous chapter was a lengthy process that took several months. As a result, the gross sample comprised $n = 1508$ experts. The structure of the gross sample as well as the case numers of the respective main and substrata are documented in Fig. 3. In the third column, it is also noted from which sample strata the experts were recruited for the 33 guided interviews.

Main stratum	Sub-stratum	Selection for expert interviews			Gross number of addresses
1	0		**Health insurances**		100
	1	x	Health insurance statutory/private	47	
	2	x	Nursing care insurance statutory/private	53	
	3		Others	0	
2	0		**Medical profession**		84
	1		Associations of Statutory Health Insurance Physicians	52	
	2	x	Medical Chambers	19	
	3		Stakeholder organisations	12	
	4		Others	1	
3	0		**Dental profession**	45	45
4	0		**Krankenhaussektor (einschließlich Patientenhotels)**		152
	1		Hospital: Medical management	24	
	2	x	Hospital: Nursing management	27	
	3	x	Hospital: Commercial management	27	
	4		Hospital operators (public, non-profit, private, ...)	0	
	5		Hospital associations	39	
	6		Quality assurance in hospitals	24	
	7	x	Patient hotels	10	
	8		Others	1	
5	0		**Care sector**		114
	1		German Nursing Council	1	
	2		Care associations	44	
	3		Nursing teachers associations	9	
	4	x	Outpatient services	36	
	5	x	Inpatient care facilities	18	
	6		Quality assurance in care	0	
	7		Others	6	
6	0		**Pharmaceutical sector**		100
	1		Pharmacists' associations	9	
	2	x	Chambers of pharmacists	10	
	3		Pharmaceutical manufacturers, wholesalers and intermediaries	43	
	4		Association of Researching Pharmaceutical Manufacturers	0	
	5	x	Medical laboratories (large-scale laboratories)	38	
	6		Others	0	
7	0		**Medical technology and information technology**		143
	1	x	Medical technology developers (medical devices)	50	
	2		Medical technology developers (medical aids)	2	
	3	x	Information technology developers	42	
	4		Medical technology manufacturers/implementeurs (strategic planning/production)	22	
	5	x	HomeCare	17	
	6		Others	10	
8	0		**Psychotherapeutic Sector**	43	43
9	0		**Education and training sector**		104
	1	x	Further education academies	78	
	2	x	German Employee Academy	7	
	3		Others	18	
10	0		**Other health occupations**		77
	1	x	Occupational therapists (e.g. ErgoAkademie)	16	
	2	x	Physiotherapists	28	
	3	x	Speech therapists	20	
	4		Others	13	
11	0		**Medical Occupations**		71
	1		Arbeitsgemeinschaft der wissenschaftlich interessierten medical-technical assistant	1	
	2	x	Association of Medical Occupations	9	
	3		German Association of Technical Assistants in Medicine	21	
	4		Midwives	27	
	5		Others	13	
12	0		**Scientific institutions**		153
	1		Chairs, scientific institutes (nursing science)	21	
	2	x	Chairs, scientific institutes (health services research)	29	
	3		Chairs, scientific institutes (occupational research)	23	
	4	x	BIBB	8	
	5	x	Chairs, scientific institutes (ageing research: German Centre of Gerontology)	22	
	6		Chairs, scientific institutes (ageing research: Cologne/Bonn Competence Network)	1	
	7		Fraunhofer Society/Institutes	7	
	8		Occupational societies	34	
	9		Others	7	

Fig. 3 Structure, strata and case numbers of the expert sample. (Source: Klaes et al. 2011, p. 60; Banz et al., 2010, p. 45)

13	0		**Administration and supervisory authorities**		55
	1		Upper federal and state authorities: Labour, health, social affairs	20	
	2	x	Upper federal and Land authorities: Education/training (e.g. responsible for training)	19	
	3		Public health service	16	
	4		Others	0	
14	0		**Representation of persons affected**		56
	2	x	Disabled people's associations (physical disability)	43	
	3	x	Consumer/patient associations	6	
	4	x	Associations of relatives (e.g. Alzheimer initiatives, etc.)	7	
	5		Others	0	
15	0		**Tariff partners**	0	65
	1	x	Employers	27	
	2	x	Employees	36	
	3		Others	2	
16	0	x	**Social work**	30	30
17	0		**Health promotion, prevention and wellness sector**		67
	1		Health promotion/prevention	15	
	2	x	Wellness	40	
	3		Health hotels	12	
	4		Others	0	
18	0		**Innovative structures and model projects**		46
	1	x	Private public health	2	
	2		Intersectoral networks	7	
	3	x	Service centre	3	
	4		Model project	34	
	5		Others	0	
19	0	x	**Further experts**	3	3
Total					**1,508**

Fig. 3 (continued)

5 Operationalisation of the Research Question

The research question was operationalised in a multi-stage process. First, the general problem was operationalised in an explorative phase on the basis of literature research, structured interviews and the first, non-standardised Delphi round. Then, scenarios were developed on this basis and extensive item lists were compiled. On this basis, the experts evaluated the occurrence of certain developments in the second, quantitative Delphi round.

5.1 Literature Research and Analysis

At the beginning of the project, a systematic analysis of publications was carried out. For this purpose, a literature search was carried out that was not only based on conventional publications. In order to be able to include as complete and current a status as possible, this also included so-called grey literature and Internet publications. The research was carried out using a keyword catalogue, which was successively (further) developed (Klaes et al., 2011, p. 32). Subsequently, the researched publications were analysed in detail. On this basis, the basic assumptions of the study were critically examined and further differentiated. From the findings of the literature research and analysis, 52 core theses were derived, which, together with the results of the guideline interviews, formed the basis for the development of the questionnaires for the Delphi surveys (see exemplary Fig. 4).

5.2 Guidelines for the Explorative Expert Interviews

On the one hand, the qualitatively designed expert interviews were intended to supplement the results of the literature analysis and the core theses derived from it, or to modify them from a the practitioners' point of view. On the other hand, the interviews were intended to explore the possibilities and limits of expertise in answering the research question. Thus, the expert survey directly supported the development of the survey instrument for the first Delphi round. For the evaluation, the expert interviews were analysed by infas and WIAD according to a coordinated analysis scheme and recorded in an ACCESS database (Klaes et al., 2011, p. 62, 63).

The guideline for the qualitative expert interviews was developed based on the operational concept for the delimitation of the research object as outlined in Sect. 2.2 and the results of the literature analysis. It is documented in Klaes et al. (2011, pp. 167–203). After a brief introduction to the study and clarification of personal expertise – respondents were asked about their professional position, involvement with the topic and other relevant functions in addition to their main job – the background and assumptions of the study on future developments in the health care system were first explained.[2] After this explanation, the respondents were asked to provide information in response to the following guiding questions:

- Which service areas of the health care system and related areas are affected by these developments?
- How will the relationship between public and private provision change?
- What are the consequences for the activities of the employees there?
- What new or changed requirements are likely to be associated with this for employees at the intermediate qualification level?

The respondents were asked to refer (initially) to the service area for which they expected the greatest developments in the next 5–7 years or for which they could best answer the guiding questions. The expected developments in the selected service area were to be answered unaided, i.e. without predefined answer categories. If predefined central aspects (e.g. causes as well as promoting and inhibiting factors for the developments described, a description of expected developments in

[2] It was explained that the qualification requirements for training occupations in the health care system and related fields are expected to change in the next 5–7 years as a result of processes of change due to demographic change, an increase in chronic-degenerative and mental illnesses and technological progress.

A. Developments in the outpatient sector	
A.1	The purely informal and privately organised care of those in need of long-term care by family carers is becoming less likely because of the prevailing social conditions.
A.2	In the future, there will be an increasing need for support structures that enable family members to provide outpatient care for those in need of care.
A.3	In particular, the service areas of comprehensive counselling of caring relatives and the corresponding management of the care processes will become more important (care counselling, case and care management).
B. Ambient Assisted Living (AAL)	
B.1	Technological innovations are increasingly giving rise to the option of making life easier in the private household by means of technical aids and of networking the household with its surroundings
B.2	In the field of outpatient care, this creates the possibility of preventing typical nursing and medical crisis scenarios by combining sensor technology and telemedicine.
C. Intercultural opening	
C.1	Due to past and future intra-European migration, but also international migration beyond this, there is a growing need to adapt health care structures to the linguistic and cultural characteristics of immigrant population groups (intercultural opening).

Fig. 4 Development of core theses from the literature review (example). (Source: Klaes et al., 2011, p. 71)

work processes, activities and qualification requirements as precisely as possible or the naming of the occupational fields and qualification areas likely to be affected) were not addressed or not answered exhaustively, the interviewers asked standardised follow-up questions. Finally, the experts were asked whether their own or other institutions were already preparing for the developments to be expected in the future through concrete plans or concepts.

5.3 Questionnaire for the First Delphi Round

In the first Delphi round, in accordance with the screening approach, expert opinions on current and future developments in the German health care system were to be collected and thus future relevant tasks and topics for the vocational training system were to be identified. For this purpose, an eight-page questionnaire was developed for self-completion. It is documented in Klaes et al. (2011, p. 204, 2013).

The questionnaire was designed as a semi-standardised survey instrument with open questions. The experts were asked to state in their own words which organisational and technical developments they expected in the health care system in the forecast period and what effects this would have on the qualification requirements of occupational activities at the intermediate qualification level. The focus was on two primary guiding questions, to each of which specific follow-up questions were asked. The two key questions were

- "How will the health care system and its related areas (e.g. nursing, geriatric care, home care) develop in the future due to sociodemographic, technological and economic change? How are the services and structures likely to change?"
- "What impact will the developments you describe have on the division of tasks, activities, and qualificationrequirements of employees at the middle qualification level over a period of five to ten years? What new or changed requirements are likely to be associated with this for employees at the middle qualification level?"

In order to better classify the developments in the health care system and the related areas outlined by the experts, the respondents were asked to assign one or more service areas when answering the first guiding question in the questionnaire. In order to enable a socio-structural classification of the participants, they were asked about their age, gender, profession and professional position in the institution at the end of the questionnaire. Finally, a brief explanation was requested of the extent to which the respondents were personally concerned with change in the health care system in the context of their professional activities. The results of the first Delphi round were evaluated by content analysis and formed the basis for the development of the standardised survey instrument for the second Delphi round (Klaes et al., 2011, pp. 64, 66).

5.4 Questionnaire for the Second Delphi Round

The second round was carried out using a full standardised survey questionnaire. In developing the questionnaire, we used the scenario technique. In a multi-stage condensation process, six development scenarios were developed on the basis of the results of literature research and expert interviews as well as the answers from the first Delphi round. The developments named in the first Delphi round and their effects on activities and qualification requirements were assigned to the scenarios and summarised in items, on the basis of which an evaluation was carried out by the experts. The qualification-relevant developments were usually stated by several persons. Lines of development that could not be classified against the background of the explorative guideline interviews and the literature analysis or that described a singular situation were excluded from the second Delphi round (Klaes et al., 2011, p. 66).

The starting point for the development of the scenarios was formed by the core theses summarised in eleven topic areas, which had been derived from the results of the literature research. These topics were then further condensed: Taking into account the results of the guideline-supported expert interviews and the mentions from the first Delphi round, **six scenarios** were derived after an extensive discussion process. These six scenarios can be regarded as central development trends in the health care system. They describe processes that were already taking place at that time, which have also shaped the further development of health care in the following years and have necessitated new qualifications in health care professions. These scenarios are briefly summarised in the following points (Klaes et al., 2011, p. 75 f.):

- New services for the care and support of elderly and very elderly people at home and in the home environment.
- New tasks for skilled employees in outpatient and inpatient care (e.g., delegation, physician-relief services, new division of tasks).
- Intensification of health promotion and prevention in all fields of activity of the health care system.
- New services in the field of wellness and fitness as well as complementary health services (e.g., medical wellness, health tourism).
- Telemonitoring and assistance systems as drivers of new supply structures and qualification requirements (e.g., eHealth, telemedicine, telecare, ambient assisted living, Smart House).
- Increased networking and growing need for process control in all areas of the health care system (e.g., integrated and cross-sectoral care).

The six scenarios were the starting point for the standardised questionnaire of the second Delphi round, which is documented in Klaes et al. (2011, pp. 214–233). They were first explained in more detail (see Table 3 for an example of the first scenario). Then, they were examined comprehensively with detailed item lists.

For each scenario, we asked about the probability that the developments associated with the scenario would occur. The probability was to be indicated on a four-point scale ("very unlikely", "rather unlikely", rather likely,"very likely"). If the experts considered the development to be rather or very likely, they were also asked

Table 3 Example of a scenario with supplementary explanation

Scenario	New services for the care and support of elderly and very elderly people at home and in the residential environment
Explanation	At present, around 70% of people over 65 in need of care in Germany are cared for on an outpatient basis. However, the so-called "pull" into residential homes means that the proportion of people in need of care who are cared for on an outpatient basis is declining slightly. Nevertheless, in the socio-political debate the phrase "outpatient prior to inpatient" has for some time been associated with the intention of shifting not only medical but also non-medical (nursing, social care and therapeutic) care more strongly into the outpatient sector. In view of the steady increase in the number of elderly and very old people, the aim of strengthening outpatient care is, on the one hand, to provide more efficient care. On the other hand, it is intended to meet the desire of those affected to be able to live at home and in their living environment for as long as possible. As a result, a significantly increasing proportion of people in need of care could be cared for at home, i.e., on an outpatient basis, in the future.

to indicate the period of time in which they expected the said development to occur ("up to 5 years", "up to 20 years", over 10 years").

The experts were then asked to assume that the scenario will occur. Under this premise, they were asked to evaluate a detailed item list of potentially changing job requirements that may be associated with the scenario. First, respondents should indicate whether they agree or disagree with the items on activity changes. If they agreed, they were asked to indicate whether such a change in job requirements would necessitate additional or different qualifications for employees compared to today's requirements. In an open question, they were also asked to name further important developments not listed in the standardised question.

Finally, detailed lists of items per scenario were used to find out which factors inhibit and promote the developments outlined. Throughout the questionnaire, the response option "cannot/would not like to assess" was offered for each item. This was done to ensure that no one would be pressured into answering if they had insufficient expertise for a specific question. The combination of "can't/wouldn't like to" deliberately left it open for which of the two reasons mentioned no assessment was given.

In Figs. 5, 6, and 7, the questionnaire is documented as an example using excerpts for the first scenario. In total, the questionnaire comprised 20 pages with over 250 items to be evaluated.

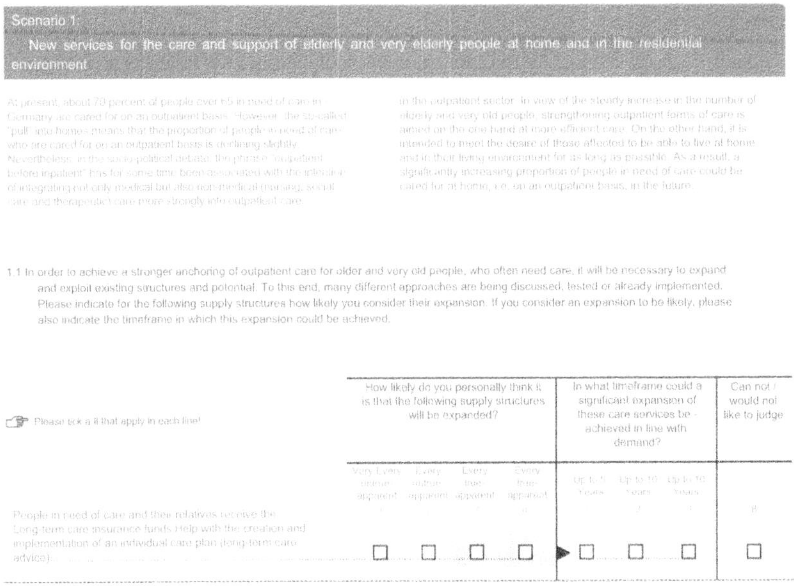

Fig. 5 Questionnaire example 1: scenario and assessment of developments

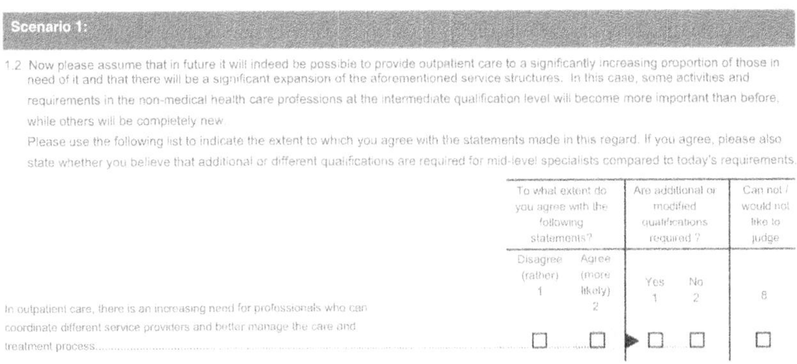

Fig. 6 Questionnaire example 2: assessment of developments in activities and qualifications

1.3 What other qualification requirements do you consider important in the course of strengthening outpatient care for older and very old people?

1.4 Whether there will be a significant expansion of outpatient care for older and very old people in the next few years depends on various factors. Please indicate to what extent you agree with the following statements.

	Agree whole heartedly 1	Vote rather 2	Rather not agree 3	Do not agree at all 4	I can't judge. I don 't know. 8
There is a lack of important legal prerequisites for the comprehensive implementation of the models mentioned in outpatient care	☐	☐	☐	☐	☐

Fig. 7 Questionnaire example 3: supplementary responses, and promoting/inhibiting factors

6 Field Course of the Delphi Rounds

6.1 First Delphi Round: Non-standardised Survey

The questionnaires of the first Delphi round were sent out in the last week of August 2010 to a total of 1508 persons or institutions of the expert sample. In the last week of September 2010, a first reminder was sent. This reminder was sent to all 1375 persons or institutions who had not yet responded to the first letter.[3] The reminder enclosed the questionnaire again; it also contained the offer to complete an online questionnaire if desired. Due to the slow response to the questionnaire, an additional, unplanned, second reminder campaign was carried out at the end of October 2010 and the field time was extended until the end of November 2010. Based on these exhaustive efforts, a response rate was finally achieved that is acceptable for a written-postal expert survey (Klaes et al., 2011, pp. 64, 65). The field statistics for the first Delphi round are presented in Table 4.

[3] If a completed questionnaire had already been received, if there had been an explicit refusal to participate, or if it had been reported back that no one in the selected institution was able to answer the question (for example, because a person had left the institution), the reminder was dispensed with.

Table 4 Field statistics for the 1st round of the Delphi survey

	Number	%
Questionnaires sent (gross)	**1512**	**100**
Neutral non-response (target person deceased, not in target group, or moved; change of address, resending requested)	141	9,3
Net sample	**1371**	**100**
Completed interviews	203	14,8
Without response	1104	80,5
Systematic non-response: target person refused to participate (in principle, not interested in the topic, not in this wave, other reasons).	64	4,7

Source: Klaes et al. (2011, p. 66)

6.2 Second Delphi Round: Quantitative Survey

In Delphi surveys, the sample of the first round is also used as a basis for the second round. In the PPH study, only an address update based on the responses from the first round and an adjustment for fundamental refusals was carried out. The questionnaires for the second round were sent to 1361 persons/institutions at the end of March 2011. Two reminder campaigns were conducted in the following 13 weeks, which included a resend of the questionnaire. By the end of the field period, 243 evaluable questionnaires had been received, representing a response rate of 18.5% (Table 5). After the end of the field phase, a further 17 questionnaires were received but could not be included in the analyses. The proportion of failures ("cannot/would not like to assess") was extraordinarily low. The quality of the data basis for the evaluations was very good (Klaes et al., 2011, p. 67).

6.3 Expert Workshops Instead of Third Survey Round

Instead of a third round of data collection, the PPH study discussed the results together with selected experts in three 1-day workshops. On the one hand, this format was chosen in order not to strain the willingness of the experts to participate in a third Delphi round. On the other hand, the workshops allowed to discuss the results in small groups in detail, to exchange comments and hints and to talk about the consequences of the identified developments for the qualification of employees of the health care system. This would not have been possible within the framework of a standardised survey.

Table 5 Field statistics for the 2nd round of the Delphi survey

	Number	%
Questionnaires sent (gross)	**1361**	**100**
Neutral non-response (target person deceased, not in target group, or moved; change of address, resending requested)	47	3,5
Net sample	**1314**	**100**
Completed interviews	243	18,5
Without response	1040	79,1
Systematic non-response: target person refused to participate (in principle, not interested in the topic, not in this wave, other reasons).	31	2,4

Source: Klaes et al. (2011, p. 68)

To ensure that the workshops were workable despite the extensive study results, these were not discussed as a whole. Instead, the three events were thematically focused on two of the six scenarios inquired about:

- Workshop 1: Telematics, Networking and Process Control in Health Care
- Workshop 2: New services for older patients and new tasks for health care professionals
- Workshop 3: Health Promotion and Medical Wellness

The selection of experts for each workshop was based on their thematic references. In preparation for the workshops, the participants received a statistical analysis of the results of the two scenarios as well as additional methodological information. 23 experts participated in the workshops. The workshops took place between 12 and 14 July 2011 (Klaes et al., 2011, p. 69).

The differentiating comments and conclusions of the participants on the survey results formed an important supplement to the results of the literature research and surveys – also from the point of view of practical feasibility – and were also included in the final report of the PPH study. Thus, even if this question was no longer part of the research assignment, general recommendations on *how* the new qualifications should be taught could be made on the basis of the quite clear votes of the experts at the workshops (Klaes et al., 2011, p. 154). This will be discussed in the next chapter after a summary of the expected new qualification needs.

7 Study Results and Conclusion

In the following sections, a highly condensed presentation of the results is provided in the sense of a general summary of the results. For the detailed, scenario-specific results, please refer to the final report of the PPH study (Klaes et al., 2011, pp. 80–148).

Table 6 summarises the probability and speed with which the experts expected a broad expansion of the respective scenario elements. It also shows the extent to which they assumed an increase in the importance of specific activities and requirements and considered new qualifications to be necessary. The ratings shown with symbols summarise the frequency and degree of agreement with the respective items (Klaes et al., 2011, p. 149).

Table 6 Distribution of the affirmative response frequencies to questions 1 (probability and speed of the expansion of the scenario) and 2 (increase in importance and additional qualification requirements) in the 2nd Delphi round in comparison of the scenarios

	Broad expansion of scenario elements		Increased importance of activities and requirements	
Scenarios	Probability	Speed	Yes	New qualification required
1. New services for the care and support of elderly and very elderly people at home and in the home environment	+	+	++	++
2. New tasks for skilled employees in outpatient and inpatient care	+	++	+	++
3. Intensification of health promotion and prevention in all fields of activity of the health care system	+	+	++	+
4. New services in the area of wellness and fitness as well as complementary health services	+	++	○	○
5. Telemonitoring, technological development and assistance systems as drivers of new supply structures and qualification requirements	○	+	+	+
6. Increased networking and growing need for process control in all areas of the health care system	○	○	++	+

Proportion and expression of approving votes: ++ very high... + high...○ medium
Source: Klaes et al. (2011, p. 150)

It turns out that in scenario 1 and 2 the experts' votes in favour of the need for new qualifications were the highest. Both scenarios are at the same time most strongly influenced by the demographic development and the associated increase in elderly, multimorbid and dementia patients (Klaes et al., 2011, p. 149). A central recommendation could be derived from the findings summarised in Table 6:

> In the sense of prioritisation, the qualification requirements resulting from scenarios 1–3 should be given priority. The new qualification requirements associated with the developments in scenarios 6 and 5 should also be tackled with high priority, followed by the requirements and new qualifications formulated in connection with scenario 4 (Klaes et al., 2011, p. 151).

Which qualification requirements were primarily addressed by this, is summarised in Table 7 for qualifications that were considered necessary across all scenarios. Only those requirements are shown which, according to the evaluators' assessment, entailed a high to very high qualification requirement in at least two scenarios. If those requirements are considered which entail new qualification requirements in all six scenarios, these are predominantly cross-sectional tasks:

- Interdisciplinary communication
- Target group oriented communication and interaction
- Health promotion and prevention
- Supply and health management
- Coordination and networking of service providers
- Quality Management
- Dealing with multimorbidity
- Electronic documentation and evaluation

This cross-sectional character also applies to a large extent to the other qualification requirements from Table 7, which do not play a role in all scenarios. However, specific requirements such as palliative care and medication management also appear alongside the cross-sectional tasks. This outlines the most important overarching areas in which modified, supplemented or even entirely new qualifications were expected for health professions for the periods surveyed. In addition, there are the additional specific qualification requirements that are only relevant in the respective scenario context. These are summarised in Table 8, where only requirements with relatively high approval ratings were included (Klaes et al., 2011, pp. 151, 153).

Overall, it emerged from the experts' assessments that specific qualifications will continue to make up a significant part of the required core competences in each health care profession in the future periods surveyed. At the same time, it was

Table 7 Cross-scenario qualification requirements in comparison of the six scenarios

Areas of activity and requirements with relatively high additional qualification needs	Scenario					
	1	2	3	4	5	6
1. Interdisciplinary communication, team orientation, multiprofessionality	●	●	●	●	●	●
2. Communication and interaction appropriate for the target group (especially with the elderly, target groups defined by settings, dementia patients, people with a migration background, people with disabilities)	●	●	●	●	●	●
3. Health promotion and prevention tailored to the needs of target groups and settings	●	●	●	●	●	●
4. Supply and health management (community or neighbourhood-based)	●	●	o	o	●	●
5. Coordination and networking of different service providers	●	●	o	o	●	●
6. Quality management	●	●	●	o	o	●
7. Dealing with multimorbidity	●	●	o	o	●	●
8. Electronic documentation and evaluation	o	●	o	o	●	●
9. Patient education and counseling	●	●	●		o	●
10. Interface management	●	●			●	●
11. Knowledge of the medical treatment chain and the intersectoral process organisation	●	●			o	●
12. Guidance for family carers	●	●	o		o	
13. Sound knowledge of settings	●		●			●
14. Palliative care, end-of-life care	●	o				●
15. Guideline-oriented action	o	●				●
16. Interdisciplinary assessments	●	●				
17. Medication management	●	●				
18. Social marketing			●	●		
19 Data security and data protection					●	●

● high to very high qualification requirement, o medium to high qualification requirement
Source: Klaes et al. (2011, p. 152)

expected that additional cross-sectional qualifications will become increasingly necessary, which will form a supplementary core area of qualifications. Against the background of the high approval rates for these developments, it was not questioned *whether* these developments would occur from the experts' point of view or which qualification areas would be affected by them. These questions were answered by the PPH study for the periods surveyed. However, the question of *how* these new qualifications should be taught was not answered. This question was also no more part of the research assignment. However, due to quite clear votes of the experts in the thematic workshops, general recommendations could be made (Klaes et al., 2011, p. 154):

Table 8 Overview of selected scenario-specific qualification requirements in the six scenarios

Areas of activity and requirements with relatively high additional qualification needs	Occupational groups
Scenario 1	
Specialised intensive care nursing skills in pain management, artificial nutrition and respiratory care to ensure outpatient intensive care.	Specialists in the outpatient sector
Deeper consideration of specific patient groups (including dementia patients, multimorbid patients, people with a migration background)	Specialists in the outpatient sector
Scenario 2	
Professional assessment of the patient's living environment, use of aids, state of health and mobility	Specialists in the outpatient sector
Functions carried out:	Clinical specialists
Life-saving measures based on new technologies	
Dialysis	
Simple surgical activities	
Radiological diagnostics on the basis of new technologies under the supervision of physicians	
Extended tasks in anaesthesia	
Scenario 3	
Enabling target persons to reflect on and take responsibility for their own health (empowerment)	Specialists in general
Professional planning and organization of events on topics of prevention and health promotion (event management)	Specialists in general
Scenario 4	
Expertise in the field of nutritional counseling	Medical and curative therapists
Expertise in the field of alternative medicine	Medical specialists
Basic knowledge of the health services offered in the field of medical wellness	Tourism specialists
Basic knowledge of medical offers in the field of medical wellness	Hotel specialists in health, sports and spa hotels
Basic knowledge of the hotel industry	Medical specialists
Knowledge of foreign languages	Specialists in the field of medical wellness
Scenario 5	
Target group-appropriate configuration of technical assistance systems (e.g. for the very elderly, dementia patients, people in need of care, older migrants)	Technical specialists

(*continued*)

Table 8 (continued)

Areas of activity and requirements with relatively high additional qualification needs	Occupational groups
Basic knowledge of the processes in nursing and medical care during the installation and maintenance of technical assistance systems	Technical specialists
Knowledge of age- and patient-specific needs and particularities in the installation and maintenance of technical assistance systems	Technical specialists
Ability to interpret the data routinely generated during telemonitoring (pre-diagnosis)	Medical specialists
Scenario 6	
Impartial advice	Coordinating and process controlling specialists
Business knowledge	
Basic knowledge of the legal framework of cooperation and the professions involved	
Determination of health and treatment status through medical interviews and the use of assessment procedures.	
Knowledge in research and application of scientific information	

Source: Klaes et al. (2011, p. 155 f)

Depending on the occupation, the new cross-sectional qualifications should be integrated with different weighting into existing training courses as well as taught in parallel to the occupation as part of continuing education and training. It was pointed out several times in the workshops that, in view of the cross-cutting nature of such extra-functional qualifications, an interdisciplinary orientation makes sense. It was also pointed out that, in addition to integrating cross-cutting competencies into existing occupations or occupations that may need to be supplemented, it may also be possible to develop new occupations that are designed in the other way round. In these occupations, cross-sectional qualifications would represent the actual core; specific qualifications could be taught in parallel to the occupation in practice as well as via continuing education and training. For example, specialists for neighbourhood management, specialists for quality management or specialists for health promotion would be conceivable (Klaes 154). In any case, the career entry phase would take on a new significance if cross-sectional qualifications were given greater weight in training. This is because the specific qualifications for the respective fields of activity would then have to be deepened in the career entry phase to the extent that they were deferred in training in favour of the new cross-sectional qualifications (Klaes et al., 2011, p. 156).

The primary goal of the PPH study was to collect expert opinions on the research question and not to establish a consensus. However, the Delphi method, in the sense of a written group discussion procedure, was at the same time well suited to illuminate different points of view and to explore room for manoeuvre.

It became clear from the study results that the elaborately compiled sample succeeded in mapping the different constellations of interests of the stakeholder groups surveyed: The study results provide differentiated information on the areas in which future developments and qualification requirements were assessed similarly across the groups of actors as well as in which areas the assessments differ according to professional background. The different interests of the groups of actors were reflected in the results with the expected clarity; the assessments of the respondents often differed between physician-based professions and non-physician health care occupations. For example, in the area of health and prevention, physicians showed almost consistently lower agreement with the qualification requirements for the non-physician health care professions than the other groups. One possible explanation is that physicians still see prevention as an original medical task and will continue to see it less as a task of other health care occupations in the future (Klaes et al., 2011, p. 112).

In terms of content, the PPH study was very broadly conceived with the topic of "Public/Private Health" in its various shades. This resulted in a broad target group of experts to be interviewed and a wide range of questions. Both led to large amounts of information that had to be bundled. Therefore, the creation of the sample, the development of the survey instruments, the analysis and evaluation of the results from the literature research and the surveys were associated with a correspondingly high effort. One particular challenge was to condense the large number of arguments from the first Delphi round in such a way that as many threads of argument as possible could be found in the standardised survey of the second Delphi round.

Overall, the chosen study design proved to be well suited to obtain the desired detailed expert assessments of future qualification needs among middle-level employees in the health care sector and related areas, despite the broad scope of the topic. However, processing the amount of information required a great deal of time and resources. For future studies of a similar nature, it is therefore recommended to critically review whether the question to be investigated is already narrowly enough defined or, if necessary, can be narrowed down even more than initially planned.

On the one hand, a stronger focus of the research question could limit the amount of information in the evaluation and the Delphi surveys. On the other hand, the group of potential experts to be included or the addresses to be researched could be more narrowly defined. Both would reduce the effort required to conduct the study without having to compromise the methodological approach outlined above.

A reduction of the expert sample without a simultaneous restriction of the questions is not recommended. The reduction in effort would possibly be bought with a loss of information. Since the dispersion of the experts' assessments is not known ex ante, there would be a risk of obtaining a systematically biased or randomly atypical picture of the experts' assessments if the sample were too small.

A similar risk could arise if experts were recruited either through an existing non-probability panel or through invitations via open online links. In both cases, the sample would be highly selective and not controllable. Although rather effortful, for obtaining robust results we recommend selecting participants through a reasoned process as implemented in the PPH study.

Literature

Banz, M., Klaes, L., Köhler, T., Leinert, J., Olthoff, C., Rommel, A., et al. (2010). *Zukünftige Qualifikationserfordernisse bei beruflichen Tätigkeiten auf mittlerer Qualifikationsebene im Bereich Public private health*. Unveröffentlichter erster Zwischenbericht für das Bundesministerium für Bildung und Forschung (BMBF), Bonn.

Häder, M. (2014). *Delphi-Befragungen. Ein Arbeitsbuch* (3. Aufl.). Springer.

Klaes, L., Köhler, T., Rommel, A., Schüler, G., & Schröder, H. (2011). Public private health. Zukünftige Qualifikationserfordernisse bei beruflichen Tätigkeiten auf mittlerer Qualifikationsebene im Bereich Public private health. Abschlussbericht. www.frequenz.net/uploads/tx_freqprojerg/Abschlussbericht_PPH_web.pdf. Zugegriffen: 26. Juni 2018.

Klaes, L., Köhler, T., Rommel, A., Schüler, G., & Schröder, H. (2013). *Public private health. Neue Qualifikationsanforderungen in der Gesundheitswirtschaft*. Bertelsmann.

Leinert, J., Rommel, A. & Schröder, H. (2019). Neue Qualifikationsanforderungen in der Gesundheitswirtschaft. Methodik und Ergebniszusammenfassung einer Delphi-Erhebung im Bereich Public Private Health. In M. Niederberger & O. Renn (Hrsg.), *Delphi-Verfahren in den Sozial- und Gesundheitswissenschaften. Konzept, Varianten und Anwendungsbeispiele* (pp. 151–185). Springer.

Niederberger, M., & Renn, O. (2018). Das klassische Delphi-Verfahren: Konzept und Vorgehensweise. In M. Niederberger & O. Renn (Hrsg.), *Das Gruppendelphi-Verfahren. Vom Konzept bis zur Anwendung* (pp. 7–25). Springer. https://doi.org/10.1007/978-3-658-18755-2.

Schüler, G., Klaes, L., Rommel, A., Schröder, H., & Köhler, T. (2013). Zukünftiger Qualifikationsbedarf in der Pflege. Ergebnisse und Konsequenzen aus dem BMBF-Forschungsnetz FreQueNz. *Bundesgesundheitsblatt – Gesundheitsforschung – Gesundheitsschutz, 56*(8), 1135–1144. https://doi.org/10.1007/s00103-013-1754-x

Modified Delphi Process to Identify Recommendations for Action for the Structural Development of Physical Activity Promotion in Germany

Hannah Gohres and Petra Kolip

Abstract

After a multitude of physical activity promoting initiatives had been launched nationally, the existing structures should be examined to determine where action is needed. For this purpose, a Delphi survey was conducted, which was prepared by expert interviews and a focus group. Subsequently, recommendations for action were developed at a workshop. Thus, elements of a traditional Delphi with those of a Group Delphi were combined. The research field has been described by previously developed theses, which were quantitatively and qualitatively assessed by 41 experts in two rounds. Priority needs for action and diverging assessments were discussed with 17 of the participants at the workshop. This enabled a multi-perspective discussion of different areas of physical activity promotion and thus offered a broader expert base compared to interviews. Questionnaire development (theses) for the Delphi survey, for which practical knowledge was required, was challenging. The preparatory expert interviews and focus group were considered useful for this purpose, but a possible bias due to a lack of perspectives cannot be ruled out.

H. Gohres (✉) · P. Kolip
School of Public Health, Bielefeld University, Bielefeld, Germany
e-mail: hannah.gohres@uni-bielefeld.de

M. Niederberger, O. Renn (eds.), *Delphi Methods In The Social And Health Sciences*, https://doi.org/10.1007/978-3-658-38862-1_8

1 Background

Physical activity is a key determinant of health. Conversely, physical inactivity is a significant risk factor for numerous diseases and premature mortality (Cavill et al., 2010; Wilson et al., 2016). Nevertheless, a large proportion of the global population is not sufficiently physically active (Hallal et al., 2012; World Health Organization, 2010, 2014). The World Health Organization (WHO) recommends physical activity of at least 2.5 h per week for adults (World Health Organization, 2010). In Germany, about half of adults do not reach this level and are therefore considered physically inactive (Finger et al., 2017). The level of physical activity decreases continuously throughout childhood and adolescence (Finger et al., 2018).

This was the reason for the adoption of the 'National Action Plan for the Reduction of Malnutrition, Physical Inactivity, Obesity and Related Diseases', which has been providing impulses for strengthening the promotion of physical activity since 2008. As part of this, the Federal Ministry of Health (BMG) funded centres for physical activity promotion, action alliances and model projects for healthy lifestyles and environments through 'IN FORM – Germany's initiative for healthy nutrition and more physical activity'. This initiative aimed to sustainably anchor physical activity and physical activity promotion in prevention and health promotion, rehabilitation, care and therapy (Bundesministerium für Ernährung und Landwirtschaft, 2017). It remains to be seen to what extent the anchoring has been successful and how the field of physical activity promotion is faring overall. As part of the project 'Structures of physical activity promotion in Germany – a Delphi study', funded by the Federal Ministry of Health, an expert-based assessment of the current situation of physical activity promotion in Germany was therefore conducted in 2015. This study aimed to identify gaps as well as duplicate structures to derive recommendations for action.

In order to assess this fragmented field of action, a multistage Delphi method was used, which was combined with other research methods. The aim was to include all relevant perspectives of actors in the field of physical activity promotion in order to outline the current situation as holistically as possible and to bundle the various needs and requirements. This article describes the methodological procedure step by step and reflects on it conclusively. It should thereby be clarified whether the method selection was appropriate retrospectively and where opportunities as well as challenges arose through the Delphi method. The results of the Delphi survey and the recommendations for action for the structural development of physical activity promotion, agreed upon during a workshop, can be found in Gohres and Kolip (2017).

1.1 Methodology

The inventory and evaluation of the structures for physical activity promotion was performed by means of a Delphi study, which was prepared with expert interviews and a focus group, and finally recommendations for action were developed (see Fig. 1). Here, the procedures of a traditional Delphi study were extended by elements of a Group Delphi (see Chap. "Real-time Delphi", in this volume; Häder, 2014; Schulz & Renn, 2009). The invited experts first answered an online questionnaire in two rounds. In order to improve consensus-building and enable a dialogical exchange, the results were discussed in a workshop afterwards. Another special aspect of the research process was the two-stage development of the Delphi survey questionnaire. The multi-stage process is described below.

1.1.1 Steps 1 and 2: Questionnaire Development

In order to avoid formulating recommendations for action on a meta-level with little practical relevance, a detailed, multi-perspective catalogue of theses was elaborated as a basis for the survey. It was important for the catalogue of theses to

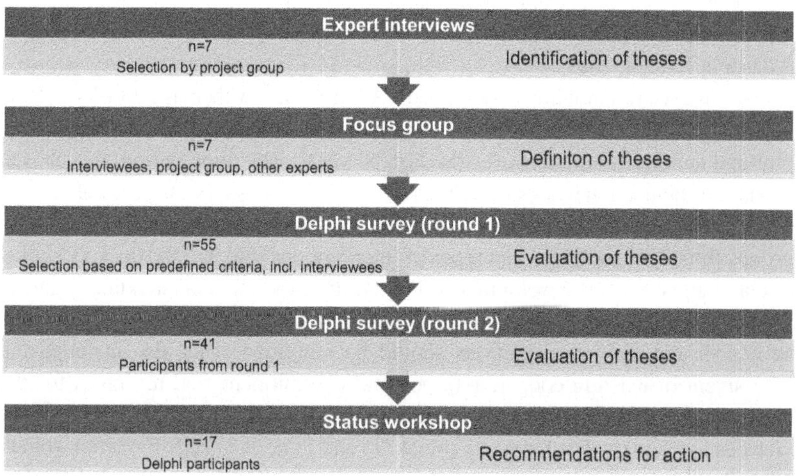

Fig. 1 Overview of the project sequence. (Source: Author)

provide the opportunity for a critical discussion and assessment of the structures of physical activity promotion. For this purpose, it was central to formulate theses that were as controversial as possible, describing the state of physical activity promotion at that time according to its progress and gaps.

In the first step of the multi-stage process, guided expert interviews ($n = 7$) were conducted to assess the status quo in the field of physical activity promotion. Expert interviews represent a field-related form of semi-structured interviews. The specific feature of expert interviews is not the methodology, but rather the target group itself. By drawing on the opinions of experts, it is possible to capture the experiences and knowledge of different stakeholders in a structured way (Kruse, 2015). For this project, experts were defined as persons who have a comprehensive overview of physical activity promotion and its recent structural development and are known for their knowledge in this field. The interviewees should represent as broad a spectrum of physical activity promotion as possible, both in terms of content and geography. Therefore, experts from the fields of prevention/health promotion, care and rehabilitation at federal, state or local level were invited. Expertise was drawn from science (health, sports and nursing science), sports federations and centres for physical activity promotion. The experts came from West, East and South Germany, while some acted nationwide. Personal interviews were chosen for the data collection as they have several advantages compared to impersonal interviewing through telephone, e-mail or internet chat rooms. Using this method, the course of the conversation can be controlled directly and visual information, such as body language, can be included. It is also assumed that a pleasant and thus more productive interview atmosphere tends to develop in a face-to-face situation (Gläser & Laudel, 2009).

The interview guidelines comprised a total of seven thematic blocks. At the beginning, the interviewees were asked to subjectively appraise the development of physical activity promotion over the last 10 years. This time period was chosen because it included the adoption of the National Action Plan in 2008. If not already addressed at the outset, the following thematic blocks addressed reaching target groups (block II) and focus and types of interventions (block III). Block IV aimed to elaborate structural developments. Firstly, the experts' understanding of structures was gathered and then structural changes, the development of sustainable structures and their preconditions should be identified. This also included the assessment of existing cooperation, political commitment, and resources for the promotion of physical activity. The subsequent thematic blocks invited the interviewees to evaluate developments (block V) and to derive needs for action (block VI). The interviews were concluded with formulating theses in block VII. The interviewees were asked to describe, as controversially as possible, the structures of physical activity promotion and related needs for action with one (or more) theses. If the interviewees were not able to do this without further instructions, they were offered sentences to complete with their assessment (e.g., 'There is a need for action in the promotion of physical activity, particularly in...'; 'Networking of physical activity promotion offers is...').

The interviews were recorded, subsequently transcribed or, in one case, paraphrased[1] and analysed according to Mayring's (2010) structuring content analysis. Qualitative content analysis was chosen because it aims to separate from the original material at an early stage in order to systematically reduce the information and structure it according to the research objective (Gläser & Laudel, 2009). Thus, it was possible to use the interview information efficiently and to depict structures of physical activity promotion. Based on the guidelines, as recommended by Schmidt (2000), a main category system was determined (deductive). Subsequently, relevant passages of the interviews were filtered out and condensed based on these criteria (Mayring, 2002, 2010). The analysis was initially carried out separately by two evaluators. The results were then compiled and discussed at a face-to-face meeting. On that basis, a first draft of the catalogue of theses was prepared. This included a large number of theses, which were summarised and shortened in several steps. For this purpose, prioritisation was carried out by all project participants.

In a subsequent focus group discussion ($n = 7$), the experts' assessments were discussed with some of the interviewees ($n = 2$), a health promotion expert ($n = 1$) and the project staff ($n = 4$) and condensed into theses that pointedly describe the structures and needs for action in physical activity promotion. Group discussions offer the advantage of ascertaining subjective structures of meanings of individuals, which are strongly linked to social contexts, and determining collective attitudes so that a multi-faceted picture on the considered topic can be drawn (Mayring, 2002; Schulz, 2012). Focus groups can be more powerful than individual interviews due to the collective body of knowledge that is obtained, and new ideas can be stimulated through group dynamics (Schulz et al., 2012). This ensured that the interview analysis provided transferable results and that the theses were comprehensible. Furthermore, the focus group ensured that the theses were not too 'harmonious' and encouraged a critical appraisal of the promotion of physical activity in the context of the Delphi survey; this was accomplished by not suggesting a consensus too early in the process.

---

[1] A seventh interviewee unexpectedly agreed to participate after the data collection and transcription phase were completed. In order to take this expert's knowledge into account, an interview was conducted but not transcribed for evaluation.

The focus group lasted 5 h and had the character of a workshop in order to enable a concrete development of theses. A presentation served as the basis for illustrating the theses identified and their underlying interview quotes in order to make the derivation process comprehensible. Based on this, a set of guidelines was created for moderation. The discourse was thus initiated and structured by the separate theses and corresponding background information. Within the individual topics, however, the focus was on openness, which also allowed the moderator to act neutrally. The procedure resembled the phase dynamics of the guidelines for the expert interviews (Kruse, 2015). The interview was recorded with a sound recorder to simplify the subsequent compilation of results. In addition, key results were protocolled to summarise the proposed changes and the consensual theses.

In the group discussion, specific proposals for reformulating theses and shortening the catalogue of theses were already made. The catalogue was then revised and sent to the participants again by e-mail to recheck the theses. After several feedback loops, the final catalogue of theses, comprised 16 theses on different areas of the promotion of physical activity and formed the basis for the actual Delphi survey in the third step. The overarching topics are 'alignment of offers and strategy' (Theses 5, 6, 11, 13 and 16), 'target groups' (Theses 1–4), 'responsibilities and resources' (Theses 10 and 12), 'networking and coordination' (Theses 7–9, 14) and 'qualification' (Thesis 15).

1.1.2 Step 3: Delphi Survey

The actual Delphi survey was conducted online, comprising two survey rounds with quantitative and qualitative elements. The standardised questionnaire was created using the software EFS Survey (Version 10.7, QuestBack). The survey was personalised, and hence only accessible to invited persons. Personal links to the survey website with appropriately pseudonymised code were sent by mail (Questback, 2015). To link the data from the two survey rounds, an identification number (ID) was created at the beginning of the survey. The ID was recorded separately from the personal data, so that linkage was not possible and to ensure the anonymity of the respondents.

In the first round, the respondents were asked to assess the theses. The second survey round served to reassess the catalogue of theses with reference to the opinions of the other participants. For this purpose, the 'average opinion' (mean and standard deviation) of all experts was presented to each participant in comparison to the personal rating from the first round (see Fig. 2). Written justifications were needed in both rounds and were also reflected back. In the second round of the survey, needs for action were additionally prioritised.

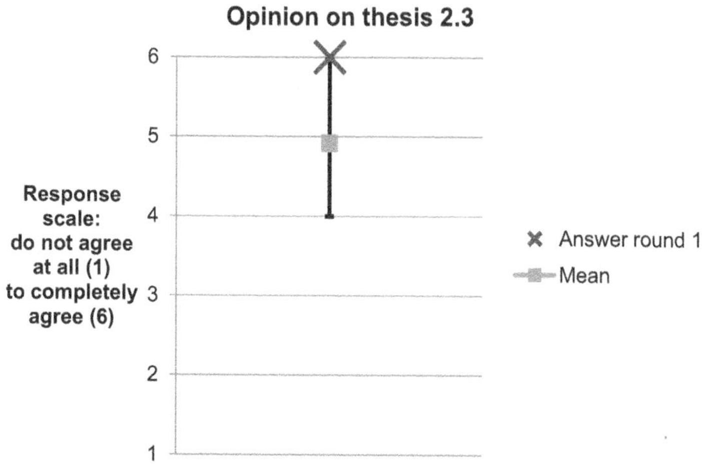

Fig. 2 Example of quantitative feedback in Delphi round 2. (Source: Author)

The questionnaire comprised the 16 theses, which should be evaluated both quantitatively and qualitatively, and was divided into five areas (see Table 1): (I) generating an identification number, (II) questions on professional background, (III) general evaluation of physical activity promotion, (IV) thesis evaluation and (V) further comments. Thesis evaluation was conducted using a six-point Likert scale (1 = strongly disagree to 6 = strongly agree) and written statements.

113 actors in the field of physical activity promotion were invited. The selection was based on the previously defined criteria, which were discussed and determined within the project group and the interview partners. Therefore, persons on the federal, state or municipal level were selected who are known for their expertise in the field of prevention/health and physical activity promotion, covering a broad spectrum of actors. Of interest was the perspective from actors with corresponding expertise from various professional fields, rather than the perspective from political decision-makers. Professional fields of the experts included coordinating centres for health of the states (incl. Centres for physical activity promotion), social insurance institutions, federations and associations, municipalities and scientific institutions. In order to assess the composition of experts, the participants were initially asked to provide their institutional affiliation (science, politics, association/federation, social insurance, other) as well as to rate their expertise (subjective competence) in the areas of prevention/health promotion, care and rehabilitation (non-specialist to high). As there was no self-assessment for each question, the potential

Table 1 Schematic description of the Delphi questionnaire (author's representation)

Section	Variables	Characteristics/content
I	Identification number	8 characters
II[a]	Subjective assessment of competence in the areas of: Prevention/health promotion Rehabilitation Care Professional background State	Assessment of expertise (six-point Likert scale: High to no expertise) Assignment to the categories science, politics, association/federation, social security, other State in which the professional activity is carried out
III[a]	Status of physical activity promotion in Germany Status of physical activity promotion in the state	General assessment (six-point Likert scale: Expandable to well established)
IV	Theses 1 to 16	Six-point Likert scale and written justification Subject areas: Target groups (theses 1–4) Alignment (theses 5, 6) Strategies and conditions (theses 7, 10–12) Networking and coordination (theses 8, 9) Care (thesis 13) Rehab (thesis 14) Qualifications (thesis 15) Effectiveness/evidence-based (thesis 16)
V	Further need for action Comments	Open question (optional)
VI[b]	Priorities	Selection of 4 priority areas for action

[a]Only in survey round 1
[b]Only in survey round 2

answer 'I cannot assess' was given for each thesis assessment, which implies a lack of expert knowledge for the specific case.

The quantitative analysis mainly utilised descriptive statistics to describe the distribution of thesis rating. Response behavior was assessed using boxplots. To determine the extent of consensus building, the change in standard deviations from round 1 to round 2 was compared. The Delphi should increase a consensus and decrease scattering (dissent), respectively (Vorgrimler & Wübben, 2003). Furthermore, rating behavior was determined to analyse the effect of the feedback based on the group mean. Giving feedback on the results from other participants can have three different outcomes: (1) the average opinion is disregarded (stable rating); (2) the rating is changed away from the average opinion to move it closer to one's own rating (contrast rating), or (3) the rating is skewed towards the average

Table 2 Categorisation of the rating behaviour between the Delphi rounds

Expression	Definition
Stable rating	No change from round 1 to 2
Assimilation rating	Change of opinion towards the mean
Contrast rating	Contrast from the mean to the original opinion (reinforcement)
New rating	First rating in round 2
Beyond average	From original opinion beyond mean
Change of mind	Opposite rating from round 1 to 2

opinion (assimilation rating) (Bardecki, 1991, cited in Vorgrimler & Wübben, 2003; Novakowski & Wellar, 2008). The ratings of the two survey rounds were compared for each thesis by the mean (paired *T*-tests; $\alpha = 0.05$) and the rating behavior was coded as depicted in Table 2. Two additional categories were observed: new ratings (no statement in round 1) and changes of mind (opposite rating from round 1 to 2). To analyse group differences between fields of activity as well as subjective competence, univariate ANOVAs or Kruskal-Wallis test with a significance level of $\alpha = 0.05$ were performed.

The qualitative analysis comprised the evaluation of the written justifications for the thesis assessments. The aim was to summarise the reasons given in order to prepare them for the second survey round to present them to the participants. This was done so that they could be taken into account in the final assessment of the theses and in answering the initial research questions. Following the summarising content analysis according to Mayring (2010), the justifications were therefore evaluated individually for each thesis. When summarising, it is important to reduce the material to the essential content. In addition, it is possible to form inductive categories. This procedure was judged appropriate for the Delphi survey. After reviewing the first justifications, the main categories were defined: Need for action, recommendations for action and criticism of the theses. According to these, the additional material was sorted and reduced to the essential contents. The result was a summary of the reasons for the thesis ratings in the form of bullet points, which allowed a further examination of the individual theses. An impression of the form of feedback in round 2 is provided by Fig. 4 in the *Results* section.

1.1.3 Status Workshop

The final step of the project was a 'status workshop' with the Delphi participants to discuss the results in more depth and to enter into an interdisciplinary exchange. The aim was to derive concrete consensual recommendations for action after the second Delphi round had not yet led to a consensus for all theses. All participants of the first round of the Delphi survey (n = 55) were invited to the status workshop. In addition, a representative of the BMG was invited as a guest. 17 experts participated; the participants represented a cross-section of the previously interviewed actors, including scientific institutions, centres for health of states (including one centre for physical activity promotion), state sports federations and the German National Paralympic Committee, social insurance agencies (health insurance), the Federal Centre for Health Education, the 'Plattform Ernährung und Bewegung' (Platform for Nutrition and Physical Activity) and the Reinhard Mohn Foundation.

The workshop lasted 1 day. After presenting the results of the theses assessment, these were discussed in thematically defined small groups. The groups were moderated by the project staff and focused on the concrete formulation of priority needs for action and possible solutions, which were then compiled and discussed in the plenary session. In contrast to the suggestion by Schulz and Renn (2009), no rotating small groups were formed to discuss and answer the questionnaire several times due to the previous written participation. The aim was to discuss theses that had been answered rather heterogeneously in the Delphi survey in order to drive consensus. The final discussion was recorded with the help of a sound recording device. The recordings, protocols and the material produced were reviewed afterwards in order to secure, supplement and elaborate the discussed recommendations for action. Following this, the elaborated recommendations were circulated again to the participants with request for reviewing to ensure a consensus.

1.2 Results: Consensus or Dissent on Structural Needs for Action in Physical Activity Promotion?

Table 3 displays the assessments of the theses in the two Delphi rounds. In the Delphi survey, many theses tended to be agreed with already in the first round (mean > 4); at the same time, the range of scales were fully used for half of the theses, indicating heterogeneous opinions. Only one thesis (9) was already not rejected by anyone in the first round (minimum = 3). Overall, after the second Delphi round, the majority of the theses rankings (7 out of 16) converged to the average opinion and the statistical variance decreased, which suggests a consensus. Many of the theses (6 out of 16), which had already been strongly agreed with before, were assessed as predominantly stable. Mean differences between rounds were significant only for Thesis 1 ($p = 0.003$). The strongest agreement (mean > 5.0) was exhibited after both rounds for

Table 3 Thesis evaluation and rating behaviour in the two Delphi rounds

Thess	*M* (SD) Round 1 (*n* = 37–55)	*M* (SD) Round 2 (*n* = 32–41)
1. Activities to promote physical activity usually reach people with an affinity for sports and physical activity	4.9 ± 0.8*	5.2 ± 0.6*
2. There is a need for action in the promotion of physical activity with regard to target group-specific strategies. I see a particular need for socially disadvantaged target groups.	5.5 ± 0.8	5.4 ± 0.8
3. There is a need for action in the promotion of physical activity with regard to target group-specific strategies. I see a particular need among people with a migrant background.	5.0 ± 1.1	4.7 ± 1.1
4. There is a need for action in the promotion of physical activity with regard to target group-specific strategies. I see a particular need for people with chronic diseases.	4.9 ± 1.1	4.8 ± 1.1
5. Most offers in the promotion of physical activity are equated with sports offers, which means that the promotion of physical activity lacks the aspect of movement in everyday life.	4.4 ± 1.6	4.5 ± 1.4
6. Physical activity promotion focuses on behavioural prevention (individual level). Environmental prevention, such as urban development or physical activity promoting schools, is missed out.	4.6 ± 1.2	4.7 ± 1.0
7. Physical activity promotion consists mainly of individual projects, but integrated, intersectoral action strategies are needed.	5.2 ± 1.0	5.2 ± 1.0
8. Physical activity promotion needs better coordination and networking structures at federal, state and local level to provide impulses.	4.8 ± 1.2	4.9 ± 1.0
9. Physical activity promotion requires coordinators who can think and act in an 'organisationally empathetic' (i.e., interdisciplinary and intersectoral) manner to work together more effectively.	5.2 ± 0.9	5.2 ± 0.9
10. Promoting physical activity at the municipal level should be a higher priority, and the corresponding responsibilities and resources must be clearly regulated and distributed.	5.2 ± 1.1	5.1 ± 1.1
11. Strengthening structures for physical activity promotion requires long-term planning strategies and a redistribution of financial resources, away from individual prevention and towards investment in environmental prevention.	4.4 ± 1.5	4.2 ± 1.4
12. Sustainable structures for physical activity promotion need stronger political support and more legal frameworks.	4.6 ± 1.4	4.5 ± 1.2

(continued)

Table 3 (continued)

Thess	*M* (SD) Round 1 (*n* = 37–55)	*M* (SD) Round 2 (*n* = 32–41)
13. In the field of care, preventing falls has become a high priority, however, it is often not thought beyond this. Therefore, the individual and environmental promotion of physical activity in nursing care must be strengthened and expanded.	5.2 ± 0.9	5.4 ± 0.7
14. The transitions of physical activity promotion within inpatient rehabilitation measures and back into people's everyday lives must be clearly regulated. To this end, the rehabilitation sector must also network more closely with other structures.	5.1 ± 1.1	5.2 ± 0.9
15. Physical activity promotion requires qualified personnel, therefore physical activity promotion must be part of the curricula of relevant training and study programmes (e.g., health professions, health and nursing sciences, teaching, educators). At present, physical activity promotion often hardly plays a role in these curricula.	5.0 ± 1.4	4.9 ± 1.2
16. The effectiveness of interventions must be ensured for structural development in physical activity promotion	5.0 ± 1.3	4.8 ± 1.2

M mean, *SD* standard deviation, *= significant mean differences, six-point scale 1 "strongly disagree" 6 "strongly agree"

- A prevention dilemma (Thesis 1),
- The need for improved target group specific strategies, particularly for socially disadvantaged target groups (Thesis 2),
- The problem of individual projects (Thesis 7),
- The need for higher-level coordinators (Thesis 9),
- Strengthening the position and responsibilities in physical activity promotion at the municipal level (Thesis 10),
- Strengthening and expanding the promotion of physical activity in nursing care (Thesis 13),
- the improvement of transitions within inpatient rehabilitation measures (Thesis 14).

For three theses, reflecting back on the results from round one led to a greater differentiation of ratings and thus to greater controversy or reduced agreement about

- The need for target group-specific strategies for people with migrant backgrounds (Thesis 3),

- Strengthening the promotion of physical activity in the curricula of relevant training courses and degree programmes (Thesis 15),
- Ensuring the effectiveness of interventions (Thesis 16).

The rating behaviour across the two Delphi rounds and the status workshop is illustrated by the third thesis 'There is a need for action in the promotion of physical activity with regard to target group-specific strategies. I see a particular need for people with a migrant background'. Most participants tended to agree with a need for action in target group-specific strategies for people with a migrant background (see Fig. 3). However, the proportion of high agreement decreased compared to round one, while rejecting ratings increased. Thus, the mean value on the response scale fell slightly from 5.0 to 4.7 ($n = 39$). The proportion of stable ratings from round one to two is lower compared to other theses (56.4%). Participants who changed their opinion mostly corrected it towards the mean (17.9%). A further 12.8% adjusted their rating beyond average in the direction of rejection or rated contrastingly (5.1%). This demonstrates a rather controversial assessment of the need for action among people with a migrant background. The ratings did not differ significantly between the fields of activity and subjective competence.

Based on the written justifications (see Fig. 4), the changed opinions and controversial assessments lead back to the attitude that a migrant background could not be identified globally as a category for a need for action, since heterogeneous groups are involved. It is necessary to strongly differentiate in the selection of target groups. It was agreed that there was a need for greater target group specificity in strategies to promote physical activity, but that individual groups should be considered in a differentiated manner. For this purpose, well-founded needs analyses

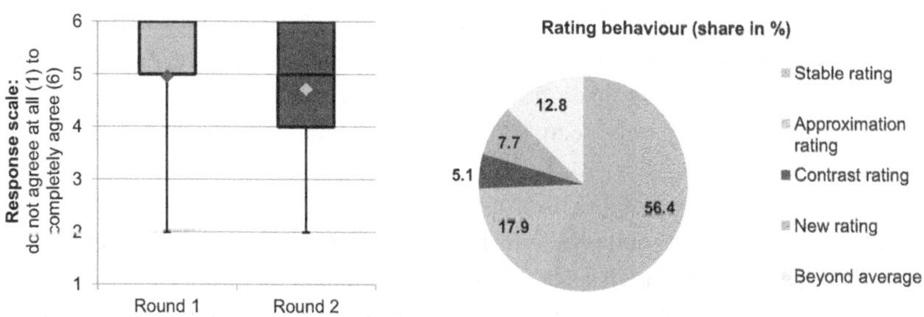

Fig. 3 Rating of thesis 3 in both survey rounds (left) as well as rating behaviour from round 1 to round 2 (right) ($n = 39$), own representation. (Explanation: The boxplots (left) show: Mean = diamond, interquartile range = box, median = horizontal line in the box and minimum/maximum = whiskers)

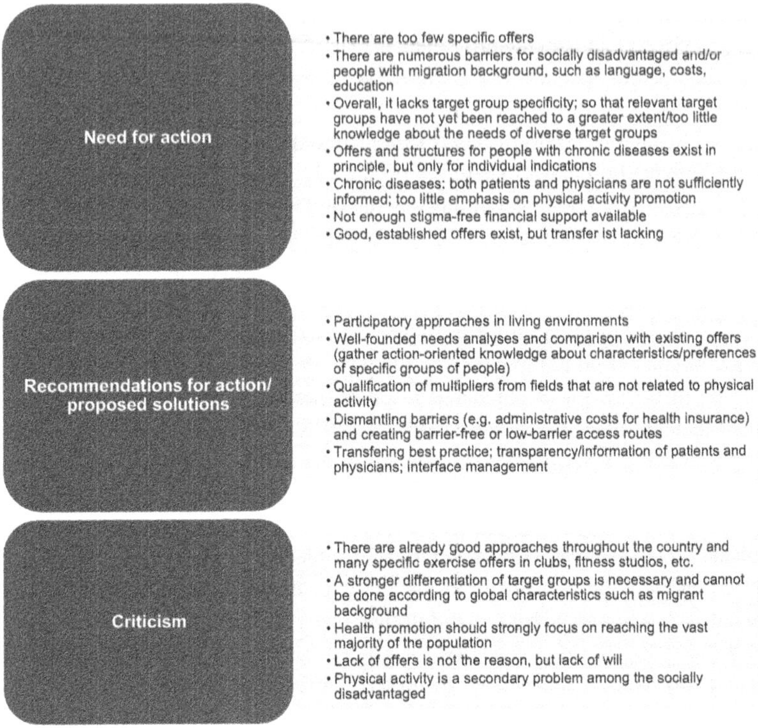

Fig. 4 Qualitative summary of the justifications for theses 2–4 on target group specificity. (Author's representation)

and a comparison with existing offers would be necessary to gain action-oriented insights into the characteristics and preferences of specific target groups. These have been largely lacking up to now. The need for socially disadvantaged target groups was most likely to be seen; setting-specific approaches were described as a possible solution.

There was also a general consensus at the workshop on a lack of target group specificity as a fundamental problem. The need for action in specific target groups must be identified on a small scale through well-founded needs analyses in order to be able to plan according to needs and requirements. A sweeping needs assessment for heterogenous groups is not possible. The goal of physical activity promotion should be to identify barriers for individual target groups and to systematically reduce them. This systematic approach is not yet in place. In order to reach diverse target groups, new target group-specific approaches should be considered. Therefore, the consensus on target group achievement is: *There is a need for action in physical activity promotion with regard to target group-specific strategies and activities. Action-oriented knowledge about the characteristics of specific groups and the associated small-scale, well-founded needs analyses are lacking. General characteristics such as a migrant background should not be an exclusive indicator for target group selection and intervention design.*

For all theses, for which a dissent had rather occurred in the second Delphi round, a consensus could be reached during the workshop. On the basis of the thesis assessments of the two Delphi rounds, priority needs for action were formulated. From the results of the Delphi survey and the status workshop, 21 recommendations for action were derived, some of which interlocked or built on each other. In the course of the discussions, strengthening of political support emerged as an overarching and fundamental element for the further structural anchoring of the hitherto rather fragmented physical activity promotion landscape. The experts called for a common national strategy to use synergies more effectively and to create sustainability. Gaps and duplications could be systematically identified and closed through an overarching strategy, as well as more coordination and networking. The participants all agreed that it would be helpful to continue to promote the exchange between experts, as was done in the Delphi project, and thus to improve cooperation structures.

Overall, the Delphi survey demonstrated that the physical activity promotion landscape is currently still fragmented. Initial positive developments can already be noted, which must be expanded and continued. However, structural anchoring must still take place or be strengthened at several levels. One challenge in this regard is the transfer and consolidation of existing offers and structures. Within the study, a diverse repertoire of possible solutions was developed, which can be used for further priority setting in the field of physical activity promotion and will require detailed discussion in the future. Some proposals, such as the development of national recommendations for physical activity (Pfeifer & Rütten, 2017), have now been implemented. However, not all of the derived needs for action and recommendations could be conclusively discussed and clarified. For example, it remained open who could set impulses for the development of long-term planning strategies. The applied methods thus entailed various strengths, but also weaknesses in addressing the initial research questions, which are discussed in the following section.

1.3 Reflection on the Methodological Approach

The study aimed to create an expert-based inventory of the structures of physical activity promotion and to derive recommendations for their further development. These goals were fully achieved. The successful implementation of the project demonstrates that the applied methods were adequate and target-oriented. Nevertheless, challenges and weaknesses emerged during the implementation, which should be taken into account for the interpretation of the results or for the planning of similar projects. Both strengths and weaknesses will be assessed step by step.

In preparation for the actual Delphi survey, a comprehensive qualitative approach was followed. To develop the questionnaire, the typical theoretically-oriented approach (Schulz & Renn, 2009) was not considered appropriate. Rather, practical knowledge was required to assess and evaluate the structures, which was bundled by the qualitative research approach in form of expert interviews and a focus group. The preparatory expert interviews were suitable to fundamentally assess the physical activity promotion landscape and to define a framework for action. Discussing and settling the theses within the focus group additionally secured the validity of the theses derived from the interviews. By including as wide a range of expertise as possible, a multifaceted view of the status quo of physical activity promotion could be ensured from the onset.

Compared to expert interviews, the Delphi survey enabled a broader expert base to be included in the assessment. The discursive character of Delphi surveys should be emphasised, as it initiated a targeted communication process and thus not only depicts individual opinions, but also captures group opinions in a consensus-oriented manner (Häder, 2014; Vorgrimler & Wübben, 2003). There are similarities to the group discussion method, although the Delphi method differs from this due to the multiple survey rounds and the anonymity of the individual contributions. In this way, group dynamic processes can be triggered while preserving the openness of the individual, while also preventing the opinion leadership of dominant participants (Döring & Bortz, 2016; Häder, 2014). Additionally, integrating quantitative and qualitative research methods increased the informational base. Due to the feedback of written justifications from the first Delphi round, a further reflection of the theses rating was often triggered in the second round in order to evaluate the approval or rejection of the average opinion. In this way, further approaches and solutions were introduced several times, which provided a basis for discussion in the subsequent workshop. Thus, a multi-perspective picture of national physical activity promotion could be drawn, so that recommendations for action could be derived and discussed within the workshop in a thesis-driven way. However, it must be noted for the evaluation of ratings that no complete objectivity can be guaranteed in the presentation, particularly for the qualitative feedback. Summaries, reformulations and selection decisions are necessary, so that not all the reasons given can be taken into account and influencing the participants opinion-forming cannot be ruled out (Vorgrimler & Wübben, 2003). However, missing contextual information could be brought up for discussion through the subsequent workshop.

In solely quantitative Delphis so many rounds of repetition are often carried out until the variance of ratings is below a defined value in order to conjecture a consensus (Häder, 2014). In this Delphi study, the results of the first round were reflected back in the second round, but it was not the stated aim to harmonise the experts' views (determined by the statistical variance), but rather primarily to qualify them. It can be assumed that some of the participants positioned themselves further in the direction of the average opinion (Vorgrimler & Wübben, 2003). Thus, after the second round of questioning, a consensus could be assumed for about half of the theses due to the reduction in variance. Contradictions and theses for which dissent was more likely to emerge after the Delphi rounds were then discussed with the participants in the workshop, and recommendations for action were developed and agreed upon. It should be noted that significant mean differences between the two Delphi rounds could only be observed for two of the 16 theses, which may be related to the overall already high level of agreement in round one.

The workshop replaced a Group Delphi. As the exemplary presentation of the assessment on one of the theses demonstrated, it was a helpful and necessary supplement to the Delphi survey. Deviations in the thesis rating as well as written justifications of individuals were discussed, so that a consensus could be reached and missing contextual information could be obtained. The advantages of the anonymity of the Delphi survey also entail the risk that the participants feel less responsible for their assessment and that they may come to a hasty, insufficiently thought-out judgement (Vorgrimler & Wübben, 2003). This effect was mitigated by the workshop within this study. Although the personal assessments from the Delphi survey remain anonymous, the value and validity of answers were discussed in the plenary session. In the course of the Delphi participants' anonymity, it was rather observed that the written justification of ratings were partly very brief. Thus, the informational gain was low for individual assessments. Furthermore, according to Vorgrimler and Wübben (2003), experts tend to make cautious judgments. Therefore, consensus building could lead to a strengthening of conservative ratings. This is confirmed by the fact that after feedbacking the results, there was often a tendency to move away from complete agreement.

For this study, elements of a traditional Delphi method were combined with those of a Group Delphi (Häder, 2014; Schulz & Renn, 2009). The version of first answering the questionnaire in two rounds in writing and anonymously and then discussing the results in a workshop has advantages, but also disadvantages. The written questionnaire enables an equal participation of the responding experts and offers them sufficient time to deal with the questions' content. At the workshop, heterogeneous ratings and priority needs for action can be discussed more effectively. At this point, there is a risk of excluding relevant aspects of the questionnaire when designing the workshop, since a consensus was assumed on the basis of the written assessment. At this point, however, misinterpretations are possible, which should be excluded by a solely personal Group Delphi (Schulz & Renn, 2009). In the context of this Delphi study, a prioritisation of the workshop contents was also carried out on the basis of the written survey. If experts had a need to discuss consensual theses, this was also taken up as far as possible. In addition, this effect is somewhat mitigated by the qualitative justifications in the written survey. However, insufficient discussion of individual theses cannot be ruled out.

The group of participants in a Delphi survey is an important factor in its validity. The aim is not to completely represent the basic population of experts, but rather 'interaction processes for knowledge generation' which are generated by the feedback (Häder, 2014). Delphi surveys are meaningful even without a large number of participants due to the targeted selection of experts in the field of interest. A broad variety of expert knowledge within the group as well as an interdisciplinary composition are critical to increasing the information gain (Novakowski & Wellar, 2008). However, the significance of the expert opinion depends not only on the expert status, but also on the willingness to participate. Thus, not all experts identified as relevant also participated in the survey. Although this is partially compensated for by the group judgement across the range of expert opinions, a comparison of goal and response is still necessary (Goodman 1987 cited in Häder, 2014). In the presented Delphi study on physical activity promotion, the aim was to cover the fields of prevention/health promotion, care and rehabilitation. Overall, many different experts from a wide range of fields were included. However, actors from the field of prevention/health promotion were overrepresented. This was already due to the recruitment process, as more inquiries were made for this area. Additionally, group comparisons were difficult due to unequally sized groups. The analyses of variance did not show significant differences for any thesis for the different areas of competence. The differences between the fields of activity were significant for two theses (thesis 5, $p = 0.024$; thesis 9, $p < 0.001$). In addition, no expert in in the field of rehabilitation could be reached, so that the results may not adequately reflect this subarea. Unfortunately, it was also not possible to recruit an expert with an urban planning or transport planning perspective. This should have been given more consideration during recruitment.

Not all of the previously interviewed persons were able to participate in the focus group, and thus the range of perspectives for the step of final thesis development was not as wide as previously envisaged. Due to the difficulty of finding a date, only three of the seven interviewees were able to keep the appointment, which was caused by the short project duration. Unfortunately, one interviewee cancelled at short notice, so that only two of the experts participated. Nevertheless, a sufficient discourse on the theses could be ensured through the qualitative elements of the Delphi survey and the concluding workshop.

However, at this point a weakness in the procedure becomes apparent. By condensing the experts' assessments into theses, some important information may have been lost. From the expert interviews, 24 theses were derived, which were further summarised and prioritised in the focus group. Aspects such as participation, the role of individual actors and the frequent coupling of the topics of physical activity and nutrition, which were previously discussed, were no longer reflected in the Delphi survey. The application of summary theses can thus remain individual aspects unexamined. Although the focus group ensured that the relevant aspects were taken up, a significant reduction took place for the design of the Delphi questionnaire. In particular, the differences between the areas of prevention/health promotion, rehabilitation and care were not fully captured within the Delphi survey. In the context of the workshop, it was noted that individual theses might have to be formulated more specifically for the different areas in order to identify specific needs for action in each case. This could not be done within this single survey. The scope of the theses to be evaluated should not be too large and the theses themselves should not be too complex. Thus, 25 theses with a length of 20 words each should not be exceeded (Parenté & Anderson-Parenté, 1987, cited in Aichholzer, 2009). With the 16 theses included in the questionnaire, some of which were, however, relatively demanding, the extent was exhausted. An increase in the number of theses or greater differentiation would probably have had a negative influence on the willingness to participate. The participants already reported a large scope of the survey when assessing the 16 theses. However, a reduction in the complexity of individual theses is recommended for similar projects.

Furthermore, a differing understanding of terms can be problematic. The expert interviews revealed different definitions of 'movement' and 'structures'. However, the theses should try to cover the dimensions mentioned (personnel, financial, material, spatial, temporal and political structures) in order to obtain a comprehensive assessment. There was often a great interest in structures of provided offers, which is why the content of physical activity promotion was also an important topic of the discussion. Due to time constraints, the workshop did not offer sufficient space for the definition of terms. One request was to take this discourse further beyond the project. In retrospect, it would make sense to extend the workshop to 1.5 to 2 days to be able to more intensively discuss areas of action identified as important. This would make it easier to continue consideration of proposed solutions, something that was ultimately neglected during the status workshop.

1.4 Conclusion

In summation, the Delphi survey can be generally evaluated as a useful instrument for the assessment of structural needs for action and the derivation of corresponding recommendations for action. The combination of quantitative and qualitative assessments of the theses led to the obtaining of useful information and allowed the elicitation of expert opinions from a wide range of actors in the field of physical activity promotion. The preparatory interviews and the focus group as well as the follow-up workshop were a useful supplement to derive recommendations for action in a discursive, multi-perspective process. However, to obtain detailed representative information about the structure of existing actors, a nationwide survey of the relevant institutions is necessary.

Literature

Aichholzer, G. (2009). Das ExpertInnen-Delphi: Methodische Grundlagen und Innovationen im Bereich Technology Foresight. In A. Bogner, B. Littig, & W. Menz (Hrsg.), *Experteninterviews. Theorien, Methoden, Anwendungsfelder* (S. 277–300). VS Verlag.

Bundesministerium für Ernährung und Landwirtschaft (2017). IN FORM Deutschlands Initiative für gesunde Ernährung und mehr Bewegung. Nationaler Aktionsplan zur Prävention von Fehlernährung, Bewegungsmangel, Übergewicht und damit zusammenhängenden Krankheiten – IN FORM Eine Zwischenbilanz (BMEL, Hrsg.). https://www.in-form.de/in-form/in-form-zwischenbericht/. Accessed 16. Juli 2018.

Cavill, N., Kahlmeier, S., & Racioppi, F. (2010). *Physical activity and health in Europe*. WHO Regional Office for Europe.

Döring, N., & Bortz, J. (2016). *Forschungsmethoden und Evaluation in den Sozial- und Humanwissenschaften*. Springer.

Finger, J. D., Mensink, G. B. M., Lange, C., & Manz, K. (2017). Gesundheitsfördernde körperliche Aktivität in der Freizeit bei Erwachsenen in Deutschland. *Journal of Health Monitoring, 2*(2), 37–44. https://doi.org/10.17886/rki-gbe-2017-027

Finger, J. D., Varnaccia, G., Borrmann, A., Lange, C., & Mensink, G. B. M. (2018). Körperliche Aktivität von Kindern und Jugendlichen in Deutschland – Querschnittergebnisse aus KiGGS Welle 2 und Trends. *Journal of Health Monitoring, 3*, 24–33.

Gläser, J., & Laudel, G. (2009). *Experteninterviews und qualitative Inhaltsanalyse – Als Instrumente rekonstruierender Untersuchungen*. VS Verlag.

Gohres, H., & Kolip, P. (2017). Strukturen der Bewegungsförderung in Deutschland. Handlungsempfehlungen zur strukturellen Weiterentwicklung als Ergebnisse einer Delphi-Befragung. *Prävention und Gesundheitsförderung, 12*(3), 203–210. https://doi.org/10.1007/s1553-017-0580-7

Häder, M. (2014). *Delphi-Befragungen. Ein Arbeitsbuch*. Springer.

Hallal, P. C., Andersen, L. B., Bull, F. C., Guthold, R., Haskell, W., & Ekelund, U. (2012). Global physical activity levels: Surveillance progress, pitfalls, and prospects. *The Lancet, 380*(9838), 247–257. https://doi.org/10.1016/s0140-6736(12)60646-1

Kruse, J. (2015). *Qualitative Interviewforschung. Ein integrativer Ansatz*. Beltz Juventa.

Mayring, P. (2002). *Einführung in die Qualitative Sozialforschung. Eine Anleitung zu qualitativem Denken*. Beltz.

Mayring, P. (2010). *Qualitative Inhaltsanalyse. Grundlagen und Techniken*. Beltz.

Novakowski, N., & Wellar, B. (2008). Using the Delphi technique in normative planning research: Methodological design consideration. *Environment and Planning A, 40*, 1485–1500.

Pfeifer, K., & Rütten, A. (2017). Nationale Empfehlungen für Bewegung und Bewegungsförderung. *Gesundheitswesen, 79*(S01), S2–S3.

questback. (2015). Enterprise Feedback Suite. EFS Survey. Version: https://doi.org/10.7/1.0.

Schmidt, C. (2000). Analyse von Leitfadeninterviews. In U. Flick (Hrsg.), *Qualitative Forschung. Ein Handbuch* (S. 447–456). Rowohlt.

Schulz, M. (2012). Quick and easy!? Fokusgruppen in der angewandten Sozialwissenschaft. In M. Schulz, B. Mack, & O. Renn (Hrsg.), *Fokusgruppen in der empirischen Sozialwissenschaft. Von der Konzeption bis zur Auswertung* (S. 9–22). Springer.

Schulz, M., & Renn, O. (2009). Das Gruppendelphi: Konzept und Vorgehensweise. In M. Schulz & O. Renn (Hrsg.), *Das Gruppendelphi. Konzept und Fragebogenkonstruktion* (S. 11–22). VS Verlag.

Schulz, M., Mack, B., & Renn, O. (Eds.). (2012). *Fokusgruppen in der empirischen Sozialwissenschaft. Von der Konzeption bis zur Auswertung*. Springer.

Vorgrimler, D. & Wübben, D. (2003). Die Delphi-Methode und ihre Eignung als Prognoseinstrument (Statistisches Bundesamt, Hrsg.) (Wirtschaft und Statistik Nr. 8), Wiesbaden.

Wilson, M. G., Ellison, G. M., & Cable, N. T. (2016). Basic science behind the cardiovascular benefits of exercise. *British Journal of Sports Medicine, 50*, 93–99.

World Health Organization. (2010). *Global recommendations on physical activity for health*. WHO.

World Health Organization. (2014). *Global status report on noncommunicable diseases 2014*. WHO.

Evaluation of Health Care Situation and Care Structures for Elderly People in the Federal State of Bremen, Germany

Results of a Delphi Study on Idea Aggregation and Strategy Development

Stefan Görres, Katrin Seibert, and Susanne Stiefler

Abstract

On behalf of the Senator for Health in the Federal State of Bremen, Germany, the Institute for Public Health and Nursing Research of the University of Bremen, conducted a study from May to October 2014 to record problem areas in the care of elderly people aged 65 years and older. The main objective was to identify the conditions for optimizing care services for the elderly in the State of Bremen, to identify starting points for optimising care in the State of Bremen. The data collection was carried out using the Delphi method. For this purpose, 87 selected experts from different areas of the Bremen health care system were invited to participate in two consecutive online surveys. After a descriptive quantitative as well as a qualitative evaluation based on content analysis of the collected data, the identified problem areas were presented to the experts in a workshop. Ideas for solution strategies were discussed by the experts with regard to their practicability and feasibility and, based on the identified problem

S. Görres (✉) · K. Seibert · S. Stiefler
Institute for Public Health and Nursing Research (IPP), University of Bremen, Bremen, Germany
e-mail: sgoerres@uni-bremen.de; kseibert@uni-bremen.de; sstiefler@uni-bremen.de

M. Niederberger, O. Renn (eds.), *Delphi Methods In The Social And Health Sciences*, https://doi.org/10.1007/978-3-658-38862-1_9

areas, results were finally summarized in an expertise. Eleven problem areas were identified, from which the four main topics of intersectoral management, geriatric care, caring neighbourhoods as well as qualification and training were derived and corresponding solution proposals were developed.

1 Health Care Situation of Older People: Background, Mandate and Objectives of the Study

Demographic change has been more pronounced in Germany than in most other European countries. High life expectancy and good overall health conditions have been made possible by improvements in medical research, hygiene, nutrition, housing, work and income. Health problems and limitations often appear only in old age and manifest themselves predominantly in multimorbidity and chronic diseases as well as mental disorders, including above all those of dementia and depression. Older people, defined in the study as people aged 65 and older, need to be treated more frequently and differently than younger people (Statistisches Bundesamt, 2011, p. 78).

Against this background – and also in view of scarce resources –, the components of health care provision for older people need to be rethought within the framework of the existing outpatient and inpatient care structures, as well as acute medical, rehabilitative, geriatric treatment strategies and psychosocial care in accordance with Book V of the German Social Code (SGB V, which regulates the statutory health insurance and its respective services), both at national and federal level.

The future health care of elderly people has to meet the following challenges when it comes to organising an efficient and needs-oriented care system despite limited financial resources:

- the reorganisation of medical care structures with a focus on the needs-oriented treatment of geriatric populations with chronic and multiple diseases in a small-scale and cross-sectoral framework;
- improving health care and prevention in old age in order to reduce or even avoid hospital admissions;
- the further development of medical and nursing guidelines for the care of older vulnerable people in outpatient as well as inpatient acute medical care (Hibbeler, 2011, p. A-14);
- the preservation of physical and mental functioning in old age in order to enable a life that is as self-determined as possible despite illness(es) and the associated physical and cognitive limitations enabling a good quality of life (BMBF, 2014);

- the nationwide expansion of outpatient and inpatient palliative medical care structures to provide comprehensive support and pain relief at the end of life for seriously ill and dying people for whom curative treatment options have been exhausted;
- overcoming segmentation in medical, nursing and social care in order to avoid disruptions in the care supply chain (BMFSFJ, 2014, p. 28);
- the integration of migrant elders into the German health care system under the premise of culturally sensitive care in the individual sectors.

These nationwide challenges also apply to the state of Bremen. Similar to most other federal states, the state of Bremen has a dense medical, nursing and therapeutic care provision network, which, supplemented by the inpatient geriatric care units that have been established and further developed since the mid-1990s, is capable of responding appropriately to the challenges of caring for older people in the state of Bremen.

However, if the generally good health care is evaluated considering the influence of the socio-economic status of older Bremen residents on health, a heterogeneous picture emerges, especially with regard to life expectancy. Particularly striking is the difference in life expectancy between Schwachhausen and Gröpelingen, two districts of Bremen that show great differences in terms of socio-economic status. For example, there is a difference of 8 years in life expectancy for men between the two districts. Schwachhausen is considered a more privileged and Gröpelingen a more disadvantaged district in Bremen regarding the socio-economic status of residents. Differences are also evident with regard to illnesses: "Socially disadvantaged people are more frequently affected by cardiovascular diseases, diabetes, lung cancer or depression than people from more privileged classes" (Landesvereinigung für Gesundheit Bremen, 2010, p. 12). The assessment rating of the subjective health status is also worse overall among socially disadvantaged persons (Landesvereinigung für Gesundheit Bremen, 2010, p. 4).

The increasing proportion of migrants and refugees poses a particular challenge to the health care system. Although the proportion of migrants in the state of Bremen who are 65 years and older is less than 10%, according to previous calculations, this is expected to increase sharply in the coming years (Landesvereinigung für Gesundheit Bremen, 2010, p. 4). Their social situation is often characterised by low income, low educational level, low language competence, information deficits, cultural differences and psychosocial factors, which can have a negative impact on health and represent an increased risk of illness for this population. A culturally sensitive organisation of health care for ageing migrants can promote the use of medical services and thus the integration into the Bremen health care system. The development of a sensitivity towards culturally different hygiene needs, taboos, boundaries of shame, rules of politeness or forms of expressing pain can help to bridge differences in the individual sectors of medical health care (Landesvereinigung für Gesundheit Bremen, 2010, p. 12).

Against this background, the question arises as to which types of solutions can and must be developed specifically for Bremen in order to adequately meet these challenges. Based on the objective to secure the health care of older people in the long term at a high quality level, the Senator for Health in the Federal State of Bremen commissioned the Institute for Public Health and Nursing Research to conduct a corresponding study. The objective was to identify existing and emerging problems in the care of older people and to identify potential solutions for optimising care. The study was conducted from May 2014 to October 2014 and based on a Delphi survey of 87 experts.

2 Research Question and Survey Method

Against the background of the need to ensure long-term, high-quality health care for older people in the Federal State of Bremen, the following questions were chosen the survey:

- Which existing and emerging can be identified in the health care provision and situation of the elderly population aged 65 and over in the federal state of Bremen?
- What possible solutions can be identified?

In line with the objectives of the funding body, the identification of problems and the search for solutions in the context of the SGB V were to be considered in particular. This means that the focus of this study was not on services and corresponding infrastructures in connection with the need for long-term care (services of Book XI of the German Social Code, long-term care insurance), but rather on those services and structures that older people in the federal state of Bremen make use of via the statutory health insurance (SGB V-services; see below: selection of experts).

As a form of highly structured group communication, the Delphi method aims to develop solutions to complex problems (Bortz & Döring, 2006, p. 261) and has the following characteristic features (Häder, 2014, p. 25; Vorgrimler & Wübben, 2003, p. 765):

- Use of a formalized questionnaire,
- Interviewing experts,
- Anonymity of individual responses,
- Eliciting a statistical group response,
- Collecting controlled feedback and
- (multiple) repetition of survey rounds.

In addition to these characteristics, which are common to all types of Delphi surveys, a specific type of Delphi (called type 1) focusing on qualitative input was applied to identify problems and elicit ideas for improving the situation. Open-ended questions were put to a panel of experts, whose selection is based on individual expertise (Häder, 2014, p. 37).

Adhering to the above mentioned characteristics as well as incorporating the high expected share of qualitative data determined the planning and implementation of the survey and evaluation steps. They described in the following paragraphs.

The recording of problem constellations and the articulation of corresponding possible solutions with regard to the health care provision and situation of older people were carried out by means of the Delphi method type 1 "Delphi survey for idea aggregation" (Häder, 2014, p. 31). The results had been generated from two successive online surveys and a concluding workshop with experts from various areas of health care in Bremen. Figure 1 shows the flow and the process of data collection and analysis of the study.

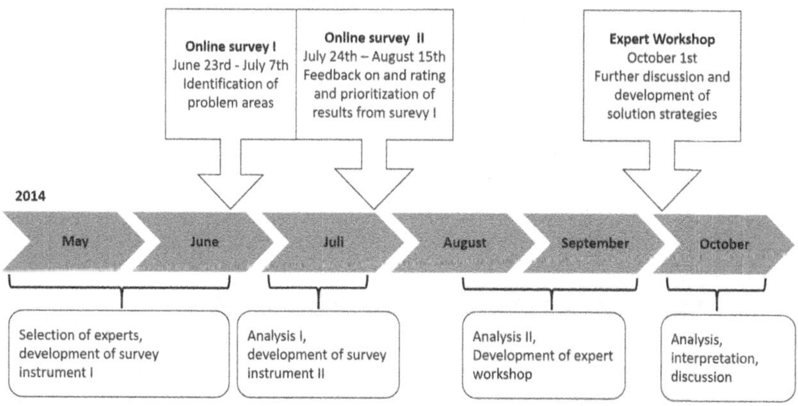

Fig. 1 Flowchart of study process and elements of data collection and analysis. (Own representation)

The first online survey was followed by another online survey soon after the evaluation of qualitative (summarizing content analysis) and quantitative data (descriptive analysis of location and dispersion measures). The second online survey included a feedback on the results from the first survey. After the renewed evaluation, the data collection ended with a workshop in which the experts discussed the results of the second online survey and developed in-depth solution strategies for the identified problems.

2.1 Selection of Experts

The selection and inclusion of suitable experts in the study was initially oriented towards the pool of experts from SGB V. Thus, experts who are considered should work in leadership positions in the areas of acute outpatient care (e.g. general practitioners), acute inpatient care (hospitals), outpatient and inpatient rehabilitation, outpatient care (nursing care services), inpatient care (nursing homes), self-help and interest groups (e.g. patient advocates, state seniors' representatives) or should have proven expertise in medical care of elderly people. In addition, persons who were in leadership positions representing service providers or politics/public affairs/administration (such as health insurance companies, health offices, senatorial authorities) were also considered for participation.

In the next step, an overview of all eligible institutions and persons was created based on an Internet search for expertise and responsibilities in the health care sector serving older people in the federal state of Bremen. In the clinical and acute outpatient sector, the focus was on specialist departments/areas in which predominantly older people are treated. Persons working in clinics with a primarily psychiatric focus and in affiliated clinics were excluded.

The final panel comprised 87 experts, who received a personalized postal information and request to support the study from the Senator for Health in the Federal State of Bremen before the actual recruitment began. Invitations to participate in the online surveys were also personalized and sent by e-mail.

2.2 Construction of the Survey Instruments

The online surveys were conducted by means of electronic questionnaires using the software Enterprise Feedback Suite (EFS) Survey 10.3. In addition to the support of a wide range of question types and formats, the data protection measures installed in the software proved to be a major argument for using this instrument, data transport is carried out using SSL encryption and the data is stored securely in a data centre certified by the German Federal Office for Information Security (BSI) in accordance with ISO 27001. Furthermore, no IP addresses of the participants are stored in the anonymous survey mode (Baltes-Götz, 2014, p. 7). The program allows the user to interrupt the survey as well as to progress in the questionnaire without being obliged to answer. The link for participation was in principle freely accessible, but was sent exclusively to the experts by e-mail.

2.3 Survey Instrument Online Survey I

In the first online survey, the focus was on identifying problems in the health care of older people in the federal state of Bremen. In contrast to other surveys, Delphi surveys have their own requirements for the survey instruments used: Usually, hardly any personal information is collected (Häder, 2014, p. 140), but due to the sometimes complex nature of the issues and topics to be assessed, it is recommended to include subjective competence questions to assess the expertise of the participating experts. In addition to the possibility of avoiding answers without sufficient expertise, competence questions signal to the participants that their answers are merely estimates (Häder, 2014, p. 133).

The questionnaire developed for this study contained introductory questions on the professional field (sector) of the respondents and on intersections with other sectors of the health care system, as well as questions on the assessment of the adequacy of health care, on the development of demand for health care services for older people, on services for older people that should be promoted more, on an assessment of the greatest problems in health care for older people, on problems to be addressed in the short, medium and long term, and on strengths of the Federal State of Bremen in health care for older people.

Both standardized questions (single or multiple choice) and open-ended questions were used. Each set of questions concluded with an assessment of the relevance of the question for the health care sector represented by the participant, as well as an indication of the frequency with which the participant dealt with the topic of the question (response options ranged from “My staff and I deal intensively with this topic, it is part of our daily work” to “Neither my staff nor I deal intensively with this topic” on a four-point scale).

A pretest of the questionnaire with regard to comprehensibility, handling, structure and required processing time was carried out with five subjects not involved in the study (a manager of outpatient nursing care, a manager of inpatient nursing care, a geriatric nurse, a nursing educator and a specialist in the field of user experience).

2.4 Survey Instrument Online Survey II

In the second online survey, participants were shown the results of the first survey. In addition, previously made statements were further concretized and approaches to solution strategies developed.

To this end, the questionnaire was based on the results of the first survey phase. In the second survey the participants were asked to concentrate on selected topic areas after viewing a graphical presentation of the initial results and to describe problems and develop potential solutions depending on the participants' expertise and own ideas.

Both standardized questions (single or multiple choice, prioritisation and ranking lists) and open-ended questions giving the option to provide a comprehensive answer were used. Questions on the subjective competence as well as the individual relevance rating was omitted in this round of questioning.

This second survey instrument was also pretested.

2.5 Development and Implementation of the Expert Workshop

Based on the results of the first and second online survey, four thematic complexes (intersectoral management, caring neighbourhoods, geriatric care, qualification and training) were identified, which were made available to the expert panel for further discussion during the workshop using discussion-guiding stimuli.

The participants were given the opportunity to familiarize themselves with the topics to be discussed and to assign themselves to one of four discussion groups according to their interests. After a short presentation on the structure, process and initial results of the study, a member of the study team moderated a group discussion lasting 75 min. During this discussion, the participants had the opportunity to assess and complement the proposed solutions and to further specify which settings, institutions or persons should be involved in implementing the proposal. The participants also considered where responsibilities should lie and, if a proposal addressed specific target groups, how these could be reached. The main focus for all proposals was the search for appropriate solutions to the problems identifies earlier.

2.6 Translation of Results

As the online surveys and the workshop were conducted in German, results were initially compiled in German and then translated to English for publication. Primary translation was performed by a third party provider and then validated by two of the authors responsible for data collection and analysis and then validated by a third author with the same institutional background, who had access to the German language results.

3 Presentation of the Results

3.1 Description of the Sample

A total of 87 experts were invited to participate in the online surveys and the concluding expert workshop. Table 1 provides an overview of participation and response in all three phases of the survey.

The participants needed a mean of 54 min 20 s (median 16 min 16 s) to complete the first online survey, and a mean of 31 min 24 s (median 25 min 50 s) to complete the second online survey. In both surveys, most dropouts occurred on the first page (greeting and entry): 35 dropouts in the first survey and 15 dropouts in the second survey. The majority of the respondents classified the topics of the study as relevant to very relevant and dealt intensively with the topics in their daily work.

Table 1 Participation and response in the study phases, own representation

	First online survey	Second online survey		Workshop
Invited (n)	87	87	Invited (n)	87
Data supplied*	94	43		
Completed	59	30	Participated	24
Return (completed/s)	67.8%	34.5%	Return (participated/s)	27.6%

The difference to the number of invited persons results from the survey mode 'anonymous' of the online survey (link to the survey was freely accessible)

3.2 Results of the Online Surveys

3.2.1 Problems Identified

Eleven problems could be identified (Table 2). A summary overview was generated from the free text responses. Quotations from the free-text responses are listed as examples in each case.

Table 2 Results of the first online survey: Identified problem areas, own representation

Problem area	Sample quotes
People with dementia	*"lack of levels of care for dementia patients"* [sequence number 18].
Health policy	*"...not a focus of health policy work regarding the older population"* [sequence number 18]. *"Lack of expertise on the part of political actors"* [sequence number 63].
Outpatient care	*"Outreach solutions oriented towards and in the living environment of people are not sufficiently supported. People have to go into the care of institutions when they have higher needs - alternative solutions related to the living environment cannot be financed by the current possibilities."* [sequence number 109]
Funding	*"The greatest problems in the health care of older people in Bremen lie, on the one hand, in the area of scarce financial resources (from the area of social long-term care insurance), which are made available to older people in need of help from the social security system."* [sequence number 21]
Medical treatments	*"Specialists do not offer home visits - specialist and dental care for care home residents - accessible medical practices"* [sequence number. 114].
Provision deficits	*"significant communication deficits in all areas of health care - also due to economic interests of health care providers » too little time in all areas of care"* [sequence number 67].
Social aspects	*"no government offers to promote fitness in old age, especially for those who cannot participate in opportunities offered due to slim pensions"* [sequence number 18].
Staff	*"On the other hand, considerable problems result from the fact that, measured against the existing need for nursing care, too few nursing professionals are available to care for the elderly"* [sequence number 21]. *"Too little geriatric knowledge among many physicians, but also among nurses"* [sequence number 71].
Intersectoral problems	*"Lack of cross-sectoral models of care"* [sequence number 25]. *"the uncoordinated juxtaposition of care structures"* [sequence number 46].
Inpatient long-term care	*"Underprovision of medically necessary nursing home services"* [sequence number 71].
Acute inpatient care in hospitals	*"insufficient places for geriatric care in acute care hospital"* [sequence number 84].

The majority of the experts ($n = 32$) answered the question "How do you assess the health care of older people in the state of Bremen in the sector you indicated?" with "underprovided", 19 participants assume adequate care conditions, and one person classifies their own sector as overprovided.

In addition to these areas, the experts also highlighted strengths that the state of Bremen has developed in the context of health care for older people or that it can draw on. These are characterized in particular by:

- good geriatric acute care,
- a high degree of cooperation and networking,
- a good accessibility of the services offered, in view of short distances,
- relatively manageable structures with many alternatives and choices
- a high quality of care through a high quota of experts and
- clearly perceptible support from politics, for example in the establishment of nursing science at Bremen universities.

In the first wave of the survey the experts were able to identify areas that they considered to be particularly problematic, the second survey provided the opportunity to the participating experts to prioritise aspects of individual problem areas - based on the free-text responses from the first survey - and to develop suggestions for solutions that the respondents considered to have the greatest chance of being successfully implemented by the Federal State of Bremen or the Senatorial Department of Health.

Based on the information provided by the experts in the first two rounds of the survey, there was a recurring tendency for thematic complexes and motifs to be taken up repeatedly and dealt with in the free text responses in particular.

3.3 Results of the Online Surveys

Based on the preceding prioritisation of problems by the participants of the online surveys, four main topics were derived, which formed the starting point for the contents to be discussed and worked on in the third survey phase – the expert workshop:

- Intersectoral management,
- Geriatric care,
- Caring neighbourhoods, and
- Qualifications and training.

These four main topics contain initial ideas for the development of solution strategies that emerged particularly from the second survey. These solution strategies were not prioritized further by the participating experts, but discussed during the expert workshop in a comprehensive manner.

4 Interpretation and Discussion of the Results

In the context of the expert workshop, the participants were asked to identify one potential solution for each of the main topics (intersectoral management, geriatric care, caring neighbourhood and qualification and training) as highly relevant for an early strategy development. These potential solutions are briefly presented and substantiated in the following section.

4.1 Specific Solutions in the Topic Area: Intersectoral Management

Figure 2 illustrates the main topic of intersectoral management according to the problems identified during the online surveys and the elicitation of potential solutions developed during the Delphi process. More specific proposals (for example, the establishment of cross-sectoral working groups) and terms that emerged in different formulations from the free-text responses (for example, case management) were also listed. Against the background of a growing diversity of actors and services in the health care system, there is a need on the one hand for clearly identifiable and accessible information on health care services for the target group of older people, and on the other hand there is the requirement for to control and manage parallel structures and to avoid the risk of duplication of services. This is exacerbated by the fact that, with an increasing workload in the outpatient and inpatient sector, the design of transition processes and the implementation of successful discharge management in particular represent a challenge for the health care professionals involved. High-quality care often fails – as also described by the experts – due to fragmented responsibilities. Improved case and care management as well as interactive case conferences seem to be suitable instruments to influence a successful cooperation of the interfaces in the care sectors.

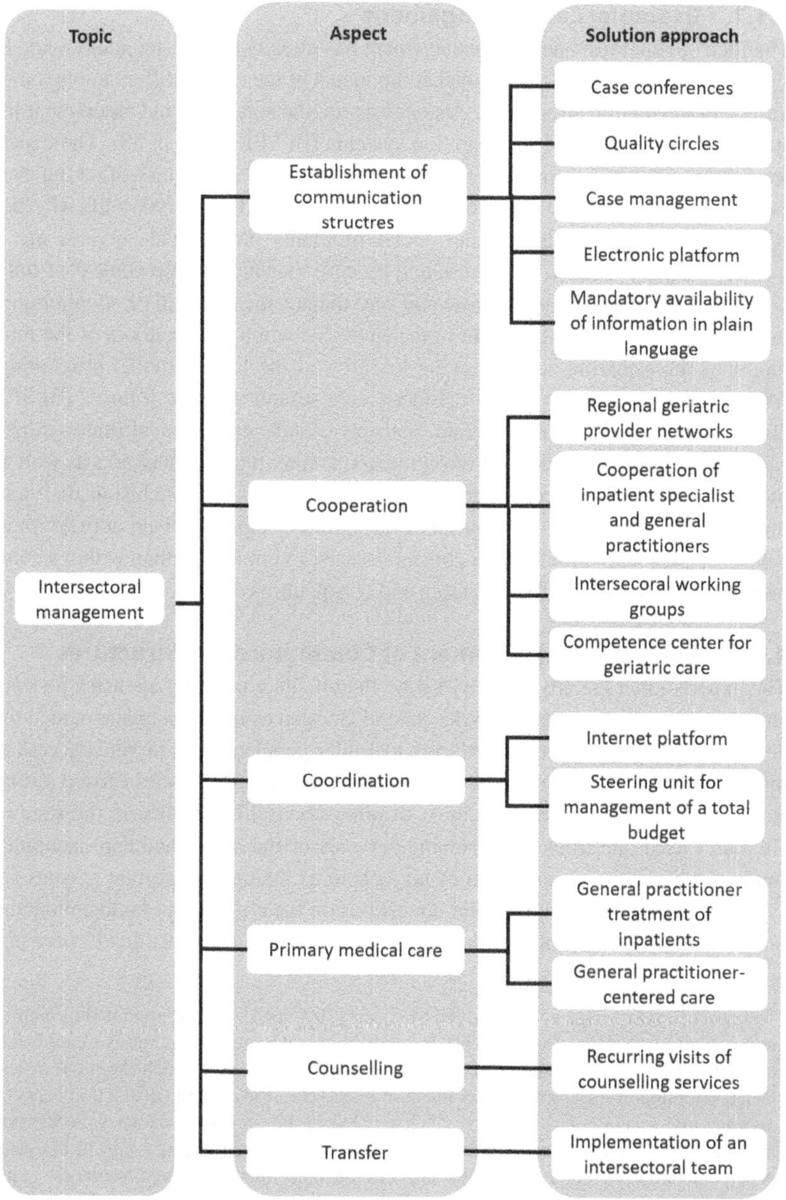

Fig. 2 Overview of discussed problems and solution strategies, workshop group of *intersectoral management.* (Own representation)

4.1.1 Example: Case Management

The idea of superordinate case management has already been tested nationwide in several pilot projects. The individual components of the design differ, among other things, in the qualification of the case managers, the screening and assessment instruments used and the documentation systems (BFSFJ, 2004, p. 58). The expert workshop opted for a neutral, not interest-driven body with the task of taking over case management both as an accompanying feature in the everyday life of older people and if specific health and social problems prevail and services are – limited[1] – by the roles to be represented by case managers in the context of individual case support. Individual case and care management should be sought rather in relation to the city district than to the state as a whole. The authors of the final report of the scientific accompanying research of the federal model programme "Altenhilfestrukturen der Zukunft (Elderly care structures of the future)" (BFSFJ, 2004, p. 63) had evaluated different concepts of case management (among them case management in the context of segment-spanning regional networks as well as individual case assistance in networks). They came to the conclusion that case management starting from institutions with an interdisciplinary team or from counselling centres with direct patient contact is easier to implement than within a comprehensive network of different actors and co-operations.

4.1.2 Example: Establishment of Communication Structures

The experts rated the advice provided by the on-site consulting agencies for care and age ("Pflegestützpunkte") in the state of Bremen as insufficient and named the need to bundle information and to provide older people a more targeted access to this information. The evaluation of the on-site consulting agencies carried out by Rothgang et al. (2012) in the context of other counselling centres in the state of Bremen raised questions the financing services of the health and care insurance funds and about the organisation of home care as the most important reasons for visiting an on-site consulting point. Questions on the criteria for classification and on the funding benefits of the health and long-term care insurance funds were pri-

---

[1] The goal of case management described by Ewers (1997, p. 315), to respond to the complex needs of mostly chronically ill people through individual and comprehensive care offers across the segmented boundaries of the care system, is achieved through the more or less clear assumption of different roles by the case managers. However, the distinction between advocacy and access control (Ewers, 1997, p. 316) in the functions advocacy, broker and gate-keeper includes varying parts of budget control and management – e.g. in the gatekeeper function (Ewers, 1997, p. 318). This circumstance makes an implementation in the sense of the interviewed experts with the involvement of a superordinate, neutral body more difficult.

marily asked by people without appropriate care level (Rothgang et al., 2012, p. 56). Among the types of care, questions on home care were ranked ahead of the offers of housing with services and inpatient care, while the topics of medical care and palliative care (SGB V) were of little relevance (Rothgang et al., 2012, p. 52). The reasons for contacting the counselling facilities assessed in the evaluation (Rothgang et al., 2012, p. 70) should be considered for bundling and processing targeted information. With regard to the further operation of the on-site consulting agencies in the Federal State of Bremen after March 2016, further development and optimisation of the information offered seems to be warranted – for example within the framework of the online presence of the on-site consulting points – can be identified here.

It appears to be more difficult to implement a link between counselling and information services and the obligation of the statutory health insurance and social long-term care insurance providers to provide education, counselling and information in the sense of §§ 13, 14 and 15 of the German Social Code, Book I, using the established documents with links to education and information campaigns on other topics.[2]

All experts agreed that a uniform transition instrument taking into account the proportion of information to be recorded is required in the outpatient and (partially) inpatient settings. The requirement for "care management, in particular to solve problems during the transition between the various care settings" is clarified in Section 11 (4) of the SGB V, as well as by the amendment of Section 39 (1) of the SGB V, by the German Statutory Health Insurance Structure Act (GKV-VStG) with the addition of "Hospital treatment also includes discharge management to solve problems during the transition to nursing care after hospital treatment". Also against the background of the national *expert standard Discharge Management in* Nursing (DNQP, 2009) developed by the German Network for Quality Development in Nursing (DNQP), the acute inpatient services in particular are asked to transfer patients to post-hospital care facilities while avoiding disruptions in care provision through an optimised exchange of information between the actors involved in the discharge process (DNQP, 2009, p. 7). Nationwide, approaches to the development and implementation of a uniform transfer instrument exist in several cities. As an

[2] At this point, the expert group also pointed out the legal obligation to provide information on the subject of organ donation. This obligation is explicitly binding in § 2 paragraph 1 of the Transplantation Act (TPG) for the bodies responsible under state law and federal authorities as well as the health insurance funds. An integration of further topics is not planned and cannot be implemented in a binding and obligatory manner without changes within the legislation.

example, the *Dresden Transition Questionnaire* can be highlighted. With the aim of ensuring continuity of care with regard to the transfer of information during transition across sectors, the city of Dresden developed an instrument that was tested in 2013 (Landeshauptstadt Dresden, 2013). The transfer instrument is supplemented by an additional questionnaire for patients with dementia/cognitive impairment (Liedtke, 2014). This additional form is suitable for depicting circumstances that are not addressed in the usual transition documents (Liedtke, 2014, p. 23). These experiences show that corresponding transition instruments are certainly suitable for improving the quality of information from the perspectives of the actors, who are asked to review and revise their positions regularly. It remains questionable whether and how positive effects of such an instrument are reflected at the level of quality of care.

4.2 Specific Approaches in the Topic Area of Geriatric Care

Figure 3 illustrates the structure of the main topic of geriatric care according to the areas identified from the results of the online surveys and the associated starting points for solution strategies. Here, both more specific proposals (for example, the employment of permanent (specialist) medical staff in geriatric care facilities) and terms that emerged in different formulations from the free-text responses (for example, geriatric day clinics) are listed in the figure.

In contrast to federal states such as Rhineland-Palatinate or Saxony, Bremen did not have a comprehensive geriatric concept[3] at the time of the study. The orientation of geriatrics as a service in the clinical sector[4] described in the hospital framework plan of the state of Bremen at the time of the study explains the neglect of geriatric facilities in the outpatient sector noted in the "Geriatrics Guidelines". High-quality care for older people is supposed to take into account a comprehensive, cross-sectoral perspective of the service providers involved.

[3]A geriatric care concept was adopted by the senatorial authority in summer 2018 (see https://www.senatspressestelle.bremen.de/detail.php?gsid=bremen146.c.303932.de&asl=bremen02.c.732.de)

[4]In some federal states such as Bremen and Hamburg, acute geriatrics is exclusively implemented as hospital treatment in accordance with § 39 SGB V, while in others such as Bavaria or Rhineland-Palatinate, it is implemented in accordance with § 40 SGB V in the form of rehabilitation facilities.

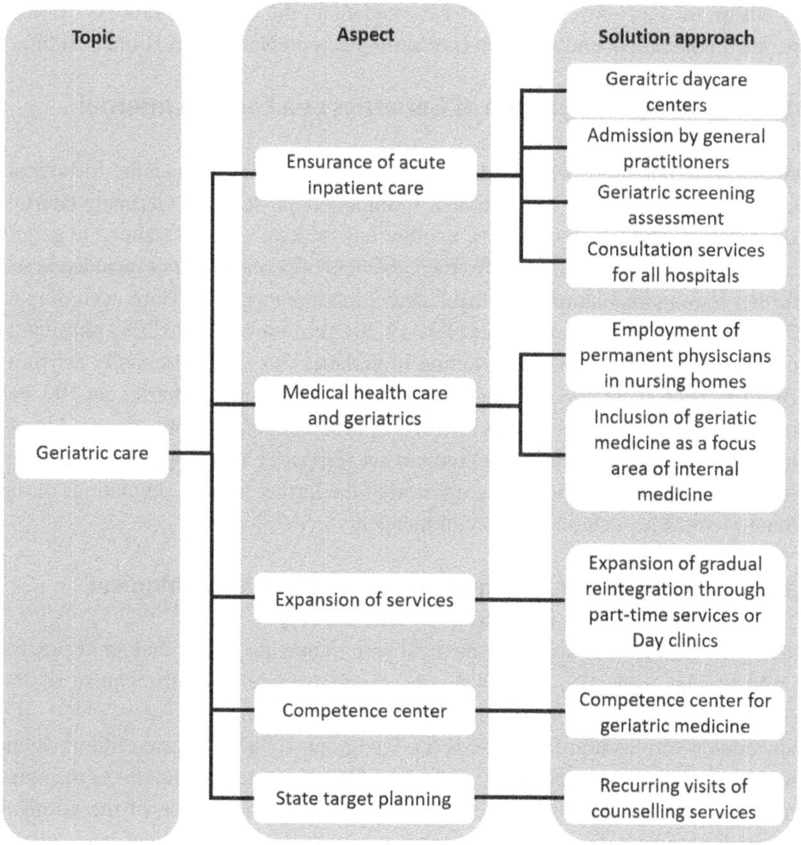

Fig. 3 Overview of discussed areas and solutions, workshop group geriatric care. (Own representation)

4.2.1 Example: Development of a Binding Geriatric Concept

It was proposed to establish a geriatric concept for the federal state of Bremen on the basis of concepts already existing in several federal states. However, differences in the organisation of geriatric care between the federal states must be taken into account. When considering the content of a geriatric concept for Bremen, it is important to consider the need, on the one hand, to give greater priority to early geriatric rehabilitation, for example by systematically identifying the rehabilitation potential of older people in GP practices or acute hospitals, and, on the other hand, to ensure the early involvement of geriatricians in the treatment process of older people in outpatient and inpatient care settings, as emphasized in Hilmer (2009).

4.2.2 Example: Inclusion of Geriatrics as a Focus of Internal Medicine

At the time the study was conducted, further training as a specialist in internal medicine and geriatrics was available in three federal states in Germany (Berlin, Brandenburg and Saxony-Anhalt). In other federal states, further training in geriatric medicine is also possible. In Bremen, the field of geriatrics is not included in the further training regulations as a focal area of internal medicine. Thus, according to Pippel et al. (2014, p. A1412 f.) as of 31.12.2012 only seven out of 2082 physicians nationwide with an additional training in geriatrics were professionally active in Bremen. Thus, there were 1.1 doctors with further training in geriatrics per 100,000 inhabitants. Bremen thus has the lowest proportion of doctors with enhanced training in geriatrics in a nationwide comparison (Pippel et al., 2014, p. A1412 f.). In order to focus on geriatric care, a revision of the further training regulations of the State Medical Association was recommended.

4.2.3 Example: Employing Permanent (Specialist) Medical Staff in Care Facilities for the Elderly

The perceived lack of specialist medical care in nursing homes and strategies for improvement were also discussed[5] on several occasions. In the course of the Nursing Care Realignment Act (Pflege-Neuausrichtungs-Gesetz – PNG), the amendments to Section 114 of SGB XI, Paragraph 1, have obligated full inpatient nursing facilities since January 1, 2014, to inform the state associations of the nursing care insurance funds immediately after a regular inspection of the arrangements for medical, specialist and dental care as well as the supply of medications

[5] In the main topic of the BARMER GEK Nursing Care Report published in 2008, Rothgang et al. (2008, p. 213) summarise the assessment of the medical care situation in nursing homes in relation to different medical disciplines: Nursing home residents have - in comparison to persons without need of care - fewer contacts with specialists from the fields of internal medicine (partly statistically significant), ophthalmology (statistically significant), ear, nose and throat medicine (not statistically significant) and orthopaedics (statistically significant) and more contacts with doctors from the fields of general medicine and neurology/psychiatry (statistically significant in each case), dermatologists (partly statistically significant). Similar numbers of contacts exist with doctors in the fields of urology/gynecology and surgery. The data of the current nursing report (Rothgang et al., 2014) focus on the dental care of the residents and also show significantly fewer doctor contacts in this area compared to people not in need of care of the same age, gender and morbidity (Rothgang et al., 2014, p. 22).

in the facilities. In particular, reference is to be made, among other things, to the conclusion and content of cooperation agreements or the integration of the facility into networks of doctors. In the Federal State of Bremen, the Act to Ensure the Rights of People with Support, Care and Support Needs in Supportive Housing (Bremisches Wohn- und Betreuungsgesetz, BremWoBeG) is intended to support residents in supportive housing facilities in asserting their interests and needs and to protect them from disadvantages resulting from the linking of housing with support services (see § 1 (1) BremWoBeG). The requirements described in § 12 BremWoBeG for the care and support facilities for the permission of operation mentioned in paragraph 2 point 4 in particular are designed to secure medical, dental and other health or therapeutic care. In the opinion of the experts, this would be a starting point at the state level to explicitly emphasise specialist medical care and to further stipulate binding proof of measures to ensure specialist medical care within the facility or affiliated to the facility.

4.3 Specific Approaches in the Topic Area of Caring Neighbourhoods

Figure 4 illustrates the structure of the thematic focus on caring neighbourhoods according to the areas identified from the results of the online surveys and the associated solutions to address these problems. This includes both more specific proposals (for example, the mandatory provision of information in easy-to-understand language) and terms that emerged in different formulations from the free-text responses (for example, the development of concepts).

Meeting the demand for *outpatient* care *before inpatient* care means promoting the development and integration of care services and structures in the neighbourhood. Here, accessibility proves to be particularly difficult for people from vulnerable groups.

4.3.1 Example: Neighbourhood Work

Neighbourhood work is intended to promote social participation in particular. There already are a number of approaches in the state of Bremen that have proven successful in practice in the integration of older people into services for social participation. Since 2008, outreach visits have been carried out in three districts in the city of Bremen – first as a model project and now as a regular service since April 2013. These so-called preventive home visits aim, on the one hand, to promote participation in society and, on the other hand, to prolong life in one's own home environment. In addition, the quality of life of older people is to be improved

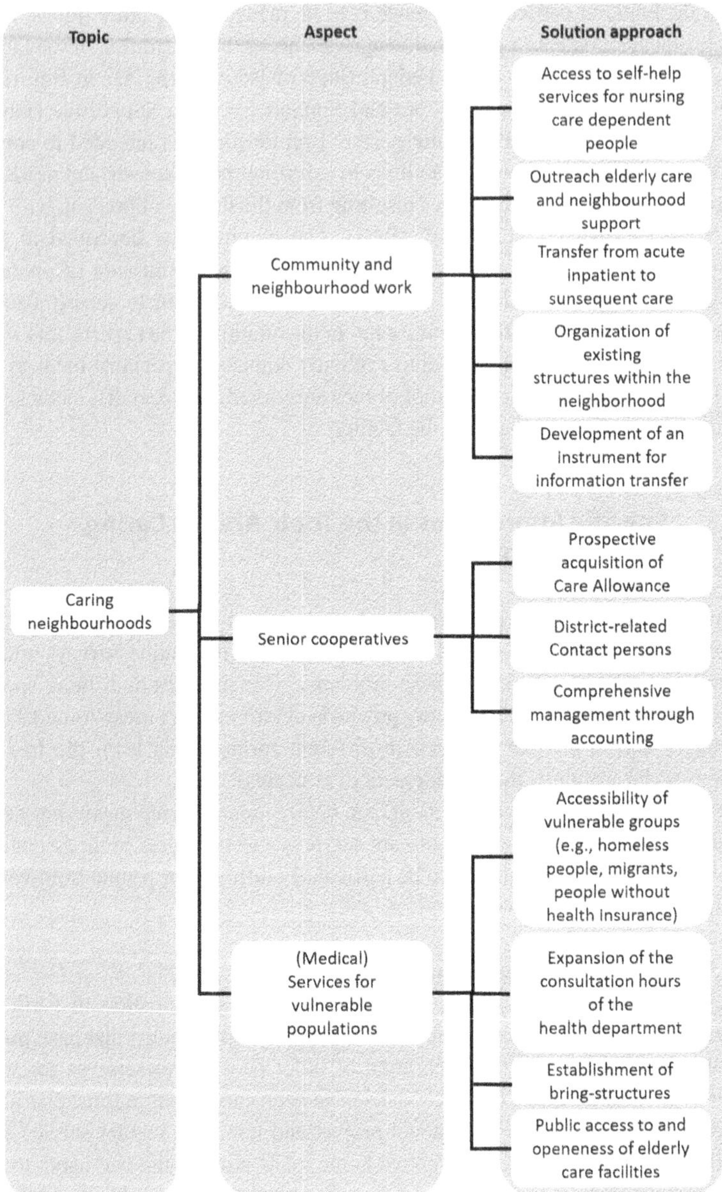

Fig. 4 Overview of discussed problems and suggested solutions workshop group caring neighbourhoods. (Own representation)

by the various actors on site. The evaluation carried out in Bremen (Habermann & Pielage, 2011) does not provide a clear answer to the question of whether the concept of preventive home visits can sustainably increase the social participation of older people.

4.4 Specific Solutions in the Area of Qualification and Training

Figure 5 illustrates the structure of the main topic of qualifications and training according to the areas identified in the online surveys and the associated solution strategies. These include both more specific proposals (for example, the recogni-

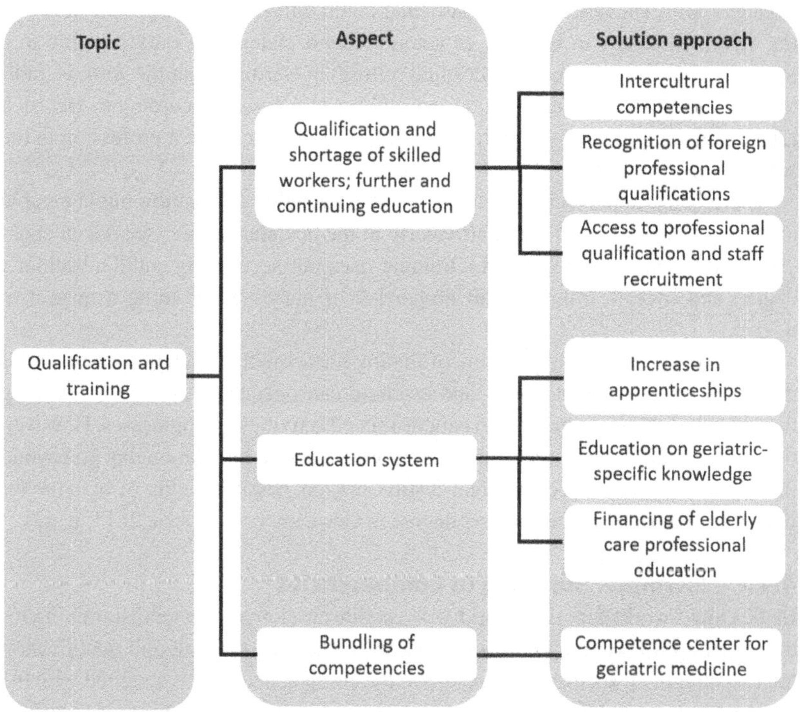

Fig. 5 Overview of discussed problems and solution strategies, workshop group qualification and training. (Own representation)

tion of vocational qualifications from abroad) and terms that emerged in different formulations from the free-text responses (for example, intercultural competencies).

In view of the challenge posed by the changes in the care needs of older and chronically ill people resulting from demographic change, questions arise as to the occupational profiles and future training paths as well as the necessary qualifications of health care professionals.

4.4.1 Example: Access Professional Qualification and Staff Recruitment

According to the experts, the task of increasing the attractiveness of the nursing profession lies in the hands of the respective institutions. If students are asked about the relevance of selected factors for their choice of profession, the factor "secure job" comes first, followed by "autonomy, independent work" (Ernst & Young, 2009). The latter point in particular could influence young people in deciding against a career in nursing, as autonomous decisions are only possible to a limited extent (especially in the hospital setting) in Germany and the work is traditionally anchored in hierarchical organisational structures. According to Hentrich (2011), high earnings are rarely a reason for trainees to choose a profession in the sector "health and care".

There is the opportunity that nurses with a bachelor's education might be able to increase the quality of care particularly in the hospital setting (see Aiken et al., 2014). In Germany, nurses' initial training does not necessarily entail a bachlor's degree and overall, only a small proportion of nurses are holding a respective degree.

The trend observed in Germany of finding nurses with a bachelor's or master's degree in science, management and teaching can only be addressed in the long term by integrating graduates into patient-related activities and processes. However, this requires nationwide concepts of employment and remuneration that go beyond initial considerations of individual institutions on possible fields of activity for nurses with a bachelors or masters degree in Germany (see Görres, 2013, p. 43).

4.4.2 Example: Bundling of Competencies

In the expert workshop, there was hardly any discussion of a generalist training for the nursing professions. However, it became clear that training and qualification are essential in all sectors. With regard to the competencies to be acquired with the training and the fields of activity that present themselves, planning of measures within the framework of a Bremen education offensive for the health care professions is gaining importance.

4.4.3 Example: Intercultural Competencies

Model projects aiming to increase the intercultural competencies of employees in the care sector appear to be successful when knowledge is imparted in a practical manner with reference to theory in the living environment of the caregivers (Multikulturelles Forum Lünen, 2006, p. 31 ff.). Particular relevance is attached to the intergenerational transfer of competencies. This does not only apply to intercultural competencies, but also to knowledge retention. Bremen already has concepts in this area[6] that could be transferred to other institutions. The prerequisite for this, however, is proof of positive effects, which can be verified by means of evaluation.

In order to ensure cross-setional care for older people, district-based support for patients by a nurse may be a viable option. In Germany, projects for the accompaniment of older people by volunteers are already being carried out, in which volunteers at neighbourhood level contribute to reducing the interface problem (Forschungsinstitut Geragogik, 2014). At this point, the use of professional caregivers instead of volunteers might be feasible due to their special expertise.

The relevance of a sustainable strategy concept on questions of qualification of health care professionals becomes clear in this thematic focus. A Bremen education initiative in this area can serve as a logical consequence for dealing with the problem.

4.5 Summary of the Discussion

In summary, for many of the solutions proposed by the experts, comparable (model) projects exist at both state and federal level, whose experience and procedures can be used to design and implement solution strategies for the state of Bremen. However, many of these projects have not yet been sufficiently evaluated - especially with regard to their effects on the actual health care situation of older people.

For the federal state of Bremen, the proposals for the development of a geriatrics concept, a uniform transition instrument and an education offensive for health care professions seem particularly suitable for optimising the cooperation in the area of interface management. This requirement has been emphasised several

[6] See, for example, the model project "Demogra-fitte Pflege" of the Krankenhaus St.-Joseph-Stift (Krankenhaus St.-Joseph-Stift (ed.) 2014).

times, and for reacting to the shortage of skilled workers in the nursing professions - and ultimately for making a contribution to improving the care situation of older people.

5 Strengths and Limitations of the Study

A particular strength of the survey is the successful integration of experts from various sectors involved in the health care of older people in the federal state of Bremen. Thus, it was possible to draw a multi-perspective image of problems and potential solutions as a means and to give different actors from the health care sector in the federal state of Bremen the opportunity to help shape solution strategies. Even if the results are not detailed enough, the procedure itself can certainly be a blueprint for other federal states.

The survey method chosen accommodates the complexity that is associated with the more general questions of the study: The Delphi survey for the aggregation of ideas was suitable to give the experts room for the development of their own ideas without restricting the discourse with too many standardized propositions. The combination of qualitative and quantitative data as well as the feedback of the results enabled the structured collection of expert knowledge and also increased the consensus building effort within the surveyed group while at the same time allowing all participants to shape the results (Elmer et al., 2010, p. 122). The Delphi method is a suitable research approach, especially in a field in which it is not primarily a matter of gathering expert knowledge for generating projections, but rather to identify real needs (Elmer et al., 2010, p. 122).

Although special, homogeneous groups (in this case experts with geriatric-specific knowledge in the Bremen health care landscape) of respondents who are directly affected by the survey topic have been more willing to participate (Jackob et al., 2009, p. 68), there were several limiting factors in the survey results caused by the time required to answer the first online survey. According to published empirical values, a response rate of 30% can be assumed in the first survey of Delphi studies (Häder, 2014, p. 118). With a response rate of 67.8% in the first survey phase, the present study is therefore considerably above the expected rate. Among the remaining participants from the first survey, a response rate of 70–75% can be assumed in the subsequent surveys (Häder, 2014, p. 118). With 50.8% in the second survey wave and 40.7% participation rate in the expert workshop, this rate[7]

[7] The data on the response rate refer to the population of persons invited to participate ($n = 87$) in all three survey phases presented.

is below the expected one. Reasons for this may lie in the chosen topic of the question or the degree of difficulty and scope of the questionnaire (Häder, 2000, p. 12).

It must also be mentioned that, due to the short duration of the study, the pretest of the instruments of the online surveys was carried out exclusively with regard to the comprehensibility and complexity of the contents, but no content-related data evaluation. The participants also had little time to take part in the survey due to the short field phases of the online surveys. The request of some participants for an extension of the field phases could not be met.

Due to the varying complexity of the discussion in the discussion groups of the expert workshop, it cannot be assumed that there was a consistently uniform procedure of moderation and written documentation. However, since tape recordings and photographic documentation of the results of the individual groups were available in addition to the workshop minutes, it was possible to reconstruct the course of the discussion and the topics dealt with by the groups without any problems.

6 Conclusions

The present Delphi survey was commissioned by the Senator for Health in the Federal State of Bremen and aimed at interviewing experts on the health care of the elderly population in the State of Bremen. Both the identification of problems in the health care of older people and the description of possible solutions were the subject of the study. The problems addressed by the experts in the course of the study and the main topics discussed make it clear that classic problems of networks and networking in the health care, in addition to questions of qualitative and quantitative control of the shortage of skilled workers in the nursing profession, turned out to be the overarching challenges and hurdles in the successful implementation of high-quality care.

The already existing strengths of the Federal State of Bremen (such as the already good accessibility and networks of the actors) in the health care of elderly people were emphasized by the experts. This lead to the expectation that efforts to deal with the problems and solution strategies identified in this study will be taken seriously by cooperation partners involved in the health care of older people.

Particularly from the solution strategies discussed by the experts in the third survey phase, recommendations for action can be formulated, taking into account approaches that are already implemented.

In the context of cooperation and participation in the design of the proposed solution strategies it is also important to include the target group to which interventions, concepts and campaigns are directed the older citizens in the Federal State of

Bremen. The inclusion of their perspective may assist responsible decision makers in the State Health System in their effort that development and survey processes can be aligned more purposefully to the needs and requirements of the elderly and can support a successful improvement of health care more sustainably.

Literature

Aiken, L. H., Sloane, D. M., Bruyneel, L., Van den Heede, K., Griffiths, P., Busse, R., et al. (2014). Nurse staffing and education and hospital mortality in nine European countries: A retrospective observational study. *The Lancet, 383*, 1824–1830.

Baltes-Götz, B. (2014). Online-Umfragen mit Enterprise Feedback Suite Survey 10.2. Zentrum für Informations-, Medien- und Kommunikationstechnologie (ZIMK) an der Universität Trier (Hrsg.), Trier Verfügbar unter: http://www.uni-trier.de/fileadmin/urt/doku/efs/efsurvey.pdf. Zugegriffen 20 Nov 2014.

BFSFJ Bundesministerium für Familie, Senioren, Frauen und Jugend (Hrsg.). (2004). *Altenhilfestrukturen der Zukunft. Abschlussbericht der wissenschaftlichen Begleitforschung zum Bundesmodellprogramm.* Hans Jacobs.

BMBF Bundesministerium für Bildung und Forschung (Hrsg.). (2014). Gesundheit erhalten – Ältere Menschen. https://www.gesundheitsforschung-bmbf.de/de/altere-menschen-6779.php. Zugegriffen: 20 Nov 2014.

BMFSFJ Bundesministerium für Familie, Senioren, Frauen und Jugend (Hrsg.). (2014). *Eine neue Kultur des Alterns – Altersbilder in der Gesellschaft. Erkenntnisse und Empfehlungen des Sechsten Altenberichts.* Berlin. https://www.bmfsfj.de/blob/93190/37cc62a3c0c978034dcdc430432c655a/6–altenbericht-eine-neue-kultur-des-alterns-data.pdf. Zugegriffen: 20 Nov 2014.

Bortz, J., & Döring, N. (2006). *Forschungsmethoden und Evaluation für Human- und Sozialwissenschaftler.* 4., überarbeitete Auflage. Springer.

DNQP Deutsches Netzwerk für Qualitätsentwicklung in der Pflege (Hrsg.). (2009). Expertenstandard Entlassungsmanagement in der Pflege – 1. Aktualisierung 2009. *Schriftenreihe des Deutschen Netzwerks für Qualitätsentwicklung in der Pflege.*

Elmer, F., Seifert, I., Kreibich, H., & Thieken, A. (2010). A Delphi method expert survey to derive standards for flood damage data collection. *Risk Analysis, 30*(1), 107–124.

Ernst & Young GmbH Wirtschaftsprüfungsgesellschaft (Hrsg.). (2009). *Studenten in Deutschland 2009 – Was sie bewegt. Wohin sie wollen.* https://blog.recrutainment.de/wp-content/uploads/2009/09/Studentenstudie_2009.pdf. Zugegriffen: 25 Nov 2014.

Ewers, M. (1997). Case Management in der klinischen Versorgung. *Zeitschrift für Gesundheitswissenschaften, 5*(4), 309–322.

Forschungsinstitut Geragogik. (2014). Patientenbegleitung. http://www.fogera.de/patienten-begleitung/. Zugegriffen: 25 Nov 2014.

Görres, S. (2013). Orientierungsrahmen: Gesellschaftliche Veränderungen, Trends und Bedarfe. (Robert Bosch Stiftung, Hrsg.) *Gesundheitsberufe neu denken – Gesundheitsberufe neu regeln. Grundsätze und Perspektiven. Eine Denkschrift der Robert Bosch Stiftung.*

Habermann, M., & Pielage, F. (2011). *Aufsuchende Altenarbeit/Hausbesuche – Wissenschaftliche Begleitung und Evaluation*. Hochschule Bremen.

Häder, M. (2000). Die Expertenauswahl bei Delphi-Befragungen. *ZUMA How-to-Reihe*(5). https://www.gesis.org/fileadmin/upload/forschung/publikationen/gesis_reihen/howto/how-to5mh.pdf. Zugegriffen: 20 Nov 2014.

Häder, M. (2014). *Delphi-Befragung. Ein Arbeitsbuch* (3. Aufl.). Springer.

Hentrich, K. (2011). Einflussfaktoren auf die Berufswahlentscheidung Jugendlicher an der ersten Schwelle. Eine theoretische und empirische Analyse. In D. Frommeberger (Hrsg.). *Magdeburger Schriften zur Berufs- und Wirtschaftspädagogik.*

Hibbeler, B. (2011). Ärztliche Versorgung alter Menschen: Reale Probleme und viel Polemik. Bundesärztekammer und Kassenärztliche Bundesvereinigung (Hrsg.). *Deutsches Ärzteblatt, 108*(1–2), A14.

Hilmer, T. (2009). Älter werden ist unser aller Zukunft. Ärztekammer Bremen (Hrsg.). *Bremer Ärztejournal, 9*(62), 4. https://www.aekhb.de/data/mediapool/baej_09_09_gesamt.pdf. Zugegriffen: 20 Nov 2014.

Jackob, N., Schoen, H., & Zerback, T. (Hrsg.). (2009). *Sozialforschung im Internet* (1. Aufl.). VS Verlag & GWV Fachverlage GmbH.

Krankenhaus St.-Joseph-Stift Bremen (Hrsg.). (2014). *Das Projekt demogra-fitte Pflege im St. Joseph-Stift*. http://www.sjs-bremen.de/de/pflege-begleitung/pflegedirektion/projekt-demogra-fitte-pflege-im-st-joseph-stift.html. Zugegriffen: 25 Nov 2014.

Landeshauptstadt Dresden (Hrsg.). (2013). Dresdner Überleitungsbogen geht in die Testphase. – Pressemitteilung vom 18. Juli 2013. http://www.dresden.de/de/02/035/01/2013/07/pm_086.php. Zugegriffen: 25 Nov 2014.

Landesvereinigung für Gesundheit Bremen e. V. (Hrsg.). (2010). Gesund alt werden in Bremen. Informationen – Erfahrungen – Praxisbeispiele. S. 4.

Liedtke, P. (2014). *Ergebnisse der Evaluation des Zusatzbogens für Patienten mit einer Demenz/kognitiven Beeinträchtigung*. Dresden. http://www.dresden.de/de/03/senioren/pflege/pflegenetz-dresden.php. Zugegriffen: 25 Nov 2014.

Multikulturelles Forum Lünen e. V. (Hrsg.). (2006). *Entwicklung interkultureller Handlungskompetenzen von Kranken- und Altenpflegepersonal*. Ergebnisse des Modellprojektes und Dokumentation. Lünen. http://www.multikulti-forum.de/fileadmin/user_upload/Download_PDF/Interkulturelle_Handlungskompetenzen_-_Dokumentation.pdf. Zugegriffen: 25 Nov 2014.

Pippel, K., Ernst, F., & Lübke, N. (2014). Weiter Bedarf an geriatrischem Nachwuchs. Vor allem im hausärztlichen Bereich werden Zusatzqualifikationen immer notwendiger. *Deutsches Ärzteblatt, 111*(33–34), A1412–A1413.

Rothgang, H., Borchert, L., Müller, R., & Unger, R. (2008). GEK-Pflegereport 2008. Schwerpunktthema: Medizinische Versorgung in Pflegeheimen. In GEK (Hrsg.) *Schriftenreihe zur Gesundheitsanalyse* (Bd. 66). Asgard Verlagsservice.

Rothgang, H., Bohns, S., Bauknecht, M., Sauer, S., Baumkötter, A., Naber, H., Francie, P., & de Vasconcelos, D. (2012). *Evaluation der Pflegestützpunkte im Kontext weiterer Beratungsstellen im Land Bremen*. Zentrum für Sozialpolitik, Universität Bremen. (Abschlussbericht).

Rothgang, H., Müller, R., Mundhenk, R., & Unger, R. (2014). BARMER GEK Pflegereport. Schwerpunkt: Zahnärztliche Versorgung Pflegebedürftiger. In *Schriftenreihe zur Gesundheitsanalyse* (Bd. 29). Asgard-Verlagsservice.

Statistisches Bundesamt (Hrsg.). (2011). Im Blickpunkt: Ältere Menschen in Deutschland und der EU; Wiesbaden. Verfügbar unter: https://www.destatis.de/DE/Publikationen/Thematisch/Bevoelkerung/Bevoelkerungsstand/BlickpunktAeltereMenschen1021221119004.pdf?__blob=publicationFile. Zugegriffen: 20 Nov 2014.

Vorgrimler, D., & Wübben, D. (2003). Die Delphi-Methode und ihre Eignung als Prognoseinstrument. In Statistisches Bundesamt (Hrsg.). *Wirtschaft und Statistik* (S. 763–774).

A Delphi Survey on Strategies of Staff Retention and Recruitment in Professional Nursing: Research Question, Operationalisation and Questionnaire Development

Nora Lämmel, Jutta Mohr, and Karin Reiber

Abstract

The care sector is in a state of upheaval: There are already too few nursing professionals today. In addition, the need will increase in the future. So what measures are facilities in Baden-Württemberg taking against this imbalance? What do the companies need in order to be able to implement measures successfully? These questions are answered by the sub-project of the University of Applied Sciences in Esslingen in the research network "ZAFH care4care - Need for Qualified Nursing Personnel in the Context of Ageing, Diversity and Satisfaction" on the basis of a Delphi survey. Centres for Applied Research at Universities of Applied Sciences (Zentren für angewandte Forschung an Hochschulen für angewandte Wissenschaften, ZAFH) are interdisciplinary and inter-university as well as inter-faculty research associations. They are funded by the Ministry of Science, Research and Arts Baden-Württemberg with EU structural funds (EFRE) over a period of 3 to 5 years. With the help of the Delphi survey, three rounds of questioning will be used to find out not only about the implemented measures and desirable ideas, but also about the neces-

N. Lämmel · J. Mohr · K. Reiber (✉)
Faculty Social Work, Education and Nursing Science, Esslingen University of Applied Sciences, Esslingen, Germany
e-mail: karin.reiber@hs-esslingen.de

M. Niederberger, O. Renn (eds.), *Delphi Methods In The Social And Health Sciences*, https://doi.org/10.1007/978-3-658-38862-1_10

sary framework conditions. The aim of the Delphi survey is to evaluate the measures implemented by nursing managers of the facilities with regard to their relevance. In the course of this process, at the end of the Delphi survey, measures for the recruitment and retention of skilled workers are presented which these members of the nursing sector assess to be relevant, effective and implementable. The following article explains the methodological procedure of the Delphi survey.

1 Introduction

The shortage of nursing staff in Germany is currently one of the most discussed topics and the pressure to act has reached a critical moment: In facilities, departments or parts of departments are being temporarily closed, scheduled interventions and examinations are being postponed, new clients (outpatient and long-term care) are not being accepted. The workload and complexity of nursing services are constantly increasing, which in turn can be detrimental to the quality of nursing care. Furthermore, it is evident that the quantitative as well as the qualitative demand for professional care will continue to increase (Rothgang et al., 2012, p. 51 ff.). The reasons for this are far-reaching and widely discussed, for example, demographic development (Ibid., p. 10), the low length of time spent in the profession (DGB Bundesvorstand, 2015, p. 10), the approaching wave of retirement (Bonin et al., 2015, p. 23), etc. How can this dramatic development be counteracted? The blanket answers – raising wages, improving working conditions and increasing job attractiveness – fall short of answering this highly complex question. Rather, different levels, responsibilities and interests, legal and operational framework conditions, path dependencies, gender issues, etc. must be taken into account in order to be able to meet the demand for skilled workers in a qualified manner.

This is the objective of the "Centre for Applied Research at Universities of Applied Sciences (ZAFH) care4care – Need for Qualified Nursing Personnel in the Context of Ageing, Diversity and Satisfaction". By using the different perspectives of the groups surveyed, ideas are generated and developed as to how nursing professionals can be retained in the profession and how new nursing professionals can be recruited. In addition, it will be investigated how the attractiveness of the nursing profession can be increased. This object of investigation requires a high degree of multi-perspectivity and a multi-methodological approach.

In this article, the Delphi survey as a method of the research network is taken into consideration. At the beginning, the research network and the sub-project of the University of Applied Sciences Esslingen are briefly outlined in order to clarify the embedding and the relevance of the Delphi survey in the overall context. Then the procedure of the Delphi survey is presented. The focus is on the methodical procedure, the research design, the evaluation and the interpretation as well as the utilisation of the results. The aim is to show the relevance of the survey method both within the project and for the nursing and health sciences, but also which prerequisites, potential stumbling blocks and methodological considerations must be taken into account when designing a multi-stage Delphi survey over the entire survey period. During the writing of this paper, the first round of the Delphi survey is taking place. Subsequent rounds are in the planning stages, with the second round scheduled for winter 2018 and the third round in early 2019. The results will be available in February 2020.

2 The ZAFH care4care Research Network

The ZAFH care4care research association, consisting of the lead University of Applied Sciences Esslingen, the Ravensburg-Weingarten University of Applied Sciences and the Institute for Applied Economic Research, located in Tübingen, is investigating three different yet closely interwoven *fields of action:*

- Field of action I: Retaining skilled workers in the nursing profession
- Field of action II: Attracting new skilled workers or tapping new potential
- Field of action III: Increasing the attractiveness of the nursing profession

The research network is supported by two practice partners: the Berufsgenossenschaft für Gesundheitsdienst und Wohlfahrtspflege and the Welcome Center Sozialwirtschaft Baden-Württemberg. The network is funded for 3 years by the Ministry of Science, Research and Arts Baden-Württemberg with EU structural funds (EFRE).

The various methodological approaches and the results of the different subprojects are triangulated throughout the entire research process and validated with nursing practice using a variety of formats. The application-oriented character of the network is intended to guarantee that the results can be implemented in practice.

3 The Sub-project of the Hochschule Esslingen

"Retaining skilled workers" and "Attracting new skilled workers or tapping new potential" are the fields of action to be addressed at The University of Applied Sciences Esslingen. In the course of this process, this sub-project focuses on the company's actions. In addition to the Delphi survey, a methodological approach was chosen that includes expert interviews and operational case studies as further survey methods. This mix of methods can ensure that the following goals are achieved:

- Adaptive strategies for systematic personnel recruitment, retention and development are developed, taking into account the necessary political and social framework.
- Adaptive strategies for dealing with professional, life-world and cultural diversity of nursing staff are developed with regard to complex and different needs, as well as demands on professional nursing.
- There are concrete indications for the further development of the nursing profession, its differentiation into different qualification levels and forms, as well as a sharpening of the professional profile in the context of interprofessional cooperation.

Before the Delphi survey is discussed in detail, the intertwining of the Delphi survey with the operational case studies and expert interviews within the sub-project is presented.

At the beginning of the project, a comprehensive literature review and explorative *expert interviews* were used to identify dimensions of action that served as a basis for the construction of the survey instruments of the Delphi survey and the operational case studies. In order to avoid moving within prefabricated topics in connection with the topic of the need for skilled nursing staff, the explorative expert interviews had the function of determining practice-saturated experiential knowledge, which, on the one hand, consists of field understanding and action routines, but, on the other hand, also of knowledge of innovative projects, which may require further verification (Meuser & Nagel, 2013, p. 460 f.). Parallel to the Delphi survey and the operational case studies, further exemplary in-depth interviews with experts will be conducted, so that certain project-relevant questions can be comprehensively included in the analysis that cannot be clarified using the other survey methods. At the end of the survey phase, further expert interviews are planned for the purpose of validation.

Within the framework of the *focused multi-perspective operational case studies,* the operational actions in relation to the need for qualified nursing staff are analysed. The aim of the operational case studies is to explore the topic of the need for skilled workers from different perspectives within several institutions. In this way, the question can be answered as to which action requirements are identified and how the need for action is communicated in everyday operational life to the places where action can and must be taken. In addition, the development and evaluation of solution strategies are analysed in the individual companies. The operational case studies thus serve to examine the concrete challenges, problems and ways of dealing with the need for skilled workers in day-to-day operations on the basis of defined topics.

The results of the expert interviews and the operational case studies flow into the Delphi survey throughout the entire research process – and vice versa. In this way, new findings can be directly linked. Figure 1 provides an overview of the methodological procedure of the project.

4 The Delphi Survey of ZAFH care4care

How do different groups in the care sector act to actively meet the demand for skilled workers? Which measures and strategies are applied and which are not? What conditions are necessary for the implementation of these measures and strategies? Which measures and strategies are considered effective for the recruitment and retention of skilled nursing staff?

These questions seem to be widely answered by various national literature (cf. e.g. Zängl, 2015; Behr, 2015) and international studies, as well as comparisons (cf. e.g. Lartey et al., 2014; Heintze, 2015; Simon & Mehmecke, 2017; Romppanen & Häggman-Laitila, 2017). However, through the expert interviews already conducted, it is apparent that the scale, scope and conceptual underpinnings of interventions vary widely across the care sector. This discrepancy plays a central role in the Delphi survey of the ZAFH care4care. Since there is no empirical evidence as to which measures and strategies of securing skilled labour are applied in the institutions of the care sector in Baden-Württemberg, experts are asked in the Delphi survey to assess this uncertain state of affairs, about which only incomplete knowledge exists, by means of a structured group communication process (Häder & Häder, 1995, p. 12). This makes it possible to analyse which measures are assessed as effective and are actually implemented and which framework conditions are necessary for this. In addition, it can be investigated which innovative ideas are

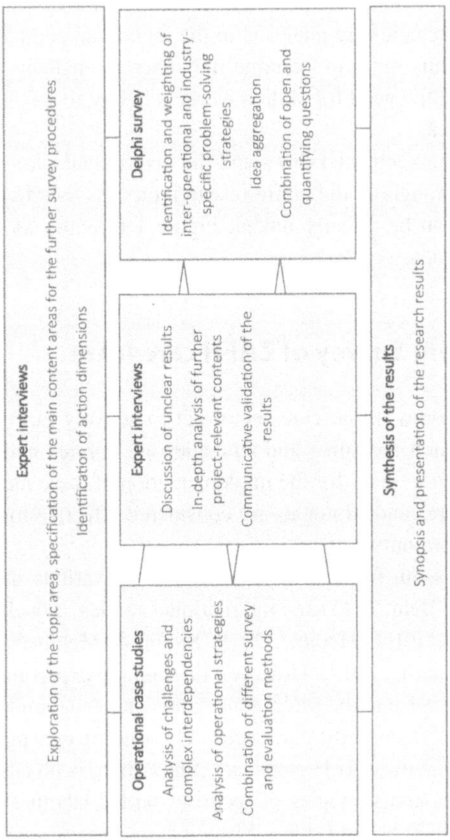

Fig. 1 Research design of the ZAFH care4care – Esslingen sub-project. (Source: Own representation, © ZAFH care4care)

practiced in the Baden-Württemberg nursing landscape – in the best case with success.

The content structure of the questionnaire follows pre-identified dimensions of action that were derived as a result of the expert interviews and the literature review (Niederberger & Renn, 2018, p. 9). These key themes form an initial blueprint of the project. They name those topics which, for nursing practice, decisively determine the everyday work of nursing professionals in the context of the nursing shortage:

- Education
- Participation
- Human resources development
- Migration
- Work organisation and leadership
- Care financing
- Intra–/interprofessional cooperation
- Sectoral cooperation

At the end of the Delphi survey, adaptive strategies and measures will therefore be discussed on the basis of the identified dimensions of action, taking into account the necessary political and social framework across companies and sectors.

This goal is based on the assumption that corporate action is determined by different participants and different logics of action. These logics of action and the associated actions can vary considerably in some cases. Even if all participants are confronted with the sector-wide need for skilled nursing staff, this can, however, be felt differently in the individual facilities - a few facilities have sufficient staff and many others struggle with the effects of the need for skilled staff. These preconditions form the basis for deriving the research guiding questions of the Delphi survey (see figure). The premises and the research questions presented in Fig. 2 show that operational action - especially the constellations of action - as well as the promoting but also inhibiting factors of this action are not sufficiently known. Accordingly, a type 3 Delphi, i.e. a "Delphi survey to identify and qualify a diffuse set of facts" (Hader, 2014, p. 33 f.), is conducted to determine this unclear state of affairs. "Expert opinions (...) are subjected to a quantifying evaluation, which means that their majority capability is presented and tested" (Ibid., p. 33 f.).

Selection and Recruitment of Experts

In order to analyse this object of investigation, nursing managers of all organisations offering professional nursing services as well as headmasters of nursing

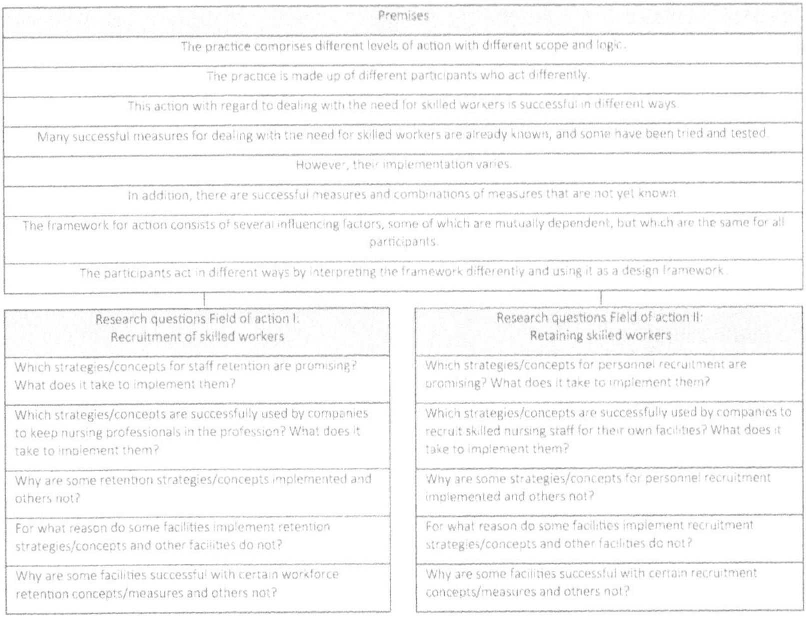

Fig. 2 Research design of the ZAFH care4care – Esslingen sub-project. (Source: Own representation, © ZAFH care4care)

schools in the Neckar-Alb region and the urban district of Stuttgart will be interviewed. Accordingly, a full survey was conducted in these regions. The Neckar-Alb region was selected because the spatial categories of the state of Baden-Württemberg are represented here on a "small scale" (Wirtschaftsministerium Baden-Württemberg, 2002). This means that both urban and rural areas can be included in the survey. The concentration on the urban district of Stuttgart as the state capital is intended to show the special features and problems of a large city. The selection of the two groups of respondents (nursing directors and school directors) is based on the fact that the nursing directors exercise the decision-making authority in the field of nursing and are thus responsible for the nursing professionals employed and (also) responsible for the recruitment of new nursing professionals. The school management of the training institutions are primarily responsible for the training of prospective nursing specialists. The sampling includes 468 institutions.

For the survey, there is deliberately no pre-selection of facilities on the basis of facility size or other structural characteristics in order to generate an image of care service providers in their diversity. Since the nursing professionals work in a very differentiated sector with heterogeneous characteristics, such as different care settings, carrier structures, legal forms, financing and tariff systems, the challenge in the construction of the design and the questionnaires is to reflect this diversity. In order to ensure a sector-wide overview across the different rounds, all experts are asked to participate in each round of the survey and not only the participants of the previous round. This procedure can possibly even contribute to increasing the response rate in the second round (Brosi et al., 2003, p. 15). The effects of sampling on questionnaire construction are explained in Sect. 4.1.

Procedure of the Delphi Survey

In concrete terms, this means that a three-stage Delphi procedure will be used to comprehensively and differentiatedly survey the operational actions of the care sector with regard to securing skilled workers and to discuss the effectiveness of these actions. In the first round, assessments of the need for skilled nursing staff in Baden-Württemberg and in the specific facility, measures for securing skilled staff within the individual facilities and a ranking of the most important topics with regard to securing skilled staff are asked. The measures are queried on the basis of the key topics identified in advance. These are used as the basis for the Delphi survey as dimensions of action, whereby the topics and areas of action were selected that can be assessed and influenced by the company. For example, the respondents cannot take any action within certain areas that are regulated, for example, due to legal requirements. These dimensions of action, which were selected for the Delphi survey, form the contextual framework. Thus, the focus of the analysis is the handling of the current nursing staff demand in Baden-Württemberg and thus also the active shaping of future nursing care, in the form of operational possibilities for action. By evaluating the effectiveness and feasibility of the measures in the survey, which is represented by a joint assessment of the experts, a selection of measures can subsequently be made available to the institutions in the care sector. These can then be adapted by the companies to the specific conditions on site. Figure 3 shows the process and the objectives of the individual rounds. This presentation serves as an initial overview. On the following pages, the methodological procedure and the conception of the Delphi survey will be explained in detail, i.e. the individual rounds will be presented with regard to their conception, justification, evaluation procedure and result utilisation, as well as challenges.

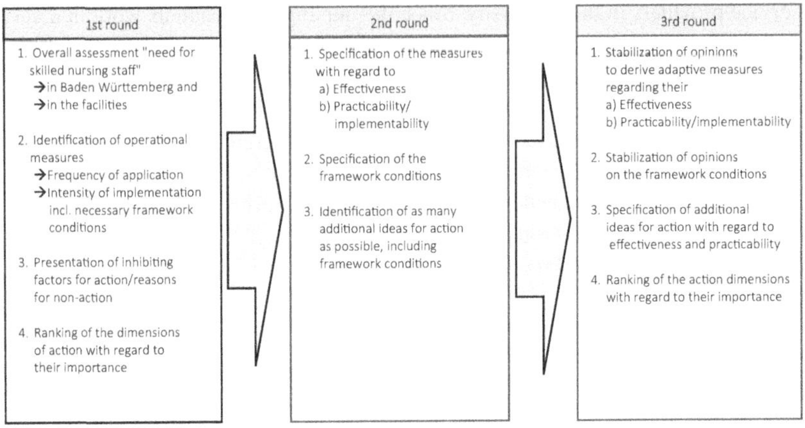

Fig. 3 Procedure and objectives of the Delphi survey ZAFH care4care. (Source: Own representation, © ZAFH care4care)

4.1 Design of the Delphi Survey

The three-stage Delphi procedure of ZAFH care4care is multi-layered: It includes qualitative as well as quantitative survey components and strives to satisfy the conditions of diversity and complexity of the care sector, but also of the object of investigation. The overall design provides for different types of questions with different objectives to be asked in each round of the survey. Nevertheless, the dimensions of action developed across all three survey rounds are to serve as structure-forming elements. Ideally, all respondents should participate in the survey across all rounds. In rounds 2 and 3, individual results of the preliminary round(s) will be presented and, if necessary, deviations and anomalies will be discussed. The Delphi survey is designed as an online survey. The traceability of the panel process is guaranteed via ID. This procedure allows that personal and institution-related data are not asked repeatedly in the following rounds, as they are only collected during the first participation in the survey.

4.1.1 Round 1

The focus of the first round is on the survey of the current situation in two respects: on the one hand, an assessment is made of the overall need for skilled nursing staff and, on the other hand, the intensity of action taken in different areas to meet the need for skilled staff is surveyed. Accordingly, the objectives of the first round are defined as follows:

- An overall assessment of the situation with regard to the "need for skilled nursing staff" has been made.
- The key themes are examined as dimensions of action with regard to their frequency of application or intensity of implementation and the framework conditions required.
- Reasons for low implementation intensity of the action dimensions are analysed.
- The dimensions of action are weighted according to their importance with regard to staff recruitment and retention.[1]

The results of the first round condition the conception of the second round of questioning. On the one hand, further aspects of questions that were sufficiently answered in the first round can be asked. On the other hand, topics that are not sufficiently saturated can be asked again. Assessments of discrepancies and deviations can also be discussed or unclear results can be fed back.

(a) **Challenges**

The implementation of these objectives in the questionnaire design is associated with some methodological and content-related challenges that have to be considered throughout all rounds – but especially in the first round. The combination of the survey of the measures with the recording of their frequency of application or intensity of implementation requires a questionnaire that couples closed parts and open questions. The design of the questionnaire for the first round thus corresponds to an extended Delphi survey, as it is neither a classic Delphi (Niederberger & Renn, 2018, p. 9 ff.) nor a purely qualitative or standardised first round of questioning (Häder, 2014, p. 91 ff.).

The *heterogeneity of the sample*, which has already been discussed, makes the creation of the questionnaire difficult. When selecting the questions, care was therefore taken to ensure that the occupational groups of geriatric nursing and health care and (paediatric) nursing in the different settings of acute care, inpatient short/long-term care, outpatient care, etc. are adequately represented. Accordingly, dimensions of action are selected that are relevant for the various occupational groups in the different care settings. In addition, the functions and types of institution (health care/nursing institution or institution for nursing education, further

---

[1]The ranking information is only a snapshot that may change in the final evaluation (Vorgrimler & Wübben, 2003, p. 773). Therefore, these results can be presented and re-performed in the further course of the survey.

education or training) of the respondents are very different. This circumstance is taken into account by appropriate filtering in the survey.

Due to the complexity and multi-layered nature of the object of investigation as well as a large number of independent variables, the *selection of key topics* and their subsequent transformation into dimensions of action are of great importance. Since the questionnaire should not be too long, the most important dimensions of action are selected, which allow the mapping of the (non-)action of the surveyed institutions. Or in other words: there are relevant variables that can influence the context of the need for skilled workers but are not included in the survey.

Another important factor for the success of the first round of the Delphi survey is the *retention of experts* across all rounds. The participation in all three rounds has the benefit for the respondents of getting an insight into the measures and strategies of the care industry as a whole exclusively before the publication of the results. If necessary, impulses for their own work can already be derived from this during the survey period. However, the data can also serve as a source of information as to which prerequisites must be met in order to implement effective measures in practice and to cover the need for skilled workers in the respective institution.

(b) **Structure and questionnaire construction**

In addition to questions about the institution and the person, the questionnaire for the first round contains three content blocks. The questions about the facility (block 1) are asked at the beginning. Here, for example, it is asked to which care sector the facility belongs. These questions are used for filtering and clustering the facilities surveyed in order to carry out individual evaluations for individual subgroups and settings. Further facility-related and personal data are asked at the end of the questionnaire (block 5). As a substitute for subjective competence questions (Häder, 2014, p. 131 ff.; Niederberger & Renn, 2018, p. 78 ff.), the participants' experience in the respective function is recorded.

Block 2: This block of questions deals with the need for nursing staff at different levels. In this way, it is analysed how the need for qualified nursing staff is assessed in Baden-Württemberg and in one's own facility. The scope of one's own measures in relation to the overall need for skilled workers is also surveyed. From this, it can be deduced whether the facilities are actively addressing the need for skilled workers and with what success they are doing so.

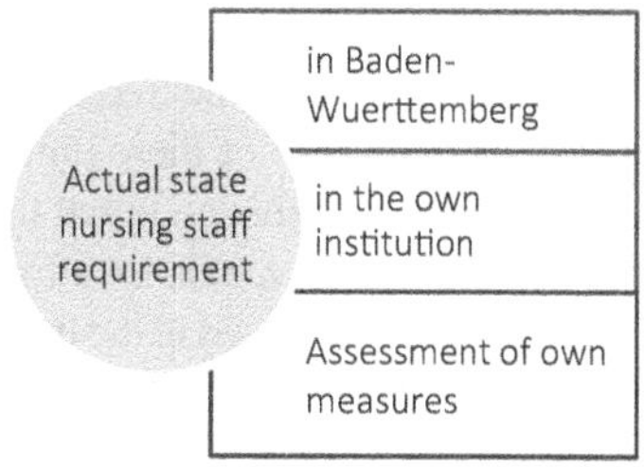

Block 3: The relevant contents of the dimensions of action form the structuring-framework of the third block of questions: training, external presentation, leadership, working conditions and work organisation, enabling career prospects as well as influence and co-determination. Within selected topics, closed questions are asked about forms of operational action. In this context, it is stated whether and to what intensity measures are taken in a certain area. If the previous question is answered positively, open questions are then asked about measures that have been successfully applied and the framework conditions required for this. In order to inquire about the reasons why no systematic planning and application of measures takes place, different answer options are presented in a closed form. These questions are asked of respondents who do not take any measures. By specifying the dimensions of action and the systematic nature of the questions, it is possible to ascertain the intensity of implementation of company action with regard to the issue of "skilled labour requirements". At the same time, the expected diversity of the open answers (due to the heterogeneous sample), which would have required a high level of abstraction in the evaluation, can be countered (Häder, 2014, p. 122).

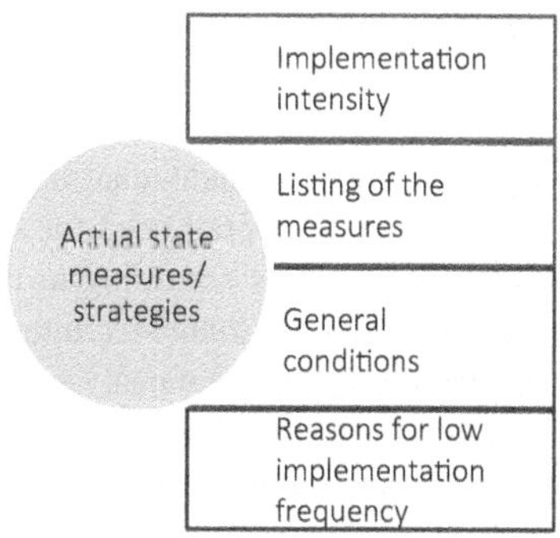

Block 4: Here, the dimensions of action are evaluated with regard to their importance for the two fields of action of personnel recruitment and retention. These questions serve to analyse the relevance of these dimensions of action in relation to the two fields of action. In addition, an initial trend is to be derived as to which topic is the most important in each case for attracting or retaining skilled nursing staff. These questions were designed in the manner of ranking questions (Niederberger & Renn, 2018, p. 69).

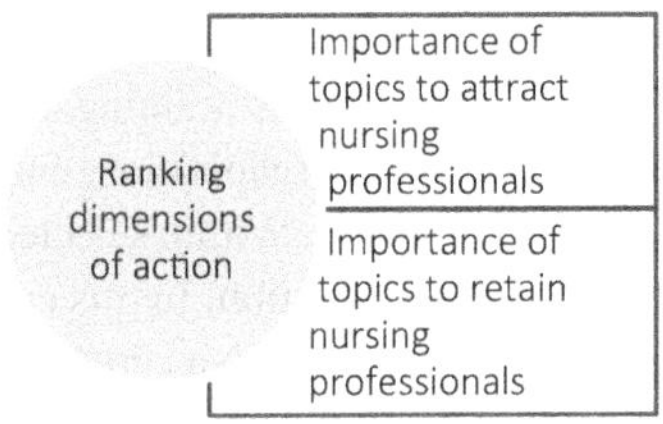

The special features of the questionnaire are the differentiated filtering and the possibility of clustering. The filtering enables the simultaneous recording of measures and inhibiting factors. Clustering offers the possibility of specific evaluations that allow conclusions to be drawn about whether, for example, different actions are taken in different settings.

(c) **Strategy for the evaluation of the results**

The questionnaire contains both qualitative and quantitative elements. Interpretative and numerical analyses are conducted (Niederberger & Renn, 2018, p. 174 f.). Thus, different evaluation methods are applied.

The closed (mostly ordinally scaled) questions are first evaluated descriptively using statistical methods. Group comparisons are then carried out, e.g. by setting and/or legal form, and individual items are tested for statistical correlations, e.g. the degree of implementation intensity of individual measures and the effectiveness of the measures in relation to the overall need for skilled workers. The key topics are weighted as action dimensions according to their effectiveness using mean value calculations with regard to personnel recruitment and retention.

The open questions are evaluated by content analysis (cf. e.g. Meuser & Nagel, 2013, p. 466 f.; Flick, 2012, p. 414 ff.) and clustered into topic areas. For this purpose, similar statements are grouped together and systematized on the basis of keywords. All answers are weighted equally; e.g. assessments of institutions with a large number of employees are not weighted more heavily than those of smaller institutions or vice versa. However, if there are noticeable differences, the results can be clustered according to the type and size of the facilities.

4.1.2 Round 2

In the second round, in addition to feedback on the results of the first round, a quantifying discussion of the measures takes place in order to determine their effectiveness and feasibility – also across sectors. This procedure aims to achieve the highest possible stability of opinions in order to differentiate the data on strategies and measures obtained in round 1. The survey will focus on the following areas:

- The effectiveness of measures within the dimensions of action is specified.
- In addition, the measures are evaluated in terms of their feasibility.
- The social and political framework conditions for the successful implementation of various measures are discussed and specified.
- Further ideas and the necessary framework conditions are generated.

(a) **Challenges**

For the second round of questioning, the focus is on the *assessment* of the *effectiveness* of the measures surveyed and their *feasibility*. Due to the diverse work contexts and settings, the effects, scope and limits of the individual measures can be assessed very differently. The presentation of all answer categories in the questionnaire serves to "trigger thought processes in the participants and thereby induce an improvement of the original judgments in the further course of the survey" (Häder, 2014, p. 200).

The *framework conditions* (e.g. legal, social and health policy requirements) are also assessed with regard to their influence in order to obtain reliable data for the necessary socio-political course settings. In the course of this assessment, the second round will specify the necessary framework conditions, which may have been mentioned in very general terms in the first round. Here, it can be helpful to give examples.

Furthermore, a high commitment of the *experts* to the survey is supported. Since the questionnaire of the first round is extensive, the respondents are informed at the beginning of the second survey wave that this questionnaire is faster to answer. Additionally, the benefit of this round for the respondents is emphasized.

(b) **Structure and questionnaire construction**

At the beginning of the survey, selected descriptive results from the preliminary round will be presented and, if necessary, specific questions will be asked about the results (block 1). The structure or structuring framework is designed analogously to the first round: In addition to the information on the person and the institution (blocks 2 and 5), which serve as filter guidance and clustering, the action dimensions will serve as structure-giving characteristics in the following blocks. The questions on the person and institution will only be asked of those respondents who are taking part in the survey for the first time.

Block 3: The experts are asked to evaluate the aggregated measures with regard to the target variables of personnel recruitment and retention in terms of their effectiveness and the aggregated framework conditions required for this. Furthermore, in this block, analogous to the evaluation of effectiveness, evaluations of feasibility are also carried out. This block of questions is particularly interesting in contrast to the items on effectiveness, since a measure can be very effective but not applicable in practice. This makes it possible to analyse the discrepancy between possible action and actual action in the area of securing skilled labour.

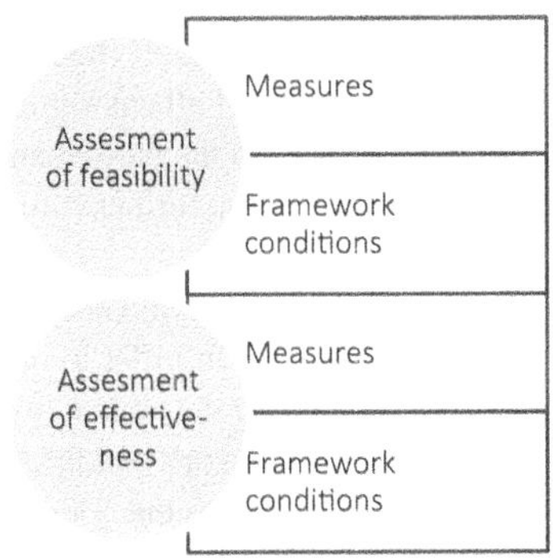

Block 4: The content block of the questionnaire concludes with the "magic wand question", i.e. if all resources were available, which measures should be taken and which (political, legislative) framework conditions would have to be changed for this. The insight interest of this block is based on the fact that par-

ticularly innovative measures are identified and can be presented and evaluated in the next round.

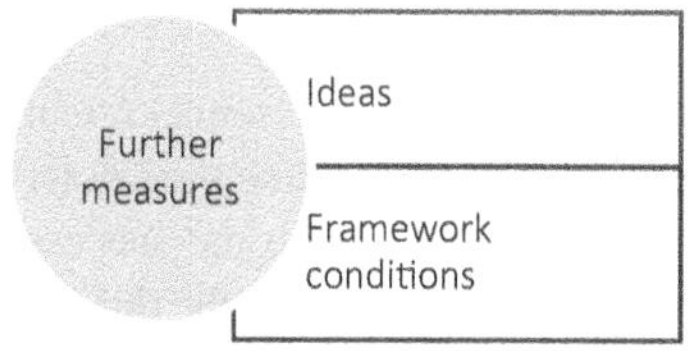

(c) **Strategy for the evaluation of the results**

The assessments of effectiveness and feasibility are evaluated descriptively. For this purpose, frequencies are listed, medians, arithmetic means and standard deviations are presented for quasi-metric data. The coefficient of variation can be used to assess whether the item is inconsistently assessed and thus should be asked again in the next round (Niederberger & Renn 2018, p. 88). In addition, special attention is paid to the correlation of feasibility and effectiveness in order to assess the participants' ability to act. The open "magic wand question" – analogous to the open questions of the first round of the survey – will be evaluated and categorised using content analysis.

Overall, it should be noted that individual measures that are not capable of gaining majority support can nevertheless be effective in practice and are included in the analysis. Here it is the task of the researchers to take these into account in the course of the content-analytical evaluation of the open questions – otherwise there is a risk that innovative ideas may be lost.

4.1.3 Round 3

The aim of the third round is to map a majority stable opinion (Häder, 2014, p. 33 f., 125) on adaptive measures and ideas for action in relation to the two fields of action. For this purpose, the topics are again processed for evaluation. Unclear or divergent results are reflected back to the participants and presented again for assessment. The desirable measures are also assessed for their feasibility and effectiveness. The ranking of the action dimensions is carried out again to check the stability of opinions.

A fourth round of questioning is not planned so as not to go beyond the time frame and the conception of the survey and not to overstrain the participants.

Experience shows that a satisfactory result can be achieved after three rounds (Häder, 2014, p. 126).

(a) **Challenges**

In order to discuss adaptive strategies of personnel retention and recruitment, it is necessary to develop effective and at the same time practicable measures. For this purpose, the information obtained so far on the successfully implemented – but also desirable – measures will be processed in the third round. In this context, particular care must be taken to ensure that, when combining the different results in the online questionnaire, the meaningfulness and *manageability* of the online questionnaire is not negatively affected due to the different levels and target variables.

Another challenge will be the *stability of opinions* regarding rankings of effectiveness and feasibility. Due to the complexity of the issue and the very heterogeneous sample, it is possible that different opinions will be generated in some topics. However, this does not necessarily mean that the measures are not suitable for a majority, but rather that it is necessary to carry out a very differentiated evaluation in order to identify possible group-specific agreements. If the assessments and opinions on individual dimensions of action do not produce uniform or group-specific recommendations overall (Häder, 2014, p. 125) or dissents (Niederberger & Renn, 2018, p. 13), this is also a result worth discussing.

(b) **Structure and questionnaire construction**

The final questionnaire of the Delphi survey again contains the questions on personal and institution-related data (blocks 1 and 4), since it is always possible that respondents participate who did not take part in a previous round. However, only these participants will receive these questions in the third round. In this way, clustering and filtering can be guaranteed across all rounds.

Block 2: Measures that were assessed as divergent are assessed again in terms of their effectiveness and practicability, taking into account the assessment of the previous round. Those measures that were not assessed as effective or practicable in the previous round are not asked again - unless an unexplainable divergence emerges in the synopsis of the responses (Niederberger & Renn, 2018, p. 89).

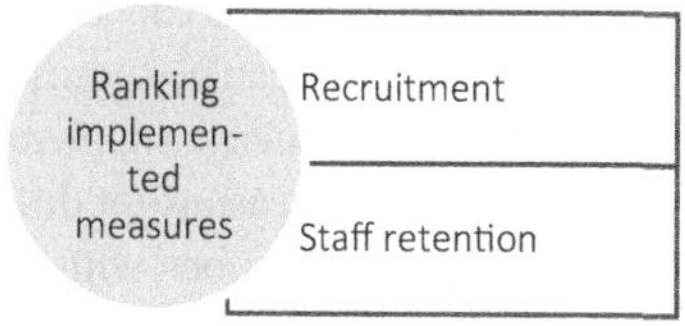

Block 3: Here, the desirable measures of the second round are evaluated for the first time with regard to their effectiveness and feasibility. Only those ideas are presented that are relevant to the subject of the study.

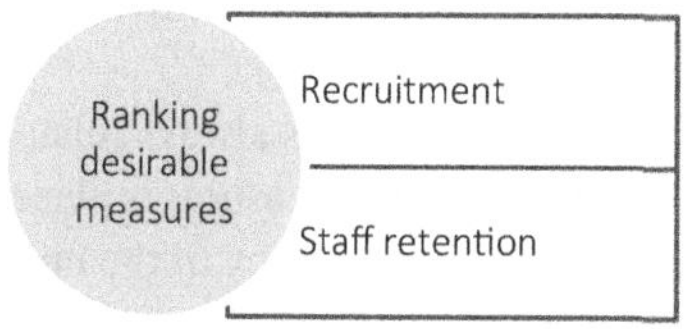

Block 4: Here, a ranking of the dimensions of action takes place again. The ranking refers in each case to the importance of the individual dimensions of action in relation to measures for personnel recruitment and retention - analogous to the ranking of the first round. This makes it possible to check whether the assessment of the rankings changes as a result of the reflection of the assessments from the first round of the survey (Vorgrimler & Wübben, 2003, p. 773) and the addition of further ideas.

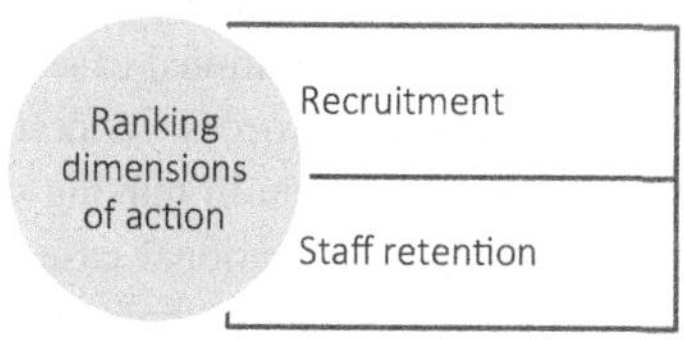

(c) **Strategy for the evaluation of the results**

Analogous to the second round, a descriptive evaluation and a presentation of the mean values and measures of dispersion will take place (Niederberger & Renn, 2018, p. 92). The results are analysed to determine whether there is consensus or dissent among the experts on the individual measures, their effectiveness and feasibility. The discrepancy about certain measures can also be an important result, as it may reveal the extent to which a measure can be successful in one institution and not in others. When analysing the discrepancies, supplementary expert interviews can be a suitable instrument to analyse the reasons for differing assessments. Here, for example, experts from umbrella organisations with a superior knowledge can become relevant. The specification of the assessments with regard to the feasibility of the measures allows forecasts about whether the implementation of individual measures can succeed.

In addition, the ranking of the dimensions for action can be used to set priorities in terms of measures to retain and recruit staff. The most important dimensions of action represent the highest need for action. These results must be interpreted in different settings, financing and tariff systems, carrier structures, etc., in order to develop adaptive strategies for the care sector.

The interpretation of all collected data is always related to further context variables. The development of strategies and measures is placed in relation to overarching aspects. These include the historical legacy of the nursing profession as a typically female profession and the general logic associated with *care work* (Friese, 2017). Furthermore, the intensification of the problematic due to demographic change and medical-technical progress as well as the increasing economization in the context of a neoliberalization (Krampe, 2015) are to be discussed. An isolated analysis and interpretation of the surveyed measures would not suffice for the diversity of the object of investigation.

4.2 Triangulation

The results of the individual rounds of the Delphi survey are taken into account in the development of instruments for the operational case studies and further expert interviews throughout the entire research process – and vice versa. In this way, the topic of personnel recruitment and retention in nursing can be discussed both in breadth (Delphi survey) and in depth (operational case studies and expert interviews), and weaknesses of one method can be balanced by the strengths of the other (Schnell et al., 2005, p. 262).

The collected measures and reasons for non-action can be discussed in depth directly in the companies of the care sector within the framework of the operational case studies and, if necessary, expanded or adapted. In addition, interesting findings from the operational case studies can be assessed by experts in the form of supplementary items in the Delphi survey. Parallel to the Delphi survey and the operational case studies, expert interviews will be conducted. These serve, among other things, to deepen or explain unclear facts from the other surveys with those active in the environment of the care sector - such as interest groups, politics, cost bearers, etc. Conversely, new findings from these supplementary interviews can flow into the Delphi survey. In the course of this process, transparent documentation is an important component of triangulation, in order to make the origin of new aspects (collected from another data source) comprehensible to the respondents.

Triangulation offers the possibility for the Delphi survey to include new contents directly and to have them assessed by experts. The multi-method approach is appropriate in view of the complexity and multi-layeredness of the topic in order to discuss the object of the study "Operational action for adaptive handling of the need for skilled workers" and to show ways how skilled workers can be recruited and retained in their profession.

5 Conclusion

According to the Nursing Thermometer 2018 (Isfort & Weidner, 2018, p. 66), there are 13,900 vacancies (in full-time equivalents) in Germany. There are hardly any other sectors with so many vacancies – even though the shortage of skilled workers has permeated all areas of the labour market. Institutions, providers, umbrella organisations, politicians and cost bearers are trying to make adjustments, but they are still not succeeding in recruiting more skilled personnel across the board and reducing fluctuation. Now it is a matter of finding concrete approaches that contribute to an improvement of the nursing staff situation. This is where ZAFH care4care comes in, with the aim of developing adaptive strategies for recruiting and retaining staff in cooperation with nursing practice.

In this context, the Delphi survey is a suitable method to generate strategies and measures of operational action from practice for practice. The success of a Delphi survey of type 3 in relation to a multi-layered object of investigation depends on many aspects. These include the design of the individual rounds, the selection of the right addressees and dimensions of action in their area of responsibility, the evaluation of the individual rounds taking into account the results of the previous rounds, as well as the interpretation of the results on the basis of different contexts and intervening variables. Accordingly, it makes sense to conduct extensive preliminary research at the beginning of a Delphi survey (in this case in the form of a comprehensive literature review and interviews with experts) in order to structure the diffuse facts in advance. The formulation of objectives is indispensable in order to define the basic population and the sampling and to make a selection of topics. In the next step, the overall design of the Delphi survey including the objectives and the possibilities of interleaving the individual rounds has to be worked out. Thereupon, the individual dimensions are operationalized and transferred into a questionnaire. The evaluation of the answers and the development of the questionnaires for the following rounds can run in parallel. Even if the individual steps are described here in a linear way, the development and implementation of the Delphi survey is a circular process, since the sub-steps are mutually dependent.

A potential risk of a Delphi study is the isolated construction of the questionnaire for one round without considering the further rounds. Furthermore, with regard to the sample, there is the general challenge of identifying suitable experts, making the benefits of the survey sufficiently transparent to them, and thus being able to win them over for participation in all survey rounds.

Due to the far-reaching consideration of diverse special features of the nursing sector and its complex questionnaire constructions, a continuous process of discussion and reflection beyond the core team is indispensable. The procedure can be described as a constant process of negotiation in order to appropriately address the subject matter, but still ensure the manageability of the survey. This Delphi procedure is basically a further development of the ideal-typical Delphi type 3 "for the determination and qualification of a diffuse issue", since here opinions are obtained on an as yet indeterminable issue, but, in addition, elements of a quantitative survey are also included. In this way, at the same time the measures themselves can be recorded and evaluated for effectiveness and feasibility, but also the intensity of implementation and conducive or inhibiting framework conditions of operational action can be presented. For the health and nursing sciences, such a complex Delphi procedure is both innovative and forward-looking.

Literature

Behr, T. (Eds.). (2015). *Aufbruch Pflege: Hintergründe – Analysen – Entwicklungsperspektiven.* Springer.

Bonin, H., Braeseke, G., & Ganserer, A. (2015). *Internationale Fachkräfterekrutierung in der deutschen Pflegebranche: Chancen und Hemmnisse aus Sicht der Einrichtungen.* Bertelsmann Stiftung.

Brosi, W. H., Krekel, E. M., & Ulrich, J. G. (2003). *Delphi-Erhebung zur Identifikation von Forschungs- und Entwicklungsaufgaben in der beruflichen Aus- und Weiterbildung.* https://www.bibb.de/dokumente/pdf/wd_65_delphi-erhebung.pdf. Accessed 25 June 2018.

DGB Bundesvorstand (Eds.). (2015). *Zwischenbilanz zum Ausbildungspakt in der Altenpflege (2012–2015).* http://doku.iab.de/externe/2015/k150423r25.pdf. Accessed 25 June 2018.

Flick, U. (2012). *Qualitative Sozialforschung. Eine Einführung* (5th ed.). rowohlts enzyklopädie im Rowohlt Taschenbuch.

Friese, M. (2017). Care Work. Eckpunkte der Professionalisierung und Qualitätsentwicklung in personenbezogenen Dienstleistungsberufen. In U. Weyland & K. Reiber (Eds.), *Entwicklungen und Perspektiven in den Gesundheitsberufen – Aktuelle Handlungs- und Forschungsfelder* (pp. 29–49). Bertelsmann. (Berichte zur beruflichen Bildung).

Häder, M. (2014). *Delphi-Befragungen. Ein Arbeitsbuch* (3rd ed.). Springer.

Häder, M., & Häder, S. (1995). Delphi und Kognitionspsychologie. Ein Zugang zur theoretischen Fundierung der Delphi-Methode. *ZUMA-Nachrichten, 37,* 8–34. http://www.gesis.org/fileadmin/upload/forschung/publikationen/zeitschriften-/zuma_nachrichten/zn_37.pdf. Accessed 25 June 2018.

Heintze, C. (2015). *Auf der Highroad. Der skandinavische Weg zu einem zeitgemäßen Pflegesystem: Ein Vergleich zwischen fünf nordischen Ländern und Deutschland; Expertise im Auftrag der Abteilung Wirtschafts- und Sozialpolitik der Friedrich-Ebert-Stiftung* (2nd ed.). WISO Diskurs Expertisen und Dokumentationen zur Wirtschafts- und Sozialpolitik. Friedrich-Ebert-Stiftung Abt. Wirtschafts- und Sozialpolitik.

Isfort, M., & Weidner, F. (2018). *Pflege-Thermometer 2018. Eine bundesweite Befragung von Leitungskräften zur Situation der Pflege und Patientenversorgung in der stationären Langzeitpflege in Deutschland.* Köln: Deutsches Institut für angewandte Pflegeforschung e. V. (DIP). https://www.dip.de/fileadmin/data/pdf/projekte/Pflege_Thermometer_2018.pdf. Accessed 21 June 2018.

Krampe, E.-M. (2015). Zwischenbilanz und aktuelle Entwicklungen in der Akademisierung der Gesundheitsberufe. In J. Pundt & K. Kälble (Eds.), *Gesundheitsberufe und gesundheitsberufliche Bildungskonzepte* (pp. 139–164). Apollon University Press.

Lartey, S., Cummings, G., & Profetto-McGrath, J. (2014). Interventions that promote retention of experienced registered nurses in health care settings: A systematic review. *Journal of Nursing Management, 22*(8), 1027–1041.

Meuser, N., & Nagel, U. (2013). Experteninterviews – Wissenssoziologische Voraussetzungen und methodische Durchführung. In B. Friebertshäuser, A. Langer, & A. Prengel (Eds.), *Handbuch qualitative Forschungsmethoden in der Erziehungswissenschaft* (4th ed., pp. 457–471). Beltz.

Niederberger, M., & Renn, O. (2018). *Das Gruppendelphi-Verfahren. Vom Konzept bis zur Anwendung*. Springer.

Romppanen, J., & Häggman-Laitila, A. (2017). Interventions for nurses' well-being at work: A quantitative systematic review. *Journal of Advanced Nursing, 73*(7), 1555–1569.

Rothgang, H., Müller, R., & Unger, R. (2012). *Themenreport "Pflege 2030": Was ist zu erwarten – Was ist zu tun?* Bertelsmann Stiftung.

Schnell, R., Hill, P. B., & Esser, E. (2005). *Methoden der empirischen Sozialforschung* (7th ed.). Oldenbourg Wissenschaftsverlag GmbH.

Simon, M., & Mehmecke, S. (2017). *Nurse-to-Patient Ratios: Ein internationaler Überblick über staatliche Vorgaben zu einer Mindestbesetzung im Pflegedienst der Krankenhäuser.* https://www.boeckler.de/pdf/p_fofoe_WP_027_2017.pdf. Accessed 20 June 2018.

Vorgrimler, D., & Wübben, D. (2003). Die Delphi-Methode und ihre Eignung als Prognoseinstrument. *Wirtschaft und Statistik, 8*, 763–774.

Wirtschaftsministerium Baden-Württemberg (Eds.). (2002). *Landesentwicklungsplan Baden-Württemberg 2002. – LEP 2002.* https://vm.baden-wuerttemberg.de/fileadmin/redaktion/m-mvi/intern/Dateien/Broschueren-/Landesentwichlungsplan_2002.PDF. Accessed 25 June 2018.

Zängl, P. (Ed.). (2015). *Zukunft der Pflege: 20 Jahre Norddeutsches Zentrum zur Weiterentwicklung der Pflege*. Springer.

Assessment of Health-Related Measures Using the Group Delphi Method

Michael M. Zwick, Marco Sonnberger, Jürgen Deuschle, and Regina Schröter

Abstract

Delphi methods are considered to be the best way to obtain scientifically based forecasts of future events and developments that are as reliable as possible. As part of a BMBF project on juvenile obesity, we used the Group Delphi method to ask experts and stakeholders to assess measures for the prevention of excess weight and obesity in childhood and adolescence in terms of their reasonableness, effectiveness and feasibility, as well as which social institutions should implement the respective measures. This article presents our implementation of a Group Delphi process in order to give the reader an idea of how such work-

M. M. Zwick (✉)
University of Stuttgart, Sociology of Technology, Risk and Environment, Stuttgart, Germany
e-mail: zwick@sowi.uni-stuttgart.de

M. Sonnberger
ZIRIUS – Centre for Interdisciplinary Risk and Innovation Studies, University of Stuttgart, Stuttgart, Germany
e-mail: marco.sonnberger@zirius.uni-stuttgart.de

J. Deuschle
Deizisau, Germany
e-mail: juergen@die-radler.de

R. Schröter
Tamm, Germany
e-mail: regina.schroeter@me.com

M. Niederberger, O. Renn (eds.), *Delphi Methods In The Social And Health Sciences*, https://doi.org/10.1007/978-3-658-38862-1_11

shops are practically applied and to demonstrate their advantages and shortcomings.

1 Introduction

Even before the turn of the millennium, excess weight and obesity were regarded as ongoing problems in Germany that received varying degrees of media coverage. Triggered by a report published by the World Health Organisation (WHO) (2000), this topic has gained considerable media, public and political attention since the start of the century and has been framed as an "obesity epidemic" (e.g. Wabitsch et al., 2005; Fankhänel, 2007).

As part of its Socioecological Research programme, the Federal Ministry of Education and Research (BMBF) funded a research project entitled "Excess weight and obesity in children, adolescents and young adults as a systemic risk" between 2006 and 2009. The aim was to scientifically research the causes of juvenile obesity, the living conditions and subjective experiences of overweight and obese children, adolescents and young adults in an interdisciplinary way,[1] and to develop bundles of measures for prevention. In accordance with this broad objective, the disciplines involved pursued a multi-method approach that included the evaluation of nutrition diaries and somatic examinations of those affected (Müller et al., 2011, p. 92), as well as a standardised, representative survey of pupils in three German states (Müller et al., 2011; Krömker & Vogler, 2011), secondary analyses of microcensus data (Helmert et al., 2011), qualitative semi-structured interviews with directly or indirectly affected persons (Peter, 2011; Deuschle & Sonnberger, 2011; Barlösius & Philipps, 2011; Schiek, 2011), expert interviews and focus groups (Zwick, 2011, p. 72).

The bundles of measures for obesity prevention that were identified during the research process on the basis of interviews with experts and focus groups (Zwick & Schröter, 2009, p. 10; 2011, p. 243 f.) were then subjected to a Group Delphi process in spring 2008. The aim was to have experts and stakeholders assessing the measures with regard to their reasonableness, effectiveness and feasibility, but also with regard to which social institutions appear suitable for launching the respective measure. The Group Delphi thereby constituted a transdisciplinary element that

[1] The disciplines involved were sociology, epidemiology, health science, philosophy, physiology, psychology, risk analysis and assessment, social policy, law and economics. (cf. Zwick & Schröter, 2009, p. 7).

was used to identify and assess measures that are practice-oriented and likely to be effective.

Why use a Group Delphi? If relevant and competent experts[2] can be recruited to take part, the Delphi method promises a maximum of assessment certainty in the clarification of complex, ambivalent and highly uncertain questions about the future. The Delphi method is primarily used for the "determination of expert judgements on topics in futurology..." and, as in our case, for "[...] policy development and priority setting" (Schulz & Renn, 2009a, p. 16 f.). Compared to the 'traditional' purely questionnaire-based variant, the particular advantage of the Group Delphi is that the expert judgements can immediately be discursively clarified, especially in the case of disagreement: Is the disagreement a matter of semantics or something more concrete? In the former case, the experts can contribute to the semantic clarification of terms and statements. In the case of factually based disagreement, the reasons for divergent judgements can be discussed and recorded ad hoc by the experts in the group. According to Schulz and Renn, the Group Delphi method has therefore proved particularly useful "for questions that require expert knowledge and an exceptional judgement, and which aim to achieve an interpretative classification of the facts" (Schulz & Renn, 2009b, p. 114).

In the following section, we will reflect on the question of how a Delphi Group may help assessing measures typical of policy advice from a transdisciplinary perspective. In the subsequent section, we will present the Delphi Group as part of our obesity project in more detail, including its structure, benefits, limitations, and results. In a final chapter, we will draw a critical conclusion.

2 The Group Delphi as a Method of Transdisciplinary Knowledge Integration

The term transdisciplinarity refers to a research principle that aims to develop knowledge about a specific social problem by involving different academic disciplines (interdisciplinarity) and non-academic actors (Brandt et al., 2013, p. 1). Transdisciplinary research is thus useful "[...] where a solely professional or disciplinary definition of problems and solutions is not possible" (Mittelstraß, 2005, p. 20). The transdisciplinary research process is divided into three phases: (a) problem identification and transformation (precise definition of the problem to be investigated as well as the translation of the problem into a research question), (b) prob-

[2] In this context, not only academics but also practitioners and stakeholders can be considered "experience-based" experts (Defila & Di Giulio, 2015).

lem analysis (generation of novel insights with regard to the object of investigation), and (c) the formulation of practice-oriented solution and action strategies (development of recommendations for action, measures, prototypes, scenarios, etc.) (Pohl & Hirsch Hadorn, 2008, p. 431; Jahn et al., 2012). All three phases of the transdisciplinary research process draw on the expertise of various relevant scientific disciplines as well as actors outside academia (e.g. from business, civil society, government administration, etc.). One of the greatest challenges here is the systematic integration of the various disciplinary and practice-related bodies of knowledge (Jahn, 2008, pp. 32–33). A distinction is made between the following three forms of knowledge: (a) system knowledge (knowledge about the origins and potential further development of a particular problem), (b) orientation knowledge (knowledge about what goals should be aimed at by changing a particular current state and the extent to which these can be regarded as desirable) and (c) transformation knowledge (knowledge about how to design the path from the current state to the target state) (Pohl & Hirsch Hadorn, 2008, pp. 431–432).

In the transdisciplinary research process, the Group Delphi is of particular importance during the third phase (formulating practice-oriented solution and action strategies), since this involves systematically relating different forms of knowledge to one another and integrating them. In other words, the interdisciplinary academic knowledge about the origin of a certain problem (system knowledge) must be translated into practice-related transformation knowledge. Alternatively, the system knowledge can be used to assess the effectiveness or impact of the transformation knowledge. Ultimately, knowledge about possible solutions must also be critically examined in terms of the social desirability (orientation knowledge) of the associated problem-solving paths. It goes without saying that the desirability of certain problem-solving paths is often assessed differently by different actors depending on their interests and positionings.

The problem of knowledge integration can be illustrated using a simple example: From a medical point of view, it is considered a proven fact that the excessive consumption of fast food makes people overweight. The social science work carried out during the project discussed here has also shown that various factors coalesce to form a set of effects that we have described as an "adipogenic environment". These factors include the effects of affluent societies with their omnipresent supply of food and drink, the advertising of high-calorie foods, their sale in educational institutions, as well as families that are disintegrated and dysfunctional with regard to health literacy, role model behaviour and social support. This can be referred to as system knowledge. This knowledge can be used to develop different options for reducing the consumption of high-calorie food and beverages (e.g. informative measures such as traffic light labels, bans on advertising of excessively sugary or fatty foods, bans on the sale of those foods in public educational institutions, etc.). This is transformational knowledge.

However these options have different levels of desirability, depending on the perspective of the stakeholder assessing them. For instance, taxing certain food ingredients certainly contradicts the objectives of economic interest groups. This is orientation knowledge. The actors involved in the transdisciplinary research process each have their own (different) body of knowledge.

The expertise of academics lies mainly in the field of system knowledge. With regard to transformation knowledge, however, academics usually lack practice-related expertise, and with regard to orientation knowledge they lack the legitimacy to determine the target dimensions of social development processes (Defila & Di Giulio, 2019). It is primarily non-academic actors experienced in the 'real-world' processing of problems (e.g. people from government administration, business or non-governmental organisations, civil society) who can provide the corresponding transformation knowledge. In representative democracies, elected representatives are solely responsible for setting binding goals for social developments. Yet stakeholders, as representatives of group interests and values, also have corresponding orientation knowledge (Renn et al., 1995). This means that orientation knowledge can be represented in the research process through the involvement of stakeholders.

The Group Delphi method makes it possible to assemble a group of different actors who, together, bring with them all three forms of knowledge, and to integrate these different forms in a discursive way. The transformation knowledge can be used to assess the feasibility, the orientation knowledge to assess the desirability and the system knowledge to assess the effectiveness of certain recommendations for action. The result of the Group Delphi is thereby an assessment of recommendations for action in terms of their effectiveness based on scientific knowledge, their feasibility based on practical experience, and their desirability or acceptability from the perspective of different social groups. At the end of the Group Delphi process, socially robust, co-produced knowledge is thus available for solving complex social problems.

3 Obesity in Childhood and Adolescence: Determining Effective Prevention Measures by Means of Group Delphi

3.1 Empirical Preliminary Work for the Identification of Measures

The decision to conduct a Delphi workshop was a response to BMBF's request to develop innovative and robust approaches to the problem of juvenile obesity. This required intensive preliminary work.

To prepare for the workshop, we first carried out an in-depth, exploratory analysis of the extensive qualitative data that had been obtained during the project in order to identify promising preventative measures.[3] This data included ten guided expert interviews on specific topics, in which, among other things, preventive measures that appeared to be suitable were discussed. The experts interviewed included various physicians who deal with the topic of obesity from a medical or psychological perspective, sports and nutrition scientists, kindergarten directors and self-help group organisers, as well as representatives from health insurance companies.

Indications of suitable prevention strategies were also found in a series of 15 focus groups conducted in the second half of 2007 with a wide variety of different participants. We had teachers and educators discuss the topic, conducted focus groups with very overweight adults, some of whom had a long history of unsuccessful diets, while participants in another focus group had lost a massive amount of weight and kept it off for several years. Yet another focus group was made up of people who were using professional help to lose weight and had already lost a considerable amount of weight by the time of the group discussion. Two further focus groups were conducted with Turkish migrants in order to find out about their perspective. Other focus groups included previously overweight adolescents who had also succeeded in losing a considerable amount of weight. In addition, we investigated the experiences of parents of very slim or obese children. Four further focus groups dealt with the specific views and proposed solutions of the food industry, the advertising industry and various actors in the health sector, as well as nutritional and fitness consultants.

[3] This chapter is based on a publication by Michael M. Zwick (2008). Passages that have been taken from that publication are not identified as such.

3.2 The Catalogue of Measures

The discussions and interviews were completely transcribed and systematically analysed for preventive measures with the aid of MAXQDA and thematic coding. In this way, it was possible to identify a total of 475 suggestions for dealing with juvenile obesity that were mentioned in the focus groups and expert interviews.

Next it was necessary to make a manageable selection for the Group Delphi using effective selection filters. For this purpose, we took a brief look at the knowledge gained during the project about the origins of obesity in childhood and adolescence. To us, this knowledge appeared to be multilateral or systemic (Zwick & Renn, 2011, p. 285). From a macroscopic perspective, juvenile obesity proves to be specific to highly industrialised, prosperous and affluent societies that make food and drink (including high-calorie foods) ubiquitous and endlessly available. At the micro level of individual preferences, decisions, and actions, those children and adolescents are most at risk of obesity who have a tendency towards "fat and sweet" tastes and at the same time pursue a sedentary lifestyle and non-physical leisure activities, often with increased media consumption (Zwick, 2011, p. 88). From a preventive point of view, in this situation (the socialising capacity of) the family is seen as primarily responsible for protecting children from some of the fat and disease-inducing temptations of industrial society, and for making them health literate and capable of taking personal responsibility. Unfortunately, however, the families of affected children often prove to be part of the problem themselves. Many of the affected children grow up in an adipogenic social environment that often lacks an awareness of the problem and the skills to deal with it, institutional accessibility and, in some cases, even interest in other family members (Zwick, 2008, p. 62 f.). For these reasons, the following catalogue of measures only contains recommendations directed at various political levels. The state takes on a parental role, so to speak, and has the task of taking preventive action where those affected and their families fail.

In the first step, we eliminated all proposals for measures that did not relate to preventive aspects of problem management in the narrow sense. In the second selection step, we only accepted preventive measures for which political responsibility and regulatory capacity (at whatever level) could exist. A further criterion was the centrality or marginality of the proposed measures: The only measures that had a chance of being submitted to the Delphi workshop were those presented by the interviewees and focus group participants as central—i.e. proposals that were addressed several times, well justified, characterised as effective, or supported by evidence.

Through this multi-stage selection process, we finally succeeded in selecting the following nine measures for the Group Delphi workshop, which formed the basis of the questionnaire we prepared for the first round of discussions:

- Include health education as a subject in the curricula of all year levels in general education schools.
- Expand the sports program in schools to two double lessons per week.
- Ban the sale of high-calorie foods (>10% sugar or > 20% fat) in schools and kindergartens.
- Expand playgrounds and sports facilities close to residential areas and guarantee free access so that children and young people have exercise-intensive leisure alternatives.
- Create agencies to coordinate anti-obesity efforts at the local, state and federal levels.
- Enforce easy-to-understand food labelling in line with the UK traffic light system.
- Enforce a ban on advertising high-calorie foods (>10% sugar or > 20% fat).
- Implement a sustainability-oriented company rating system, with increasing capital procurement costs for risk-producing companies (that might influence obesity in children and adolescents).
- Conduct studies on how children and adolescents in problem groups can be reached (e.g. through their media use) (Zwick & Schröter, 2009, p. 66).

3.3 The Questionnaire Design

The individual measures should be assessed by the experts according to how *reasonable* they are from an institutional point of view (orientation knowledge), how *effective* they appear in terms of problem-solving capacity (system knowledge) and to what extent they are considered *feasible* (transformation knowledge) by the experts. In the questionnaire, we presented the items in the form of rating scales with an interval scale from one to ten points. For the assessment of the effectiveness of measures, we additionally surveyed how certain the participants felt about their decisions from 'very uncertain' to 'very certain' on a four-point ordinal scale. After asking participants about the reasonableness of the individual measures, we added an open question about whether any relevant measures had been forgotten that were worth including in the catalogue and if so, which ones.

Beyond the three dimensions mentioned above, we wanted to use the Delphi method to find out which of the institutions mentioned in the following should take primary responsibility for implementing each of the measures: the federal government, states, municipalities, industry, charities, health insurance funds or insurers, 'nobody' and—asked openly—'who else'? As an icebreaker question, the questionnaire was preceded by a question about how serious the participant considered childhood and adolescent obesity to be compared with nine other problems facing Germany in the next 5–10 years. Once again, rating scales between one and ten points were used.[4]

3.4 The Selection of Experts

Häder describes the search for and recruitment of suitable experts for a Delphi as a crucial but extremely complicated and demanding task (2002, p. 96 f.). These problems are even more pronounced in a group Delphi, when compared to a conventional, web-based Delphi. After all, it is necessary to gather the selected experts together for a workshop on a certain day and at a certain place. This involves a long and time-consuming search for dates, for which we used an internet-based scheduling platform.

The selection of experts was greatly simplified in our case: The work of our obesity project was accompanied by a project advisory board with 20 actors from thematically relevant institutions. Its members represented a wide range of institutions, which were familiar with the research question, project design, theoretical and methodological orientation from the beginning of the project and discussed interim project results with the interdisciplinary team of researchers on a regular basis. Since the members of the advisory board were on the one hand professionally involved with the topic of obesity and on the other hand familiar with the project results, it made sense to recruit the Delphi participants from this group of experts. A total of 13 experts from our project advisory board agreed to participate and met on 5 May 2008 at a conference hotel in Stuttgart (Germany) for the group discussion. The experts' institutional backgrounds included insurance companies, ministries, administrative bodies, associations, food producers and universities or research institutions.

[4]The complete questionnaire is printed in the appendix of the publication by Zwick and Schröter (2009).

In his remarks about the Delphi method, Häder also problematises the appropriate size of the group of experts. His evaluation of the literature reveals an enormous range of recommendations, ranging from seven to an open number of participants; a Japanese Delphi process conducted in 1996 had no less than 4196 experts (Häder, 2002, p. 94 f.). The optimal number of experts depends on several factors, including the scope of the task and the number of relevant institutions and stakeholders involved. However, compared to the numbers mentioned by Häder, for purely practical reasons much narrower limits are set for the size of a Group Delphi: In order to strengthen the discursive element, we intended to have the participants discuss and complete the questionnaires together in small groups of three to four experts, and then have divergent results discussed in plenary. The conference hotel was able to provide us with five rooms, a large one for the plenary discussions and four smaller seminar rooms where the expert groups could fill out the questionnaire. In our case, this procedure proved to be useful and practicable. Based on our experience, we consider four to six groups with three to four participants each to be optimal. On the one hand, this ensures that all experts can sufficiently present their views in the working groups and plenary. On the other hand, the evaluations can be carried out in a reasonably short time.

3.5 The Implementation of the Group Delphi Process

The Group Delphi follows the logic of an iterative, two- or multi-round discourse, which in principle pursues three goals: The assessment of issues using standardised, metric scales in small groups of experts and the subsequent discussion of strongly divergent opinions in the plenary, with the goal of a (successive) convergence of the expert opinions in one or more subsequent rounds of processing. In this process, all items on which there is a broad consensus among the experts are shelved and in each subsequent round of processing only items that are still disputed among the experts are discussed. If the first goal of establishing consensus among the experts is not achieved, the discussions in the plenary open up the possibility of deciding whether the continuing disagreement is semantically based in the formulation of the item or in the subject matter. In the case of semantic ambiguities, items can be discussed immediately, clarified and further processed in an optimised form. In the case of disagreement, the method offers the opportunity to discursively obtain detailed justifications, which give rise to different assessments, and to record those justifications. This is an essential benefit of the Group Delphi approach.

Since we anticipated great problems in engaging experts for more than one workday, we planned our Group Delphi as a one-day workshop in which we envisaged two processing rounds. One group work phase was held in the morning and a second was held in the afternoon, followed by an ad hoc evaluation of the results and a detailed discussion of differing opinions in the plenary.

After two brief introductory speeches—one by the moderator on the Group Delphi method and another by a member of the project team on the content and the questions—and some organisational information, we formed four mixed working groups of three or four participants for each of the two Delphi rounds and gave them the questionnaires. The advantage of having the questionnaire filled out in four small groups rather than individually was to strengthen the discursive element in the processing of the questionnaire, but also to limit the overall workload, since only four completed questionnaires had to be subsequently evaluated.

The decision to have the plenary discussions led by a moderator who is particularly experienced in Group Delphi workshops also proved to be very successful. If the moderator is to enjoy the respect of the invited experts, she or he must not only have an appropriate social status, but also a high level of social and communicative competence and impartiality. It is advisable to take great care in the selection of a suitable moderator, because her or his abilities will to a large extent determine the success or failure of the group discussion (cf. Schulz & Renn, 2009b, p. 115). In our case, the qualities of the moderator turned out to be decisive for the success of the workshop. The institutional logic of the stakeholders in particular led to massive disagreements in the working groups and the plenary session.

The first group work phase took a good hour and a half. During the following lunch break, our team, consisting of two researchers and two assistants, carried out the evaluation of the four questionnaires. Considering the small number of questionnaires, it was relatively easy to do the evaluation using paper, pens and calculators. Due to the targeted selection and the small number of experts, we had to limit the evaluation to basic descriptive statistics (mean and range) (Sahner, 2005, p. 133), whereby we accepted deviating scores up to a maximum of three points as sufficiently "consensual".

The questionnaire was available in the form of an Excel file, into which we transferred the results for the presentation of the results. At the same time we prepared the printing of the questionnaire for the second processing round.

3.6 The Results

The results of the Group Delphi workshop have already been published in detail (Zwick & Schröter, 2009, 2011). In the following, they will only be taken up insofar as they can be used to illustrate the mode of operation, effect, advantages and limitations of the Group Delphi approach.

During our workshop there was no lack of intense and also controversial debates. We made an audio recording of the debates for our evaluation and also prepared the minutes. The analysis of the text material with the help of MAXQDA was based on paraphrases. These were created by refining, supplementing and indexing the minutes using the recordings of the plenary discussions in such a way that, if necessary, it was possible to switch directly to the original sounds of the recordings and extract quotations from them. For the publication of the Group Delphi results, this procedure proved to be extremely successful.

The differences of opinion among the experts were already evident in their answers to the ice-breaker question, which asked them to assess obesity among children and adolescents compared to nine other social problems. The most serious problem assessed by the experts—with a mean score of 7.0 points on a scale of one to ten—was the problem of financing the healthcare system, closely followed by unemployment and global climate change (6.8 points each) and securing Germany's energy needs (6.0). Obesity came next, with an average score of 5.6, followed by securing pensions (5.5) and the problem of 'new poverty' (5.3). Bringing up the rear were youth violence, right-wing extremism and terrorism, each with a score of 4.8. Not a single one of these problems was evaluated by the experts in a consensual manner.

In the assessment of the severity of the social consequences of obesity, the judgements made after the group discussions ranged from three to nine points and also prompted a dissenting opinion. This was due to the direct and above all indirect costs triggered by secondary diseases, which are difficult to quantify. In addition, the consequences of excess weight and obesity "have not been sufficiently scientifically proven either quantitatively or in terms of their severity" (Zwick & Schröter, 2011, p 246).

In the plenary, a long and intense discussion developed about the dramatic nature and severity of the consequences of juvenile obesity with the positive effect that the range of scores reduced from six to four points, with a slightly lower average assessment of the social effects (5.3 compared to 5.6 points in the first round). The harmonisation of the judgements and the intensive justification of their variability took a considerable amount of time, which meant that the remaining questions in the second round could no longer be completely processed by all the working groups. For this reason, we will also restrict the following analysis to the aspect about the "reasonableness of the prevention measures", for which the most information was generated in both rounds. In addition, we found that the experts' opinions on the reasonableness and effectiveness of the measures almost completely coincided. The contributions to the workshop discussions strengthened our impression that, in the case of preventive measures, "reasonableness" in the true sense of the word refers to "effectiveness". Based on this experience, we would recommend that other studies limit the questionnaire design to semantically distinct dimensions.

For those who want to host a one-day Group Delphi workshop with intensive discussions, we recommend the following measures: The questionnaire for the first processing round should be limited to the absolute minimum of distinct and indispensable items and dimensions. In addition, the two introductory presentations can be dispensed with if the questionnaires for the first round, together with a concise, informative cover letter, are sent digitally in the run-up to the Group Delphi workshop. We further recommend that those questionnaires be filled out and returned in advance, so that the data can be evaluated before the Group Delphi workshop and the event can begin directly with the presentation of the results and subsequent plenary discussion. Although this means the first round will not involve any group discussions, in retrospect this seems to be a favourable compromise because it saves time and avoids the problem of having to cut short the processing of the questionnaires in the second round (as was the case with our workshop).

Let us return to the reasonableness of the preventive measures proposed. Table 1 offers some interesting insights. First of all, a clear majority of the measures scored over 5.5 points on average and were thus judged to be extremely reasonable. Nevertheless, a look at the range of the scores shows that there was disagreement among the experts about the reasonableness of the measures. The only exception to this was the strong preference for the expansion of playgrounds and sports facilities for children and young people close to residential areas, presumably because there were no local politicians on the expert panel.

The three measures designed to restrict or control foodstuffs in some way were the main source of conflicting assessments and heated debates. Two of these three options even provoked dissenting opinions in the first round while the working groups were processing the questionnaires. In the plenary, these items were subject of a controversial debate that lasted more than an hour, and the discontinuation of the Delphi Group was only averted due to the exceptionally skilled moderator.

If one compares the expert judgements of these three items in the first and second rounds, then it also becomes clear how fruitful such debates can be despite distinct institutional views and individual logics, and that—to take up a thesis by Jürgen Habermas (1972)—in a well-moderated, transparent and fair debate, better arguments develop persuasive power and are able to create at least a rudimentary consensus. With regard to all three measures, the range of expert judgements decreased significantly in the second round, i.e. after the plenary debate. In the case of an advertising ban on high-calorie foods, the range shrank from eight to five points and the dissenting opinions disappeared. In relation to the labelling of foodstuffs in accordance with the British ‘traffic light system’ the range went from eight to three points, and in the case of the ban on selling high-calorie foodstuffs in schools and kindergartens the range decreased from eight to only one point. Similarly, when it came to the accessibility of children and adolescents in problem groups (measure “conduct studies on how children and adolescents in problem groups can be reached”), it was possible to reduce the range of expert assessments from nine to three points and thus to establish a broad consensus. In light of the contrasting attitudes towards these options at the beginning of the workshop, the very considerable and discursively achieved convergence of the experts’ opinions in the second phase provide, in our opinion, convincing evidence for the effectiveness of carefully moderated, fair discourse as well as for the Group Delphi method as such.

Table 1 points to another advantage of the Group Delphi process. In the first plenary discussion it became clear that more health education in general education schools was essentially desirable. However, the previous introduction of a special school subject for this purpose proved to be counterproductive, which is why the measure was considered highly controversial overall and scored an average of only 5.8 points. In the plenary discussion, this option was adapted on the fly to become “the inclusion of theoretical and practical health promotion as a cross-sectional task in teaching at all schools” and was immediately included in the questionnaire for the second round. The new item achieved consensus (now differing by two points) and was upgraded from 5.8 to 8.5 points with regard to its reasonableness. For a further three items, no scores were available due to time constraints in the second round (n/a in Table 1).

To sum up, we believe that the Group Delphi was a success, despite obvious shortcomings that were mainly due to the time pressure that arose. Our results from Table 1 convincingly document the consensus-building power of well-moderated discussions, which—to draw on Jürgen Habermas once more (1981)—can indeed be suitable for refuting the validity claims of strategically acting protagonists, for working towards consensus, but also for producing semantic clarification and content-related specification processes in only a short amount of time. Hence it seems worthwhile to conduct controversial debates about specific subject matters in a highly regulated and moderated form. A Group Delphi is, as should have become clear, an extremely effective method for discourse and analysis, since on the one hand, at the end of the workshop the majority of the results are well documented in the form of completed questionnaires. On the other hand, the audio recording and minutes allows the arguments made during the discussions to be processed and analysed in just a few days.

Table 1 How reasonable are the following preventive measures?

Measure	1st Delphi round			2nd Delphi round		
	Mean	Range	Dissenting opinion	Mean	Range	Dissenting opinion
Expand playgrounds and sports facilities close to residential areas and guarantee free access so that children and young people have exercise-intensive leisure alternatives	9.0	0[a]	No	–	–	–
Expand the sports program in all schools to two double lessons per week	7.0	4	No	n/a	n/a	–
Create agencies to coordinate anti-obesity efforts at the local, state and federal levels	7.0	5	No	n/a	n/a	–
Ban the sale of high-calorie foods (>10% sugar or > 20% fat) in schools and kindergartens	6.6	8	Yes	8.7	1	No
Enforce easy-to-understand food labelling in line with the UK traffic light system	6.0	8	No	8.5	3	No
Include health education as a subject in the curricula of all year levels in general education schools	5.8	8	No	–	–	–
New: The inclusion of theoretical and practical health promotion as a cross-sectional task in teaching at all schools	–	–	–	8.5	2	No
Enforce a ban on advertising high-calorie foods (>10% sugar or > 20% fat)	5.4	9	Yes	5.0	5	No
Conduct studies on how children and adolescents in problem groups can be reached (e.g. through their media use)	5.3	9	No	7.7	3	No
Implement a sustainability-oriented company rating system, with increasing capital procurement costs for risk-producing companies (that might influence obesity in children and adolescents)	4.0	4	No	n/a	n/a	–

Source: Zwick and Schröter (2011, p. 249)

[a]Consensual items were eliminated after the first round. *n/a.* not available

4 Summary

The Group Delphi example presented here involved the transdisciplinary evaluation of recommendations for tackling juvenile obesity. Of course, the Group Delphi method—like the 'traditional' purely questionnaire-based Delphi method—can be used in a variety of different contexts. As the previous section has already shown, the method has specific strengths and weaknesses which one should be aware of if one intends to conduct a Group Delphi workshop. Therefore, we would now like to conclude with a critical appraisal of the method.

The following points in particular should be emphasised as strengths of the Group Delphi method:

- Proven and effective procedure for identifying appropriate intervention measures, even in institutionally controversial fields.
- Appropriate strategy for reducing uncertainty in predictions about future events.
- Suitable for clarifying and reducing disagreement among experts.
- Clarification of whether disagreement among experts is semantic or based on diverging facts.
- Rapid, discursive and competent identification of reasons for divergent expert opinions.
- Fast and inexpensive procedure; the actual group procedure is completed in 1 to a maximum of 2 days; the results are available in a short time after the workshop.

In our opinion, the method's weaknesses or particular challenges are related primarily to the following points:

- The preparation phase involving the identification and recruitment of relevant experts and the selection of a suitable date is usually long and labour-intensive.
- Selecting and engaging the services of a professional, experienced moderator; for high-conflict issues, the success of the workshop may depend significantly on her or his skills.
- The high time pressure associated with running a one-day workshop and intense debates.
- High organisational stress due to ad hoc evaluations as well as the redesigning and preparing of questionnaires for the next round.

- Wider social preferences are ignored, since only experts and stakeholders are involved in the workshop, while the public is excluded.
- The frustration of those involved when, despite a great deal of effort, expertise and considerable results, none of the measures that were identified as suitable are implemented practically.

All in all, we believe that the Group Delphi is a suitable method for identifying socially robust recommendations for action in a transdisciplinary manner. The particular charm of the Group Delphi lies in its combination of a very systematic, standardised procedure with discursive elements.

Literature

Barlösius, E., & Philipps, A. (2011). Die Gesellschaft und das Selbst der 'Dicken'. Wie Kinder und Jugendliche gesellschaftliche Haltungen und Erwartungen in ihre Selbstkonstitution hineinnehmen. In M. M. Zwick, J. Deuschle, & O. Renn (Eds.), *Übergewicht und Adipositas bei Kindern und Jugendlichen* (pp. 181–201). Springer.

Brandt, P., Ernst, A., Gralla, F., Luederitz, C., Lang, D. J., Newig, J., et al. (2013). A review of transdisciplinary research in sustainability science. *Ecological Economics, 92*, 1–15.

Defila, R., & Di Giulio, A. (2015). Integrating knowledge: Challenges raised by the "inventory of synthesis". *Futures, 65*, 123–135.

Defila, R., & Di Giulio, A. (2019). Eine Reflexion über Legitimation, Partizipation und Intervention im Kontext transdisziplinärer Forschung. In M. Ukowitz & R. Hübner (Eds.), *Partizipation und Intervention. Wege der Vermittlung in der transdisziplinären Forschung* (Interventionsforschung) (Vol. 3). Springer.

Deuschle, J., & Sonnberger, M. (2011). Zum Stereotypus des übergewichtigen Kindes. In M. M. Zwick, J. Deuschle, & O. Renn (Eds.), *Übergewicht und Adipositas bei Kindern und Jugendlichen* (pp. 161–180). Springer.

Fankhänel, S. (2007). Epidemie Adipositas. Jahrestagung der Deutschen Adipositas-Gesellschaft. *Ernährung – Wissenschaft und Praxis, 1*(9), 418–420.

Habermas, J. (1972). *Vorstudien und Ergänzungen zur Theorie des kommunikativen Handelns*. Suhrkamp.

Habermas, J. (1981). *Theorie des kommunikativen Handelns* (Vol. 1). Suhrkamp.

Häder, M. (2002). *Delphi-Befragungen. Ein Arbeitsbuch*. Springer.

Helmert, U., Schorb, F., Fecht, C., & Zwick, M. M. (2011). Epidemiologische Befunde zum Übergewicht und zur Adipositas bei Kindern, Jugendlichen und jungen Erwachsenen. In M. M. Zwick, J. Deuschle, & O. Renn (Eds.), *Übergewicht und Adipositas bei Kindern und Jugendlichen* (pp. 49–70). Springer.

Jahn, T. (2008). Transdisziplinarität in der Forschungspraxis. In M. Bergmann (Ed.), *Transdisziplinäre Forschung. Integrative Forschungsprozesse verstehen und bewerten* (pp. 21–37). Campus.

Jahn, T., Bergmann, M., & Keil, F. (2012). Transdisciplinarity. *Between mainstreaming and marginalization. Ecological Economics, 79*, 1–10.

Krömker, D., & Vogler, J. (2011). Übergewicht und Adipositas – Eine Diätgeschichte. Ergebnisse einer bundesweiten Befragungsstudie mit Kindern und Jugendlichen aus psycho-sozialer Sicht. In M. M. Zwick, J. Deuschle, & O. Renn (Eds.), *Übergewicht und Adipositas bei Kindern und Jugendlichen* (pp. 115–135). Springer.

Mittelstraß, J. (2005). Methodische Transdisziplinarität. *Technikfolgenabschätzung – Theorie und Praxis, 14*(2), 18–23.

Müller, C., Roscher, K., Parlesak, A., & Bode, C. (2011). Systemische Risikofaktoren relativieren den alleinigen Einfluss von Ernährung und Bewegung bei der Entstehung von Übergewicht und Adipositas bei Kindern und Jugendlichen. In M. M. Zwick, J. Deuschle, & O. Renn (Eds.), *Übergewicht und Adipositas bei Kindern und Jugendlichen* (pp. 91–114). Springer.

Peter, C. (2011). Essen ohne Maß? Zu Formen der Essensorganisation in Familien mit 'dicken Kindern'. In M. M. Zwick, J. Deuschle, & O. Renn (Eds.), *Übergewicht und Adipositas bei Kindern und Jugendlichen* (pp. 137–159). Springer.

Pohl, C., & Hirsch Hadorn, G. (2008). Core terms in transdisciplinary research. In G. Hirsch Hadorn, H. Hoffmann-Riem, S. Biber-Klemm, W. Grossenbacher-Mansuy, D. Jove, & C. Pohl (Eds.), *Handbook of transdisciplinary research* (pp. 427–432). Springer.

Renn, O., Webler, T., & Wiedemann, P. M. (1995). The persuit of fair and competent citizen participation. In O. Renn, T. Webler, & P. M. Wiedemann (Eds.), *Fairness and competence in citizen participation. Evaluating models for environmental discourse* (pp. 339–668). Kluwer.

Sahner, H. (2005). *Schließende Statistik.* Springer.

Schiek, D. (2011). Körper von Gewicht. Zur Geschlechterdifferenz in den Ernährungs- und Körpernormen. In M. M. Zwick, J. Deuschle, & O. Renn (Eds.), *Übergewicht und Adipositas bei Kindern und Jugendlichen* (pp. 203–218). Springer.

Schulz, M., & Renn, O. (2009a). Einleitung. In M. Schulz & O. Renn (Eds.), *Das Gruppendelphi* (pp. 7–21). Springer.

Schulz, M., & Renn, O. (2009b). Diskussion der Befunde. In M. Schulz & O. Renn (Eds.), *Das Gruppendelphi* (pp. 111–117). Springer.

Wabitsch, M., Hebebrand, J., Kiess, W., & Zwiauer, K. (Eds.). (2005). *Adipositas bei Kindern und Jugendlichen. Grundlagen und Klinik.* Springer.

WHO. (2000). *Obesity: Preventing and managing the global epidemic.* Report of a WHO Consultation (WHO technical report series 894). http://whqlibdoc.who.int/trs/WHO_TRS_894.pdf. Accessed 12 Mar 2018.

Zwick, M. M. (2008). Maßnahmen wider die juvenile Adipositas. In Interdisziplinärer Forschungsschwerpunkt Risiko und nachhaltige Technikentwicklung der Universität Stuttgart (Eds.), *Stuttgarter Beiträge zur Risiko und Nachhaltigkeitsforschung* (Vol. 9). http://michaelmzwick.de/UPLOAD/ab09_zwick.pdf. Accessed 20 Mar 2018.

Zwick, M. M. (2011). Die Ursachen der Adipositas im Kindes- und Jugendalter in der modernen Gesellschaft. In M. M. Zwick, J. Deuschle, & O. Renn (Eds.), *Übergewicht und Adipositas bei Kindern und Jugendlichen* (pp. 71–90). Springer.

Zwick, M. M., & Renn, O. (2011). Adipositas im Kindes- und Jugendalter – Ein systemisches Risiko? In M. M. Zwick, J. Deuschle, & O. Renn (Eds.), *Übergewicht und Adipositas bei Kindern und Jugendlichen* (pp. 279–287). Springer.

Zwick, M. M., & Schröter, R. (2009). Begrenzter Konsens. Präventions- und Therapiemaßnahmen von Übergewicht und Adipositas im Kindes- und Jugendalter. Analyse eines Expertendelphi. In Interdisziplinärer Forschungsschwerpunkt Risiko und nachhaltige Technikentwicklung der Universität Stuttgart (Ed.), *Stuttgarter Beiträge zur Risiko- und Nachhaltigkeitsforschung* (Vol. 11). http://www.michaelmzwick.de/UPLOAD/ab011.pdf. Accessed 14 Mar 2018.

Zwick, M. M., & Schröter, R. (2011). Wirksame Prävention? Ergebnisse eines Expertendelphi. In M. M. Zwick, J. Deuschle, & O. Renn (Eds.), *Übergewicht und Adipositas bei Kindern und Jugendlichen* (pp. 239–259). Springer.

Delphi Study on the Promotion of Safety and Health Competence at Work

Clarissa Eickholt

Abstract

A Delphi study was carried out in order to identify approaches for the promotion of safety and health competence in companies. This Delphi study focused on the question of which safety and health competencies are important in small and medium-sized enterprises (SMEs) and aimed to derive measures and determine the necessary contextual factors. It was commissioned by the Federal Institute for Occupational Safety and Health (Bundesanstalt für Arbeitsschutz und Arbeitsmedizin) as part of a funding project on the promotion of safety and health competence through informal learning carried out in the process of work and faced the challenge of generating specific conditions from the temporary work and care sectors in addition to general statements. The experts from science and operational practice came from different health and social science disciplines as well as technicians, engineers and physicians. In particular for the evaluation of the second survey wave, the sector to which the experts related their answers played a predominant role.

C. Eickholt (✉)
Systemkonzept GmbH, Cologne, Germany
e-mail: Clarissa.Eickholt@systemkonzept.de

M. Niederberger, O. Renn (eds.), *Delphi Methods In The Social And Health Sciences*, https://doi.org/10.1007/978-3-658-38862-1_12

1 Delphi Study on the Promotion of Safety and Health Competence at Work

The Delphi study described below was carried out as part of the project "Safety and health competence through informal learning in the work process". The project was commissioned by the Federal Institute for Occupational Safety and Health (Bundesanstalt für Arbeitsschutz und Arbeitsmedizin BAuA, research project F2141 – Hamacher et al., 2012).

The project was essentially intended to provide an inventory of existing studies and models on safety and health at work in the context of learning and competence development. In addition, the aim was to develop a concept for the work process-oriented promotion of safety and health, including the starting points for dissemination and implementation. The latter was to be done for small and medium-sized enterprises (SMEs) in two sectors. The subsequent selection of the temporary employment and care sectors was obvious due to the BAuA's priority programmes at the time, as it was precisely in these sectors that needs were identified due to changes in working conditions and thus in the stresses and strains on employees. SMEs, i.e. companies with fewer than 50 or 250 employees, were of particular interest for the project, as formalised personnel development structures are less common here (especially in small companies).

While the inventory of existing studies and models was primarily based on literature analyses and secondary analyses, the Delphi method was selected as the basis for concept development.

The project started with the search for low-threshold opportunities for operational competence development on safety and health. This was important because the economic success of companies also depends on efficient and willing employees. Performance and willingness to perform are inconceivable without health, and corresponding competencies for maintaining health resources are necessary.

1.1 Research Questions of the Delphi Study

The overall aim of the Delphi study was to develop approaches for promoting safety and health competence through informal learning in the process of work. Two questions were formulated for this purpose:

1. What are the safety and health learning needs in SMEs?
2. Which measures and framework conditions in the company are suitable to enable informal learning on safety and health in the process of work?

1.2 Method Selection

Since the facts were delimited, but still not objectively determinable, the choice fell on the Delphi method. The aim was to give the survey of experts from science and practice a methodological system. In addition, the method enables a form of (indirect) group communication with which the substantive questions can be dealt with in depth, even though there is initially uncertain and incomplete knowledge about the issues (Häder, 2014; Häder & Häder, 1995).

In the literature, different types of Delphi surveys can be distinguished. In the study conducted, a two-stage procedure was chosen, along the lines of type 3 according to Häder (2014), i.e. with the aim of determining expert statements. In the first wave, (open) responses from the experts were generated in a qualitatively oriented survey. In the second wave, the findings of the first wave were transferred into a standardized questionnaire and evaluated with regard to selected criteria.

1.3 Selection, Approach and Participation of Experts

The selection of experts was based on various criteria. On the one hand, experts from research were to be recruited who had (scientific) expertise in at least one of the relevant content areas. On the other hand, open-minded practitioners were sought in order to be able to capture the expertise on corporate reality. Thus, on the one hand, authors of relevant publications were identified and, on the other hand, experts from (good) practice were selected, for example via the pages of the Initiative Neue Qualität der Arbeit (INQA). Due to the response rate (see below), additional recruitment was carried out for the second survey wave. In this phase, the research was extended to relevant professional associations and contacts via professional associations. In total, more than 530 experts were researched.

The interviews with the experts took place in writing. Participation was decentralised, i.e. the experts did not come together for a workshop or something similar and were not able to communicate directly with each other. About one third of the experts received the documents in electronic form upon request or via a follow-up action. Participation was always anonymous.

The experts were primarily approached by post. The questionnaire was already sent with the first contact, as well as a pre-paid and pre-addressed return envelope. A follow-up to the first wave took place after just under 6 weeks by e-mail with an attached questionnaire and the option of electronic submission. For the second wave, all experts of the first wave were contacted again (except for those who explicitly did not want to participate) and additionally the newly researched experts were contacted with a delay of about 4 weeks.

Of the 130 or so experts initially contacted, 15 took part in the comprehensive and complex first wave (response rate of 11%). Multiple responses were possible to the question about the perspective of the response. The answers from a supra-company perspective were predominantly answered by scientists (n = 8), two of whom also answered from their position as managers. Experts from management consultancies (4) and occupational health and safety actors (employers' liability insurance associations (2), occupational health and safety specialists (1)) claimed the company perspective for themselves, but in some cases also gave the inter-company perspective as multiple answers. The internal view came primarily from managers (4), employees (2) and company occupational health and safety actors (2), as well as another company actor.

In addition to the 130 experts from the first wave, around 200 further experts from the care sector and the temporary employment sector were recruited for the second wave. In the end, a total of 44 experts participated in the second wave (response rate approx. 8.3%). The sector perspectives were thus adequately represented: Care sector with 19 participants (43.2%), temporary employment sector with 16 participants 36.4%) and a further nine overarching experts, mainly with a scientific background. Overall, the focus shifted – intentionally – to the company perspective (for further details see Hamacher et al., 2012).

1.4 Structure of the Questionnaire

The questionnaires are structured in the same way for both survey waves and consist of two parts (see Table 1). The first part focuses on questions about the learning needs for safety and health (in SMEs), while the second part deals with measures and framework conditions in SMEs which, according to the previous literature analyses and evaluation of examples of good practice, are suitable for enabling informal learning in the process of work.

1.4.1 Questionnaire of the First Survey Wave

In the first wave of the survey, the participating experts were encouraged to answer questions based on their expertise and experience.

- Part I: View of employees in SMEs (their sector), competences, skills, knowledge and knowledge content. The categories were derived with reference to

Table 1 Components of the surveys

	Wave I	Wave II
Part 1	Recording of necessary competences on safety and health in SMEs	Assessment of safety and health competence needs of employees in SMEs
Part 2	Identifying approaches to promote the safety and health competences of employees in SMEs through informal learning	Assessing the practicality of approaches to promoting safety and health competence in SMEs

Hamacher et al. (2012)

Lenartz's (2011) structural model in order to roughly prescribe various competence dimensions. These include:

- Safety and health-related knowledge and basic skills on safety and health at work
- Competences in dealing with one's own person (self-control and self-awareness) in safety and health-relevant work contexts
- Competences for taking responsibility with regard to own safety and health at work and relevant issues in the company
- Competences in dealing with information relevant to safety and health in the context of work (procuring information, evaluating it, making it useful for oneself, etc.).
- Competences for safety- and health-related communication and cooperation in the context of work
- Further competences for maintaining individual health resources related to safety and health factors in the context of work

The experts were asked to give as many answers as they liked and to stay with the individual questions until their expertise and experience - in their opinion - was exhaustively represented.

- Part II: View of favourable aspects for informal learning processes on safety and health competence from an expert's point of view. The questionnaire was structured as follows: "What possibilities do you see for promoting informal learn ing on safety and health in small and medium-sized enterprises?
  - ... in general?
  - ... through the design of work tasks, work organisation, technology and the working environment?
  - ... by shaping the social conditions in the company and the corporate culture?

– ... by shaping leadership behavior and human resource management?
– ... through the design of corporate structures and corporate development?
– ... by linking them to measures of formal continuing education (training, education and training, etc.)?
– ... through individual support measures?
– ... by other measures within the company?"

Also in this part the number of answers was open.

1.4.2 Questionnaire of the Second Survey Wave

For the second survey wave, the questionnaire was completely generated from the results of the first survey wave. For this purpose, the results of the first wave were grouped together and double entries were eliminated. The objective of this second wave was to evaluate the entirety of the collected statements with regard to the learning needs of employees for safety and health competence and to assess the collected framework conditions and measures. In this second wave, a standardized questionnaire was presented to the experts.

- Part I: Assessment of 71 items on aspects of safety and health literacy (skills, knowledge, etc.), in the following categories:

Item groups and criteria in Part II of the second wave. (Own representation).

	Criterion I Importance	Criterion II Existence
(1) Knowledge and basic skills on safety and health at work General knowledge (13 items) Company-specific knowledge (5 items) Job-specific knowledge (7 items)		
(2) Competences in dealing with oneself (12 items)		
(3) Competencies for taking responsibility (10 items)		
(4) Competencies for safety- and health-related communication and cooperation (14 items)		
(5) Dealing with safety and health-related information in the context of work (10 items)		

- Part II: Assessment of approaches and contextual factors for promoting safety and health competence in the workplace with regard to their practical relevance along 81 framework conditions and measures, in the following categories:

Item groups and criteria in Part II of the second wave. (Own representation).

	Criterion I Suitability	Criterion II Degree of implementation
(1) Measures and contextual factors at the level of the organisation (17 items)		
(2) Measures and contextual factors of corporate culture (10 items)		
(3) Measures and contextual factors for personnel development and learning culture (12 items)		
(4) Measures and contextual factors of leadership behaviour (11 items)		
(5) Measures and context factors for information and communication in the company (12 items)		
(6) Measures and contextual factors of work design and work environment (11 items)		
(7) Continuing education (4 items)		
(8) Health services (4 items)		

Criterion I: How suitable is the measure or contextual factor for improving informal learning on safety and health in small and medium-sized enterprises? (1 = not at all, 2 = somewhat, 3 = well, 4 = very well)
Criterion II: How high do you rate the current degree of implementation of the measure or context factor in SMEs in your chosen sector? (1 = not at all, 2 = somewhat, 3 = well, 4 = very well)

In both waves, additional information about the person, in particular about the profession or the technical background, as well as the perspective (company or inter-company) were asked in order to be able to classify the opinion of the experts and their point of view in a better way.

1.5 Evaluations

Due to its qualitative orientation, the first wave provided open responses. These first had to be recorded and clustered. In a second step, the redundancies within the clustered answers were cleaned up and linguistic smoothing was carried out, but only where it was necessary for comprehensibility – in addition to the correction of spelling mistakes. – This time-consuming step was taken to ensure that the second wave represented the totality of the responses as accurate as possible, but also that a final set of items was available that was manageable (and reasonable) without sacrificing content. Out of the original 300 items, 71 items were included in Part I and 81 items entered Part II of the standardized questionnaire for the second wave.

The statistical analysis of the second wave was limited to descriptive frequencies, differentiated by items, scales and branches.

Step 1: Consideration at scale level

All items of an item group were assessed on a one-dimensional scale, so that it was possible to view them as a scale. For all items of an item group, the scale mean (M – mean) was formed and the standard deviation was considered; since no gross outliers could be determined for most items, further work with the mean was preferred to the median. For each scale, the difference was formed out of the responses of the two initial questions. Thus, in Part I of the questionnaire between the importance of the respective competences for safety and health in SMEs and their existence among employees and in Part II between the suitability of the measures and framework conditions for SMEs and their implementation to date.

In principle, the Likert scaling method was followed, except that instead of the more frequent use of a 7-point scale, a 4-point scale was used. The theoretical expected value of a 4-point Likert scale is 2.5, which means that values below 2.5 tend to be less important and values above 2.5 tend to of high importance.

Step 2: Consideration at item level

At item level, the mean and standard deviation were also calculated for each item. Here, too, two mean values are obtained for each questionnaire part. In Part I, the need results from the assessment of the importance of individual competence aspects in contrast to the estimated presence. (Importance - presence = (learning) need).

The relevance of operational approaches or framework conditions resulted from the suitability of the proposed measure or framework condition in relation to the assessment of the implementation status to date (suitability – implementation in SMEs = relevance to action).

Since no objective or normative criteria for assessing the strength of differences are possible through purely linguistic interpretation, a ranking was formed from the items of each scale. The higher an item is ranked, the greater the need for learning or action.

Step 3: Industry-specific evaluation

In addition to the overarching evaluations in steps 1 and 2, sector-specific observations were made. The focus was then on the renewed evaluation of the sector-specific differences per item, including the formation of specific rankings for the care and temporary employment sectors. In this way, it was possible to observe deviating rankings which characterise the respective need for competences or measures and framework conditions.

1.6 Selected Results from the Delphi Study

The most important findings are briefly presented below. The results can be read in detail in the research report by Hamacher et al. (2012 – see bibliography for link), which is freely available online.

In the first part, the experts' assessment gives indications of a clear need in all the competence areas surveyed. A consistently high assessment of importance (with slight fluctuations in individual items) meets a critical assessment of the competences in the SMEs. For the sectoral analysis, important accents with regard to the need for learning emerged:

Temporary Work

For employees in the temporary employment sector, it can be stated that there is a need for support in achieving consistent behaviour with regard to safety and health (at work in the user enterprise), promoting the use of health resources and increasing knowledge about mental hazards. The company's work system and relevant work techniques must be better known and mastered. Temporary agency workers should be enabled to speak up confidently when addressing relevant occupational health and safety aspects in the user enterprise and they should be fully informed about existing occupational health and safety measures in the user enterprise. Furthermore, they need support in using safety and health-related information in their company practice.

Care

In very simplified terms, it was stated that employees in care should be made aware of basic business management interrelationships in occupational safety and health: "To what extent is a given additional expense due to occupational safety and health measures economically sensible and necessary?" In care, the promotion of self-discipline and consistent behaviour in matters of safety and health is called for. In this context, it is particularly important to encourage employees to recognise the negative consequences for the company of behaviour that is contrary to safety and is detrimental to health. More support is needed for employees in dealing constructively with conflicts and in overcoming them. Knowledge of the safety and health offers available in the company must be improved, and the knowledge relevant to the job of designing workplaces in a healthy and ergonomic manner must be promoted. This also applies to the ability to independently obtain information relevant to safety and health.

In the second part of the study, i.e. the recording of the suitability of named measures and the assessment of the implementation status, the relevance for action could be derived. In all areas of design, a number of measures were classified as suitable for promoting informal learning. However, the degree of implementation was consistently assessed as very low. There is a clear need for action here and corresponding potential for promoting informal learning on safety and health competence in SMEs. However, the need for more formal further training measures was also mentioned. The following picture emerged specifically for the sectors:

Temporary Work

For the temporary employment sector, the experts' statements point to a resource-preserving approach to employees. Further training measures – i.e. formal further training – also promote informal learning processes to a considerable extent, create knowledge or activate and raise awareness of this. In order to promote learning processes at the workplace, great importance is attributed to an appropriate tolerance of errors and an open, constructive approach to dealing with errors. Partnership-based forms of learning are regarded as particularly helpful, as are methods of organising work and working hours that promote learning and development. The experts attribute a high development potential to concrete offers for safety- and health-oriented behaviour at the workplace, e.g. in a healthy food offer, relaxation rooms and exercise. According to the experts, it is essential that the topic of "safety and health" is highly visible and present in the company, as well as a personnel policy that builds up the competencies of employees in the long term and binds them to the company.

Care

In the care sector, the evaluation of implemented health and safety measures has the highest relevance for action, which can be interpreted as an indication that previous measures are critically assessed in terms of their implementation and scope and that an evaluation could initiate a qualitative improvement. Consideration of aspects that do not directly add value in the design of workplaces is also regarded as highly relevant to action. As in the temporary employment sector, the experts attach great importance to the visibility of the topic of "health and safety". A close contact of the company to actors in further education on safety and health is seen as helpful. Such contact allows, for example, further training measures to be specifically adapted to the situation and needs of the company and thus to initiate informal learning in the long term. In the care sector, individual and group-related advisory offers on safety and health are assumed to be highly effective, e.g. offers tailored to employees on nutrition, exercise or stress. A qualification of the managers in questions of safety and health is seen as very helpful for the informal learning of the employees. Finally, an open and constructive approach to mistakes is also needed in the care sector. Just as the promotion of collegial learning promoters and caretakers in the company is seen as beneficial by the experts.

Integration of the Results in the Overall Project

The empirical results of the Delphi study were incorporated into the correlation model for informal learning on safety and health in small and medium-sized enterprises developed in the project. This represents an essential result of the project (see Fig. 1). With the help of the experts' statements, concrete statements on framework conditions for the promotion of informal learning on safety were made for the

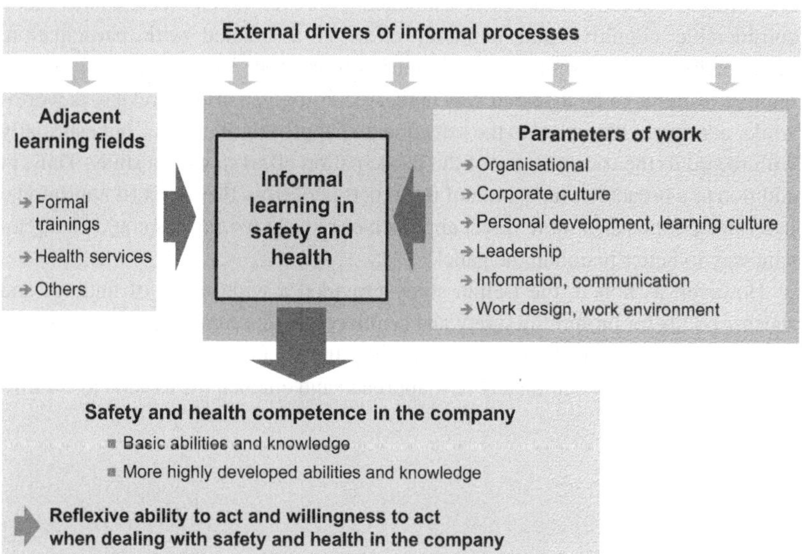

Fig. 1 Empirically formulated correlation model for informal learning on safety and health in the process of work. (Own illustration)

two sectors investigated. At the same time, related fields of learning were defined for specific sectors. Together, the design fields for informal learning on safety and health were worked out. With a view to the target size of this learning process, the findings of the study provide overall information on which specific skills, abilities and knowledge are important in small and medium-sized enterprises in the respective sectors and where the greatest need for learning is to be seen.

In the project, the design approaches elaborated were further underpinned with a series of examples of good operational practice in connection. The practice-oriented processing of the results resulted in two sector-specific manuals as well as a guideline for the creation of further sector-specific action aids.

1.7 Review of the Delphi Study

During the organization and implementation of the study, it became apparent that panel mortality was much higher than expected and could only be counteracted by recruiting additional participants. Participation in the first wave can be classified as quite time-consuming for the experts. How much time they ultimately spent answering the questions cannot be estimated. However, it is unquestionable that a considerable cognitive and temporal effort is associated with participation. Participation in the second wave of the survey took about 30 minutes, but again the number of items to be assessed was high. Accordingly, a critical review is worthwhile, not only with regard to the selection and approach of experts, but especially with regard to the transparency of the participation effort in such a study. Thus, in addition to a broader composition of the expert pool from the outset (if appropriate in terms of content), a more direct approach or request for experts could be a relevant way to better maintain the panel.

However, as hoped, the Delphi study provided a wide range of findings and starting points for promoting safety and health competence through informal learning. In addition, the Delphi study as a procedure in an "occupational safety and health" project was a completely new approach and enabled the experts to contribute in detail.

Literature

Häder, M. (2014). *Delphi-Befragungen. Ein Arbeitsbuch* (3. Aufl.). Springer.
Häder, M., & Häder, S. (1995). Delphi und Kognitionspsychologie. Ein Zugang zur theoretischen Fundierung der Delphi-Methode. *ZUMA-Nachrichten, 19*(37), 8–34.
Hamacher, W., Eickholt, C., Lenartz, N., & Blanco, S. (2012). Ansätze zur betrieblichen Förderung von Sicherheits- und Gesundheitskompetenz durch informelles Lernen im Prozess der Arbeit. In Bundesanstalt für Arbeitschutz und Arbeitsmedizin (Hrsg.), *Projekt F2141*. BAuA https://www.baua.de/DE/Angebote/Publikationen/Berichte/F2141.pdf?__blob=publicationFile&v=1. Zugegriffen: 1 Oct 2021.
Lenartz, N. (2011). *Gesundheitskompetenz und Selbstregulation. Modellbildung zur Gesundheitskompetenz unter besonderer Berücksichtigung selbstregulativer Kompetenzen*. V&R.

Delphi Methods in Health Promotion. Results of a Systematic Review

Marlen Niederberger, Ann-Kathrin Käfer, and Laura König

Abstract

Delphi methods offer great potential in the field of health promotion because they take into account expert opinions across disciplines and allow the integration of evidence-based and real-life knowledge. They are mainly used in health promotion to collect different expert opinions and as consensus processes. However, to date there has been no systematic overview of the use of Delphi methods in health promotion. For this reason, a systematic review was conducted based on publications in relevant international journals. The aim is to identify research practice with a special focus on the aspects of research purpose, expert selection, research design and presentation of results.

1 Introduction

Delphi methods are used in numerous disciplines and for various topics. The potential for application encompasses areas such as technology and environmental research, work and organisational development, and nursing and health sciences (see Cuhls et al., 1998; Jorm, 2015; Jung & Bleyer, 2017; Linstone & Turoff, 1975).

M. Niederberger (✉) · A.-K. Käfer
University of Education Schwäbisch Gmünd, Schwäbisch Gmünd, Germany
e-mail: marlen.niederberger@ph-gmuend.de; ann.kaefer@ph-gmuend.de

L. König
Münster, Germany

M. Niederberger, O. Renn (eds.), *Delphi Methods In The Social And Health Sciences*, https://doi.org/10.1007/978-3-658-38862-1_13

Delphi methods also offer great potential in health promotion. Health promotion combines various scientific disciplines (including psychology, sports science and nutrition science) and is applied by practitioners (e.g. by schools and councils), especially in the development and evaluation of health-promoting interventions. Delphi processes can support the consideration and integration of discipline-specific thought patterns and real-life expertise.

However, to date there has been a lack of both a systematic overview and a critical reflection on the use of Delphi methods in health promotion. For this reason, a systematic review was conducted on the basis of publications in relevant international journals. The aim of this review is to analyse the Delphi methods used with regard to the research question, the selection of experts, the procedure, and the presentation of results.

2 Background: Delphi Methods in Health Promotion

Health promotion is defined as the process of enabling people to have a greater degree of self-determination over their health, thereby empowering them to improve their health. The concept starts with the analysis of the health resources and potentials of people as well as at all levels of society. Aspects of social science, psychology, sport, nutrition and economics play an important role (WHO, 1986, pp. 1 ff.).

In order to identify, develop, implement and evaluate appropriate interventions as an interface between science and practice, health promotion needs concepts with empirical evidence, subject-oriented approaches and participatory instruments. In this sense, qualitative and quantitative research methods as well as inter- and transdisciplinary perspectives play an important role in health promotion.

Delphi methods appear to be an important survey method for health promotion, especially from the perspective of inter- and transdisciplinary knowledge integration. They allow the integration of knowledge from different disciplines and take into account theoretical and real-life expertise. However, Delphi methods are eminence-based methods, which are by definition subordinated to evidence-based methods in the health sciences (to which health promotion also belongs) (see Table 1). Interpreted in this way, Delphi methods are relevant above all when methods of a higher evidence level (such as randomised controlled trials (RCTs)) are not possible (Steurer, 2011, p. 960).

Detailed and systematic reviews of the specific use and potential of Delphi methods in the various fields of health sciences are few and far between. Those that

Table 1 Evidence classes

Class Ia: Evidence based on at least one meta-analysis on the basis of methodologically high-quality RCTs
Class Ib: Evidence based on at least one methodologically high-quality RCT
Class IIa: Evidence based on at least one high-quality controlled, non-randomised study
Class IIb: Evidence based on a high-quality quasi-experimental study (quasi-experiment)
Class III: Evidence based on methodologically high-quality, non-experimental descriptive studies, e.g. correlation study (correlation), case-control study
Class IV: Evidence based on systematically integrated expert opinions; descriptive studies
Class V: Case series or one or more expert opinions

Evidenzbasierung (2018)

do exist include the palliative care field (Jünger et al., 2017), radiology (Steurer, 2011), health care (Boulkedid et al., 2011) and nursing science (Keeney et al., 2001, 2006). For health promotion, in particular, a corresponding analysis is lacking. This gap prompted the undertaking of a systematic review on the use of Delphi methods in health promotion. The procedure and the results of this review are presented below.

3 Delphi Methods in Health Promotion: A Systematic Review

Research Question

Delphi methods allow a wide range of questions to be addressed. Methodological discourses attest to the relevance of the procedure and its potential for application (Aengenheyster et al., 2017; Diamond et al., 2014; Häder, 2014; Linstone & Turoff, 2011; Niederberger & Kuhn, 2013; von der Gracht, 2012). To date, there is no systematically developed evidence on the areas of application and research practice in health promotion. This question is addressed in a systematic review, in which international Delphi studies from the field of health promotion are analysed on the basis of articles. The focus is on the following research question:

How are Delphi methods used in health promotion research practice?

The methodological procedure for the review is presented below. This is followed by the presentation of the results.

3.1 Search and Selection of Delphi Studies

Delphi studies were searched for using the PubMed database. The keywords used were '*delphi*' AND '*health promotion*' and '*delphi*' AND '*Gesundheitsförderung*'. The search was limited to English- and German-language articles in the period from 2012 to 2016. A total of 107 articles were returned. For all hits, the titles and abstracts were read and used to identify relevant articles. Articles that met all of the following criteria were included in the review: empirical implementation of a Delphi method, application in a field of health promotion, and publication in English or German (see Table 2). Excluded were articles that did not conduct their own Delphi procedures, but referred to such procedures or planned them. In addition, pure literature reviews as well as conference contributions were excluded. In total, 16 articles did not meet the inclusion criteria.

Subsequently, the full texts of the remaining articles were reviewed and examined again with regard to the inclusion criteria. If the full texts were not freely accessible, they were ordered via interlibrary loan from the university library. During the review of the full texts, a further eight articles were excluded. In the end, 84 Delphi studies were included in the analysis. The complete process of study selection is shown in Fig. 1.

3.2 Analysis Grid

The analysis of the articles is concerned with the recording of research practice. Accordingly, aspects were recorded that capture the role of the Delphi method in the research process and the typical procedure of Delphi methods. To ensure comparability with other reviews of Delphi procedures, these were taken into ac-

Table 2 Inclusion and exclusion criteria. (authors' representation)

Inclusion	Authors' Delphi study
	Topic from field of health promotion
	Published in English or German
Exclusion	Planned Delphi study or not authors' Delphi study
	No description of the Delphi procedure, only mentions
	Purely methodological articles
	Conference or congress papers
	Literature reviews

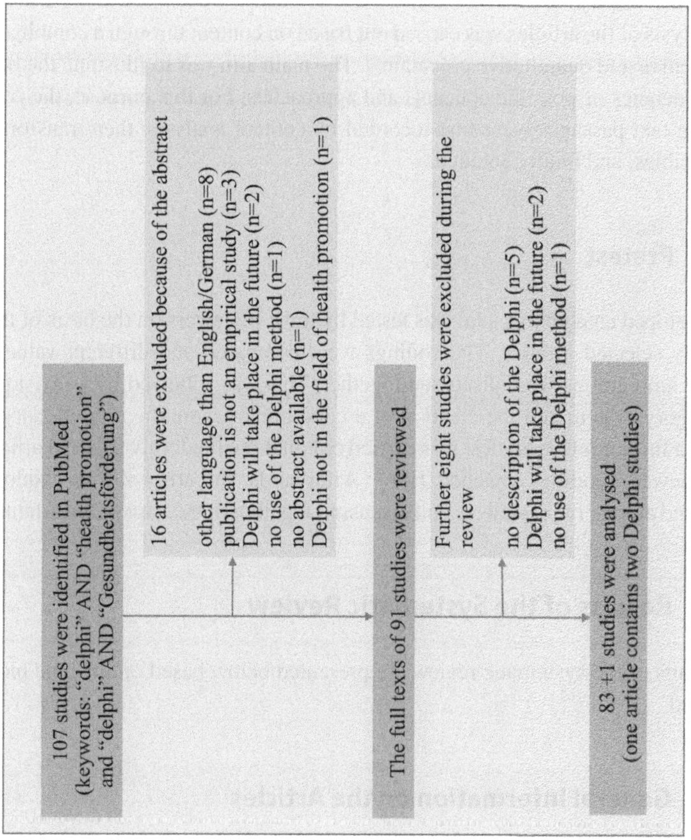

Fig. 1 Process of study selection. (Own representation)

count in the development of the analytical grid (see Boulkedid et al., 2011; Jünger et al., 2017). In total, 82 items were grouped into nine question blocks. A detailed overview of the dimensions and items examined is shown in Table 3.

3.3 Evaluation

The analysis of the articles was carried out based on content through a combination of qualitative and quantitative procedures. The main aim was to illustrate the range and frequencies of possible concepts and approaches. For this purpose, the corresponding text passages were first recorded by content analysis, then transformed into variables, and finally counted.

3.4 Pretest

The developed category system was tested by three reviewers on the basis of three randomly selected articles. The codings were compared and different values or possible ambiguities were discussed together. This was followed by a revision of the category system and the creation of a code book. Using the revised category system, a further reliability test was carried out on three randomly selected articles. The reviewers' codings matched 100%. Afterwards, the articles were randomly distributed among the reviewers and discussed together in the case of uncertainties.

4 Results of the Systematic Review

The results of the systematic review are presented below based on the nine blocks examined.

4.1 General Information on the Articles

Most of the articles are in English. There are two articles in German. The number of authors varies between one and 31, with an average of six authors per article. The number of participating institutions is correspondingly broad. On average, authors from five different institutions are involved in one article. They also frequently represent different disciplines. The average number of disciplines involved is three. In 60% (n = 50) of the articles it is stated that the Delphi study was externally funded.

Table 3 Topic blocks and dimensions of the systematic review. (authors' representation)

Topic blocks	Relevant dimensions
1. General information on the article	Number of authors References to institutions and disciplines Publication year
2. Information on the subject and objective of the Delphi procedure	Topic of the Delphi Goals of the Delphi (consensus building, idea aggregation, expert opinions, prediction) Justification for the use of the Delphi method
3. Conceptual information on the Delphi method	General definition of Delphi method Notes on the type of Delphi (e.g. traditional written or online Delphi, real-time, policy, group or hybrid Delphi) Recording of modifications to the procedure Aims of the Delphi procedure Information on the limitations of the procedure
4. Information on the general research process	Combination with other research methods Importance of the Delphi in the research process Duration of the research process
5. Composition of the expert panel	Definition of the concept of expert (self-perception and perception by others) Institutional affiliation of the experts Number of invited experts Method of recruitment Recording of sociodemographic data of the experts (gender, age and profession) Response rate between the Delphi rounds Anonymity of the experts
6. Procedure of the Delphi method	Number of Delphi rounds and their respective purpose Type of feedback between Delphi rounds Termination criterion of the Delphi process
7. Notes on the survey instruments	Survey instrument of each Delphi round Question wording (open or closed) Information on the development of the questionnaire Scope and design of the questionnaire
8. Notes on consensus building	Definition of consensus Method of recording Percentage of items with achieved consensus
9. Presentation of results	Representation in a flowchart Type of statistical analysis (descriptive or interference statistics) Use of statistical measures for analysis (e.g. median, mean) Graphical processing of the results Dealing with open statements (e.g. verbatim quotes) Focus of the evaluation (on qualitative or quantitative data)

Table 4 Year of publication. (authors' representation)

Publication year	Frequency	In per cent
2012	8	9.5
2013	11	13.1
2014	20	23.8
2015	24	28.6
2016	21	25.0
Total	84	100

The Delphi studies examined are employed around the world (including in China, Ireland, Australia and Finland). Some of them are also designed transnationally. Eight Delphi studies (10%) are carried out as transnational projects within the EU (ID6, ID13, ID19, ID22, ID69, ID75, ID83) and a further eight globally (ID2, ID9, ID24, ID49, ID68, ID73, ID89, ID90). For Germany, two Delphi studies could be identified (ID33, ID91). The analysis of the year of publication shows that Delphi methods were regularly published between 2012 and 2016, with a slight upward trend (Table 4).

Conclusion The general data of the articles show that Delphi methods are used internationally in health promotion. They are carried out as interdisciplinary research projects with several institutions and are scientifically presented in publications.

4.2 Information on the Subject and Objective of the Delphi Procedure

Delphi methods are used for different topics in the articles examined. Delphi methods are used to develop or identify indicator systems for the analysis of specific outcomes (e.g. ID10, ID39), competence profiles for specific occupational groups (e.g. ID90), success criteria or 'do-not' criteria of interventions (e.g. ID44, ID64), structural or organisational framework conditions (e.g. ID15), recommendations for politics or decision makers (e.g. ID82), priority research or activities (e.g. ID13) and new measurement tools (e.g. ID7). Delphi methods are also used to identify health promotion strategies or interventions (e.g. ID31, ID54). On an aggregate level, health promotion Delphi studies are often concerned with the development of guidelines and new standards (50%, n = 42), followed by questions related to the development of specific research foci or activities (e.g. in intervention development) in the field of health promotion (25%, n = 21).

The Delphi studies examined show the importance of consensus processes. Examined according to the four goals of Delphi processes identified by Häder (2014), it becomes clear that 76% (n = 64) of the Delphi studies are explicitly designed as consensus processes or define consensus as the central goal of the Delphi process (see Table 5). Nineteen per cent (n = 16) of the Delphi studies are used for the collection of expert opinions. Three studies fall under 'other'. These are Delphi procedures for the validation or confirmation of research results from previous surveys or a questionnaire (ID3, ID12, ID60). One study uses the Delphi method for prediction (ID25). For idea aggregation as proposed by Häder (2014), no Delphi studies can be found in the articles under investigation.

Fifty-four per cent (n = 45) of the articles examined explicitly justify the use of the Delphi process. The reasons include:

- Delphi methods are innovative, systematic and reliable (e.g. ID28).
- The experts are interviewed anonymously and group effects that arise in personal interactions are prevented (e.g. ID2, ID8, ID49, ID64, ID91).
- Delphi methods allow the involvement of a large number of experts (e.g. ID1, ID14).
- Experts from different, even distant regions can be included (e.g. ID23, ID43, ID44, ID49, ID 61, ID75).
- Delphi methods allow the identification of consensus (e.g. ID72).
- Delphi methods can be used to fill gaps in knowledge, especially when too little empirical data are available or none can be collected (e.g. ID20, ID42, ID57).
- Delphi methods are suitable for complex topics that require interdisciplinary perspectives (e.g. ID31, ID49).

Table 5 Reported Delphi type according to Häder (2014). (authors' representation)

Primary objective of the Delphi	Frequency	In per cent
Consensus	64	76.2
Forecast/prediction	1	1.2
Recording of expert opinions	16	19.0
Other	3	3.6
Total	84	100

- They are relatively inexpensive methods (e.g. ID2).
- Delphi methods enable experts to revise or consolidate their opinions (e.g. ID61, ID87).
- They can investigate and validate the legitimacy and acceptability of the results of previous studies (e.g. ID85).

Central arguments for the implementation of Delphi methods are the involvement of a larger number of experts, who can be interviewed anonymously and geographically remotely. The authors often give several reasons for using the Delphi method (e.g. ID2, ID49, ID61), which indicates a conscious and reflexive use of the method.

Conclusion Delphi methods in health promotion are mainly used to establish consensus and to collect expert opinions. They are often used for the development of guidelines and standards. According to the authors, they are a suitable method for interviewing a large number of experts from different disciplines and geographical areas. The choice of method is reflected on and justified in the publications.

4.3 Conceptual Details of the Delphi Procedure

The Delphi method is defined in 61% (n = 51) of the articles examined. In doing so, almost all articles refer to other literature sources (with the exception of six articles: ID6, ID9, ID27, ID29, ID64, ID65). Linstone and Turoff (2002, n = 9) and Hasson et al. (2000, n = 6) are referred to most frequently for a definition (see Fig. 2). Linstone and Turoff (2002) understand a Delphi process as a structured group communication process to investigate aggregated expert opinions on a complex phenomenon. Hasson et al. (2000) additionally emphasise the consensus aspect.

In most studies, Delphi procedures are associated with four characteristics: (1) expert consultation, (2) consensus process, (3) questioning in several rounds and (4) the possibility of feedback. Overall, it is noticeable that Delphi procedures are often defined by the process and the goal, and less by epistemological or paradigm-specific lines of argumentation or the survey instrument (e.g. qualitative or quantitative; see Table 6).

The analysis of the type of Delphi procedures shows a clear tendency: most articles are based on a classic Delphi procedure (70%, n = 59). These are conducted online or as a written survey. The second most common (15%, n = 13) are so-called hybrid Delphis, in which qualitative and quantitative survey instruments are combined. Typically, the first wave is designed as a qualitative interview study and the

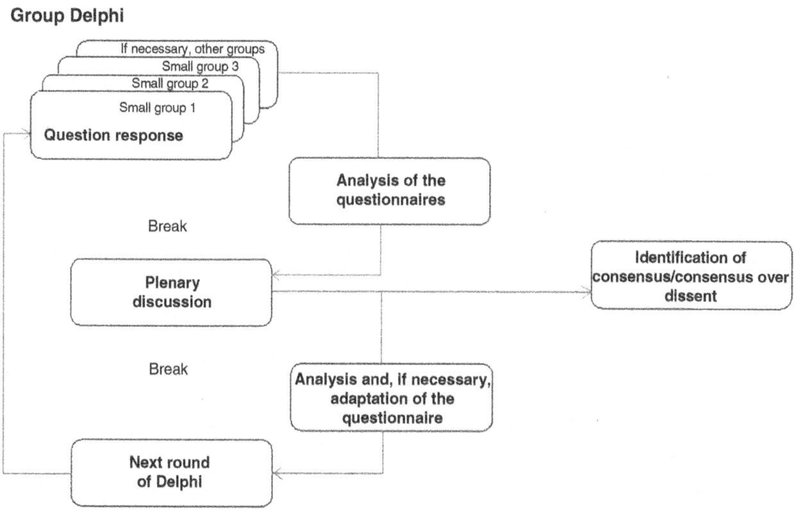

Fig. 2 The most frequently used Delphi definitions in the articles examined. (Own representation)

results are used to develop a standardised questionnaire, which is then used for the following Delphi rounds (e.g. ID7, ID42, ID43, ID44). Other Delphi methods such as the policy Delphi (to capture a range of statements, n = 3, ID36, ID87, ID90) or group Delphi methods (n = 2, ID67, ID78) are the exception.[1]

In most articles (64%, n = 54) limitations of the chosen Delphi method are explicitly discussed. Limitations include aspects about which the authors cannot make a statement with their study. Explicit limitations of the authors mainly refer to the transferability and generalisability of the results. The limitations are explained by:

- A small sample size, for example, due to low response rates or drop-outs (e.g. ID31, ID36, ID43, ID81).
- A specific selection of experts (e.g. ID1, ID55).
- Geographical aspects or specificities (e.g. ID7, ID46).
- Language restrictions (e.g. process in English – experts of other languages could not participate, ID2, ID25).
- The specifics of survey dates (e.g. Delphi survey was conducted years ago, ID42, ID44).

[1] For the definition of the different Delphi variants, please refer to other chapters in this book.

Table 6 Reported key features of Delphi procedures in the articles examined. (authors' representation)

Feature	Frequency	In per cent (n = 84)
Experts	38	45.2
Consensus process	33	39.3
Questioning in several rounds/iterations	30	35.7
Integration of feedback	20	23.8
Anonymity of respondents	14	16.7
Quantitative method	11	13.1
Quantitative and qualitative method	4	4.8
Qualitative method	3	3.6

Conclusion In health promotion, Delphi methods which follow the traditional design with a repeated written survey of the experts are mainly used. More than half of the articles define the Delphi methods and discuss their limitations with regard to the quality, scope and transferability of the results. However, these points are not addressed in more than a third of the articles.

4.4 Information on the General Research Process

Delphi methods are also used in complex research processes in combination with other survey methods. In 43% (n = 36) of the articles examined, Delphi procedures are combined with other procedures. In almost 40% (n = 14) of these studies, the Delphi survey represented the central research method. In the same number of studies they are instead used to deepen previous research findings. Delphi methods are only used as a preliminary study in exceptional cases (see Table 7).

Forty per cent (n = 34) of the articles examined indicate the duration of the Delphi process. The range is from 1 to 4 years (recorded in years). Of these, almost 80% (n = 27) indicate a duration of 1 year.

Conclusion Delphi methods can be used flexibly in the research process and can be combined with other survey methods. When they are combined in health promotion studies, they are usually the central survey instrument or are used downstream to deepen previous studies. Delphi processes can last up to several years.

Table 7 Reported relevance of Delphi procedures in combined research processes. (authors' representation)

Relevance of the Delphi	Frequency	In per cent
Pre-study	5	13.9
Central	14	38.9
Deepening	14	38.9
Other	3	8.3
Total	36	100

4.5 Composition of the Expert Panel

The term 'expert' is defined very differently in the methodological literature (Bogner et al., 2014; Niederberger & Renn, 2018). In the sociology of knowledge, the term 'expert' is associated with specific social positions, specialist knowledge and institutional affiliations. The attribution of who is and who is not an expert is usually made by the researchers (Bogner et al., 2014). In Delphi procedures, the underlying understanding of the concept of 'expert' is particularly central because they are, by definition, the ones who participate in the procedure.

The term 'expert' is operationalised very differently in the articles examined. Definitions were identified via institutional affiliation or professional position (e.g. ID14, ID36), the number and topics of publications (e.g. ID31, ID54), academic title (e.g. ID3), personal involvement (e.g. ID36) and professional experience, sometimes measured in years (e.g. ID42, ID44, ID55). But the willingness to participate (e.g. ID49) and the assumed knowledge also play a role (e.g. ID7, ID46). Most articles define experts by their assumed expertise (defined by subject knowledge or experience, 43%, n = 35), followed by institutional or organisational affiliation (41%, n = 34) and academic factors such as title, number of publications, or professional or academic degree (18%, n = 15). A combination of characteristics is also frequently given (29%, n = 24, e.g. ID39, ID81).

With regard to institutional affiliation, it is evident that the experts involved often come from both science and practice (44%, n = 36). In some studies, representatives of certain affected groups or institutions (e.g. patients) are also integrated (13%, n = 11, e.g. ID7, ID25, ID36, ID49; see Table 8).

Most of the articles indicate how the experts were identified and recruited (71%, n = 58). Typically, the experts are selected consciously according to the underlying definition. Experts are identified by:

Table 8 Reported composition of the expert group. (authors' representation)

Expert group	Frequency	In per cent
Science	13	15.9
Practice	22	26.8
Science and practice	36	43.9
Science and target group	1	1.2
Practice and target group	8	9.8
Science, practice and target group	2	2.4
Total	82[a]	100

[a]Two articles do not specify

- Third-party recommendations, snowballing (e.g. ID2, ID7, ID29, ID71, ID81).
- Research in scientific databases, such as Google Scholar, PsycINFO or PubMed (e.g. ID20, ID31).
- Institutional affiliation or membership in an organisation (e.g. ID31, ID42, ID44, ID54, ID55, ID57, ID64, ID68, ID77, ID81, ID85).
- Academic evidence, such as a specific H-index[2] or relevant publications (e.g. ID2, ID19, ID35).

Only once each were the experts identified by a random selection (ID58) or a theoretically based selection procedure (ID91).

The attribution of the status of expert in the Delphi studies examined is thus carried out by the researchers. Only in one of the articles examined is it reported that the experts addressed were asked about their self-perception before the survey (ID88, p. 1063: 'All authors had to agree that the invited persons were "experts" in the field'). During the Delphi survey, 6% (n = 5) of the studies integrate questions on the self-perceived judgemental reliability or competence of the experts. In most cases, however, it is not examined whether the persons involved also see themselves as experts on the topic.

The number of experts contacted varies greatly. In the articles that indicated the total number, the range is from five to 731 persons. On average, 94 experts (standard deviation = 19, n = 52) were asked for their support in a Delphi study. The median, i.e. the middle of the distribution, is with 39 invited experts significantly below the mean. This indicates that the number of invited persons varies considerably. An examination of the correlation of the number of experts with the Delphi type shows a strong effect (eta = 0.760). The most experts are invited in traditional

[2]The H-index is an indicator of the reputation of scientists. The index is based on the number of citations of publications in other publications.

online Delphi procedures. The largest number is found in a Delphi on forecasting in the field of information and communication technologies in health promotion (ID25). The smallest number is found in an online Delphi with two rounds for the validation of an evaluation instrument of health promotion measures in the school setting (ID60). Twelve per cent (n = 10) of the articles indicate 'all eligible' for the total number of experts.

In 70% (n = 57) of the articles, the level of response is addressed. The response rate is on average 72% in the first wave, 83% in the second wave and 89% in the third wave (each measured against the number of cases in the previous round). The results highlight two aspects:

1. The response rate for Delphi procedures is higher than for German representative population surveys. In the latter, the phenomenon of declining willingness to participate has been discussed for years and response rates of over 15% have been described as high (Ramm, 2014).
2. If experts participate in a Delphi procedure, they are also to a large extent willing to participate in several survey waves. However, a decreasing response per survey wave is to be expected.

Corresponding to the different numbers of invited experts, the number of involved experts also varies greatly (see Table 9). The concrete number ranges from low single-digit figures to several hundred persons. It is noticeable that, measured against the average, the number of experts involved per Delphi round increases. This shows that the composition of the expert group can differ for each round (e.g. ID1, ID22). In some of the Delphi procedures studied, different groups are deliberately selected or the last round is conducted with a larger number of experts. In some cases, the survey instruments also differ for each Delphi round, which has an impact on the number of participants. For example, some Delphi procedures are based on qualitative interviews in the first round and only in the second round are standardised interviews conducted (e.g. ID42, ID43, ID44). In another study, a form of policy Delphi was carried out in which a questionnaire was used first,

Table 9 Overview of the reported number of participating experts per Delphi round. (authors' representation)

Number of participating experts	Number of cases	Range	Median	Mean value	Standard deviation
First round	81	5–255	26	40	5
Second round	77	5–270	26	40	5.1
Third round	41	6–331	23	43	8.7

followed by a group discussion, and then a written survey again in the third Delphi round (ID75). In rounds one and two different experts were involved and in the third Delphi round both groups of experts were integrated in order to validate the results.

In all the articles examined, the experts are treated anonymously. However, in some cases aggregated information on the sociodemographics of the expert panel is provided. Just over a quarter (n = 21) indicate the gender of the experts and 20% (n = 16) the age. Information on profession or occupation is much more frequent (78%, n = 64).

In conclusion, the following tendencies with regard to the underlying definition of experts in Delphi procedures in health promotion can be seen:

- The attribution of expertise is done by the research team. Only in exceptional cases is it validated by the experts themselves or other persons.
- In the Delphi studies examined, experts are defined very differently, on the one hand by objective factors such as title or number of publications, and on the other hand by the expertise attributed to the respective topic.
- In the Delphi processes, persons with theory-based and persons with practical expertise are often integrated. With the help of Delphi processes, this allows the inclusion of different types of knowledge.
- The experts are usually identified and approached through their institutional or organisational affiliation.
- The number of invited and actually involved experts varies greatly and depends on the type of Delphi procedure. Sometimes all contactable persons are interviewed. The effects of the sample size on the scope and quality of the results, however, are rarely established or reflected on.
- The composition of the expert group can change between the Delphi rounds. For example, sometimes people with different expertise are integrated in subsequent Delphi rounds or additional people are recruited.

4.6 Procedure of the Delphi Process

Delphi procedures are usually carried out with several rounds of questioning. Previous reviews of Delphi procedures indicate that two Delphi rounds are usually applied in research practice (Nowack et al., 2011, p. 1611). Similarly, in the health promotion studies reviewed an average of two to three rounds are conducted. The

Table 10 Reported number of Delphi rounds. (authors' representation)

Number of Delphi rounds	Frequency	In per cent
2	33	42.3
3	42	53.8
4	1	1.3
5	2	2.6
Total	78	100

range extends up to five rounds (see Table 10). The fact that a previously defined consensus was reached was the criterion for termination in 15% (n = 13) of the Delphi studies examined. In most Delphi studies, however, pragmatic research reasons for termination were cited (63%, n = 53).

Specific objectives of the different Delphi rounds are given in the articles. The first round often serves the identification of central aspects and the development of a standardised questionnaire. In the subsequent rounds, the aim is to obtain standardised judgements, to minimise dispersion, to increase validity, and often to gain consensus or dissent. The procedure thus corresponds as far as possible to the methodological procedure in a classic Delphi process (Linstone & Turoff, 2002, pp. 5–6).

Example of the Purpose of the Delphi Rounds (ID14, p. 2665)

1. 'In the first stage, basic questions were sent (via email or fax) in an unstructured or open-ended format for the sample population, and they were asked to brain storm and express their ideas freely and then return their responses …
2. In the second stage, we used a structured questionnaire, and the responses that were received were sent to people who were asked to rate the responses using a Likert scale.
3. In the third stage, the results of the second phase were sent to the participants, and they were asked to review the responses again and to revise their comments and judgments, if necessary, and to mention their reasons for the lack of consensus and grade their importance considering the mean and median scores.'

The type of feedback between the Delphi rounds was also recorded in the review. Previous studies show that this usually takes the form of quantitative, aggregated group responses (Boulkedid et al., 2011, p. 6). In health promotion Delphi procedures, experts are also typically fed back the aggregated and anonymised group responses (60%, n = 50). This is often integrated in the questionnaire (46%, n = 39) or in extra reports (8%, n = 7). Only in exceptional cases are the individual answers also fed back (11%, n = 9, e.g. ID35, ID38, ID48a, ID48b). How the opinions of the experts change – whether they confirm, revise or radicalise their answers, for example – is not addressed in any of the Delphi studies examined. Statements about possible changes of opinion are therefore not possible.

According to the information in the articles examined, the experts rarely receive feedback on the overall results of the Delphi process. Only in seven of the examined Delphi studies (8%) is a form of communicative validation explicitly stated.

In conclusion, Delphi procedures in health promotion are usually conducted with two to three rounds. The number of rounds is usually not justified on the basis of theoretical aspects, but rather seems to be a result of pragmatic research considerations. The procedures used in Delphi studies in health promotion largely correspond to the findings from other reviews. However, individual feedback is reported significantly less frequently (Boulkedid et al., 2011, p. 6). Statements about possible changes of opinion of experts through repeated questioning with feedback are not possible on the basis of the articles analysed.

4.7 Notes on the Survey Instruments

The typical data collection instrument of a Delphi process is a questionnaire combining open and closed questions (Boulkedid et al., 2011; Niederberger & Renn, 2018). The analyses of the health promotion Delphi studies reviewed also rely on the use of questionnaires. According to the information provided in the articles, 85% (n = 71) use a questionnaire in the first round, 85% (n = 71) in the second round, and 51% (n = 43) in the third round. The increasing use of questionnaires per Delphi round shows that in some cases a qualitative instrument (interviews or workshop) is used first and quantitative instruments are only used in a second round (e.g. ID7, ID36, ID42).

According to the information in the articles, the development of the questionnaires is mostly based on literature research (36%, n = 30) or previous empirical analyses (32%, n = 27). In some Delphi procedures, the items are formulated on the basis of the findings of a first qualitative Delphi round. The quality of the questionnaire is not reflected on in the articles studied, neither by means of theoretical concepts or models nor by means of measurable quality criteria. All in all, the process from the formulation of the research question to the identification of the most important items and the development of the questionnaire resembles a black box which is hardly discussed in the articles examined. There is a widespread lack of information on systematic and comprehensible procedures for questionnaire development.

In 89% (n = 75) of the articles it is clear that mainly closed questions are used. However, open questions are also found very frequently (75%, n = 63). In 71% (n = 60) of the articles it is explicitly stated that the questionnaire contains open and closed questions. The length of the questionnaires varies greatly. Questionnaires with up to 311 items are reported. On average, each questionnaire contains 44 items. Most studies use five-point Likert scales (42%, n = 35; e.g. ID2, ID14, ID29, ID39, ID42). The scales range from two to eleven points. It can be seen that the number of points is related to the definition of consensus (see Sect. 4.8). If the intention is for a certain percentage of experts to agree with an item, scales with fewer points are used (e.g. ID36, ID70); if, on the other hand, a measure of dispersion is strived for, a greater number of points are used (e.g. ID89). These decisions are presumably based on statistical considerations about the appropriateness of the measurement level and statistical evaluation.

In conclusion, unique questionnaires are developed for each application of Delphi methods, based on analyses of literature studies or other surveys. With an average of over 40 items, they are usually relatively extensive questionnaires using a combination of open and closed questions. The wording of the questions and use of scales is influenced by the aim of the Delphi process. This indicates a conscious and reflective development of the questionnaires. The exact derivation of the items as well as the quality of the survey instrument are, however, hardly reflected on in the articles.

4.8 Notes on Consensus Building

Many of the examined Delphi studies in health promotion are designed as consensus processes (see Sect. 4.2). Ideally, this means that no further questioning of the experts takes place if a previously defined consensus has been reached. Therefore, at this point we will take a closer look at what the authors understand by consensus.

In the methodological literature on Delphi procedures, different definitions of consensus are proposed (Keeney et al., 2011; von der Gracht, 2012). Various authors propose the use of a five-point Likert scale and define consensus when at least 75% of the experts agree with a certain value on this scale (Jirwe et al., 2009; Keeney et al., 2006; Witt & de Almeida, 2008).

Table 11 Examples of definitions of consensus in the Delphi studies examined. (authors' representation)

About percentages
ID70, p. 107
'The participants were asked to score each item using [a] five-point Likert scale (extremely important = 5, very important = 4, moderately important = 3, slightly important = 2, not important = 1). .... We defined consensus as at least 80% of the participants in the Delphi team ticking the same answer category (e.g. 5 "extremely important") and no more than 15% ticking an answer category two or three categories away (e.g. 2 "slightly important" or 1 "not important").'
About interquartile range (IQR or IQD)
ID68, pp. 191–192
'A nine-point Likert scale was used to evaluate the importance: a score of 9 is considered to be critical, and a score of 1 is of limited importance to patient care. ... An IQR of ≤2 in the second round was pre-specified to indicate consensus from the first round.'
About standard deviation
ID33, p. 4
'The same experts are sent the proposed item versions to rate on a 5-point Likert scale with regard to their meaning apart from the perspective (1 – no conformity with regard to contents, 5 – total conformity with regard to contents). … for all items with at least one version with a mean ≥ 3, the item version with the highest mean is included in the final version of the questionnaire. All item versions with a mean lower than three are revised by the study team (under consideration of the comments by experts from step 4).'
About complex definitions
ID23, p. 53
'It was decided that consensus on descriptions was reached if a similar concept name was chosen by ≥70% of the experts with an IQD of ≤1.'

In the present consensus studies (n = 64), a specific consensus criterion is also given in most cases (81%, n = 52) (examples in Table 11). In the largest number of cases (42%, n = 27), consensus is defined by a specific percentage. Alternatively, consensus is defined by ordinal (14%, n = 9) and by metric measures (6%, n = 4). In some cases, several criteria are combined, such as the specification of a percentage agreement with a measure of dispersion.

The number of items achieving consensus varies greatly. Measured against the total length of the questionnaire, values between 10% and 100% are given. On average, according to the reported responses, a consensus is reached between the experts for over 60% of the items. According to previous experience, the likelihood of reaching a consensus is related to the topic, the selection of experts and the empirical data, among other factors (Hart et al., 2009; Vidgen & Gallegos, 2011, p. 6). In the articles studied, the achievement of a consensus correlated with the definition of consensus (eta = 0.558, n = 41) and the number of points on the scale (eta = 0.584, n = 40). In contrast, the number of Delphi rounds (r = −0.101, n = 45) and the number of experts involved in the first round (r = 0.104, n = 45) had hardly any effect on consensus.

Jünger et al. (2017, p. 702): Recommendations for the Presentation of Results
'Reporting of results for each round separately is highly advisable in order to make the evolving of consensus over the rounds transparent. This includes figures showing the average group response, changes between rounds, as well as any modifications of the survey instrument such as deletion, addition or modification of survey items based on previous rounds.'

In conclusion, most consensus studies give a concrete criterion. However, consensus cannot be established for all items at the end of a Delphi process. The contexts for diverging opinions are hardly reflected on. However, there are indications that especially the definition of consensus and consideration of measurement theories are relevant here. The definitions of the Delphi researchers thus have a decisive influence on the outcome of the procedure.

4.9 Presentation of Results

The study also investigated how Delphi processes are reported in the field of health promotion. This is of interest because there are to date no binding guidelines, as there are, for example, for the presentation of results of systematic reviews (see PRISMA according to Moher et al., 2009). However, recommendations are made in various studies, including for the presentation of results (Boulkedid et al,. 2011; Jünger et al., 2017). It is recommended to present survey instruments and results in rounds in order to make changes between rounds transparent.

In the articles examined, the focus of the presentation is clearly on the final results. In most cases, contrary to the recommendations mentioned, neither the survey instruments nor the results per Delphi round are presented (see Table 12).

The presentation of results is mostly based on quantitative findings (n = 58, 76%; see Table 13). Statistical findings are presented via descriptive analyses (90%, n = 76), often in the form of frequency tables (n = 54, 64%). Inferential statistical analyses are the exception (n = 8, 10%).

Table 12 Type of reporting on Delphi processes. (authors' representation)

Round-by-round presentation of the results		
	Frequency	In per cent
Yes	31	36.9
No	53	63.1
Total	84	100
Round-by-round presentation of the survey instruments		
Yes	1	1.2
No	83	98.8
Total	84	100

Table 13 Focus of reporting. (authors' representation)

Focus of reporting	Frequency	In per cent
Quantitative	58	76.3
Qualitative	10	13.2
Quantitative and qualitative	8	10.5
Total	76	100

In the studies with a qualitative focus, anonymised verbatim quotes from the experts are always included. In the studies that present qualitative and quantitative findings, half (n = 4) use verbatim quotes from the experts.

The Delphi process itself is presented in just under one in three publications (n = 27) via a flowchart showing the individual work steps. In the other studies, however, the process is often described very imprecisely and is therefore difficult to comprehend. This can be seen in articles where the focus is on other analyses carried out in the project (e.g. ID4, ID47), but also in articles where the Delphi procedure played a central role in the research process (e.g. ID38, ID41).

In conclusion, it is noticeable in the reporting that the Delphi procedures are presented very differently and procedures are sometimes presented very briefly. The information is presented very briefly in just over a quarter of the articles examined (n = 23). This sometimes makes it difficult to understand procedures, decision-making processes and possible modifications of the Delphi procedure (e.g. if more experts are integrated in a subsequent Delphi round than before).

5 Conclusion

Delphi methods are used around the world in health promotion. They are mainly used to develop consensual guidelines or standards with the help of experts. But they also play an important role in the collection of expert opinions. To date, they have hardly been used for prognoses or future studies in the field of health promotion, although they have become established in these areas and are part of the standard repertoire of methods (Cuhls, 2012; Rowe & Wright, 2011).

As a rule, the Delphi methods examined follow the procedure of a classic Delphi method. The results of the systematic review show that the variants of Delphi procedures developed in the methodological discussion are received very differently in health promotion. The real-time Delphi and the group Delphi are used rarely or not at all. Instead, a 'culture of modification' has established itself. In other words, individual modifications that take the research assignment into account are developed and used. Thus, there is a multitude of variations with regard to the number of rounds, the composition of the expert panel, the survey instrument and the definition of consensus. These variations prove the flexibility of the Delphi procedure, but they also make it difficult to comprehend the processes and results on the basis of publications.

These modifications also mean that the original constituent features of Delphi procedures are becoming increasingly variable. This concerns, above all, the term 'expert' and the concept of iteration.

- Some authors have explicitly distanced themselves from the term 'expert'. For all intents and purposes, anyone who has specific practical knowledge can be an expert. Accordingly, they instead refer to the integration of users, patients or informed citizens (e.g. ID36, ID 49, ID54, ID82).
- The concept of iteration has changed, especially due to the frequent combination of qualitative and quantitative survey instruments. Whereas originally the questionnaire was reduced with each round to the controversial or unclear items, the expert opinions of the first qualitative round are now increasingly used to develop a standardised instrument which is used in the following round (e.g. ID42, ID43, ID44). However, the concrete process of questionnaire development remains unclear. Moreover, in some Delphi procedures different experts are involved in each Delphi round, so that effectively no iteration is possible (e.g. ID55).

In some of the examined Delphi methods, however, the procedure is largely incomprehensible because information is simply missing on the number of rounds, on the definition of experts and consensus, or on the feedback design (e.g. ID46, ID59). With regard to the way Delphi methods are presented in publications, binding guidelines or standards appear to be essential, not least to ensure a consistent approach and a certain level of comparability.

Appendix: Articles Analysed

ID	*Note: Missing numbers are sources that did not meet the inclusion criteria.
1	Abidi, L., Oenema, A., Nilsen, P., Anderson, P. & van de Mheen, D. (2016). Strategies to overcome barriers to implementation of alcohol screening and brief intervention in general practice: a Delphi Study among healthcare professionals and addiction prevention experts. *Prevention Science, 17(6)* (pp. 689–699). https://doi.org/10.1007/s11121-016-0653-4.
2	Amir, L.H., Ryan, K. & Barnett, C. (2015). Delphi survey of international pharmacology experts: an attempt to derive international recommendations for use of medicine in breastfeeding women. *Breastfeeding Medicine, 10(3)* (pp. 168–174). https://doi.org/10.1089/bfm.2014.0144.
3	Anbari, Z., Mohammadbeigi, A. & Jadidi, R. (2015). Barriers and challenges in researches by Iranian students of medical universities. *Perspectives in Clinical Research, 6(2)* (pp. 98–103).
4	Anderson, L. A., Slonim, A., Yen, I. H., Jones, D. L., Allen, P., Hunter, R. H., Goins, R. T., Leith, K. H., Rosenberg, D., Satariano, W. A. & McPhillips-Tangum, C. (2014). Developing a framework and priorities to promote mobility among older adults. *Health Education & Behavior, 41(1S)* (pp. 10–18).
6	Barry, M.M., Battel-Kirk, B. & Dempsey, C. (2012). The CompHP core competencies framework for health promotion in Europe. *Health Education & Behavior, 39(6)* (pp. 648–662).
7	Bing-Jonsson, P.C., Bjørk, I.T., Hofoss, D., Kirkevold, M. & Foss, C. (2014). Competence in advanced older people nursing: Development of 'Nursing older people – competence evaluation tool'. *International Journal of Older People Nursing, 10(1)* (pp. 59–72). https://doi.org/10.1111/opn.12057.
8	Birko, S., Dove, E.S. & Özdemir, V. (2015). A Delphi technology foresight study: Mapping social construction of scientific evidence on metagenomics tests for water safety. *PLoS ONE, 10(6)*. https://doi.org/10.1371/journal.pone.0129706. eCollection 2015.
9	Bloomfield, S.F., Rook, G.A., Scott, E.A., Shanahan, F., Stanwell-Smith, R. & Turner, P. (2016). Time to abandon the hygiene hypothesis: New perspectives on allergic disease, the human microbiome, infectious disease prevention and the role of targeted hygiene. *Perspect Public Health, 136(4)* (pp. 213–224). https://doi.org/10.1177/1757913916650225.

ID	*Note: Missing numbers are sources that did not meet the inclusion criteria.
10	Camps, C., Albanell, J., Antón, A., Aranda, E., Carrato, A., Cassinello, J., Castellano, D., Cruz, J.J., Garrido, P., Guillem, V., Grávalos, C., López, G., Llorente, C., Lorenzo, A., Lluch, A., Ignacio, E. & Díaz-Rubio, E. (2016). Quality Indicators to Assure and Improve Cancer Care in Spain Using the Delphi Technique. *National Comprehensive Cancer Network, 14(5)* (pp. 553–558).
11	Chang, Y.K., Chuang, K.Y., Tseng, J.M., Lin, F.C. & Su, T.S. (2013). Hazardous workplace review program in Taiwan. *Industrial Health, 51(4)* (pp. 432–442).
12	Chen, F.L. & Lee, A. (2016). Health-promoting educational settings in Taiwan: development and evaluation of the Health-Promoting School Accreditation System. *Global Health Promotion, 23(1)* (pp. 18–25). https://doi.org/10.1177/1757975916638286.
13	Elfeddali, I., van der Feltz-Cornelis, C.M., van Os, J., Knappe, S., Vieta, E., Wittchen, H.U., Obradors-Tarragó, C. & Haro, J.M. (2014). Horizon 2020 priorities in clinical mental health research: results of a consensus-based ROAMER expert survey. *International Journal of Environmental Research and Public Health, 11(10)* (pp. 10915–10939).
14	Emadzadeh, A., Moonaghi, H.K., Bazzaz, M.M. & Karimi, S. (2016). An investigation on social accountability of general medicine curriculum. *Electronic Physician Journal, 8(7)* (pp. 2663–2669). https://doi.org/10.19082/2663.
15	Fakhri, A., Harris, P. & Maleki, M. (2015). Proposing a framework for Health Impact Assessment in Iran. *BMC Public Health, 15(335)*. https://doi.org/10.1186/s12889-015-1698-1.
17	Fernandes, L., Hagen, K.B., Bijlsma, J.W., Andreassen, O., Christensen, P., Conaghan, P.G., Doherty, M., Geenen, R., Hammond, A., Kjeken, I., Lohmander, L.S., Lund, H., Mallen, C.D., Nava, T., Oliver, S., Pavelka, K., Pitsillidou, I., da Silva, J.A., de la Torre, J., Zanoli, G., Vliet Vlieland, T.P. & European League Against Rheumatism (EULAR) (2013). EULAR recommendations for the non-pharmacological core management of hip and knee osteoarthritis. *Annals of the Rheumatic Diseases, 72 (7)* (pp. 1125–1135).
19	Forsman, A.K., Wahlbeck, K., Aarø, L.E., Alonso, J., Barry, M.M., Brunn, M., Cardoso, G., Cattan, M., de Girolamo, G., Eberhard-Gran, M., Evans-Lacko, S., Fiorillo, A., Hansson, L., Haro, J.M., Hazo, J.B., Hegerl, U., Katschnig, H., Knappe, S., Luciano, M., Miret, M., Nordentoft, M., Obradors-Tarragó, C., Pilgrim, D., Ruud, T., Salize, H.J., Stewart-Brown, S.L., Tómasson, K., van der Feltz-Cornelis, C.M., Ventus, D.B., Vuori, J., Värnik, A. & ROAMER Consortium (2015). Research priorities for public mental health in Europe: recommendations of the ROAMER project. *European Journal of Public Health, 25(2)* (pp. 249–254). https://doi.org/10.1093/eurpub/cku232.
20	Francis, C.E., Londmui, P.E., Boyer C., Andersen, L.B., Barnes, J.D., Boiarskaia, E., Cairney J., Faigenbaum, A.D., Faulkner, G., Hands, B.P., Hay, J.A., Janssen, I., Katzmarzyk, P.T., Kemper, H.C., Knudson, D., Lloyd, M., McKenzie, T.L., Olds, T.S., Sacheck, J.M., Shephard, R.J., Zhu, W. & Tremblay, M.S. (2016). The Canadian Assessment of Physical Literacy: Development of a Model of Children's Capacity for a Healthy, Active Lifestyle through a Delphi Process. *Journal of Physical Activity and Health, 13(2)* (pp. 214–222). https://doi.org/10.1123/jpah.2014-0597.

ID	*Note: Missing numbers are sources that did not meet the inclusion criteria.
22	Galatsch, M., Moser-Siegmeth, V., Blotenberg, B., Große Schlarmann, J., Schnepp, W. & Team des Internationalen Family Health Nursing Projektes (2014). Family Health Nursing – a challenge for education and training? Results of an European project. *Pflege, 27(4)* (pp. 269–277).
23	Gevers, D.W., Kremers, S.P., de Vries, N.K. & van Assema, P. (2014). Clarifying concepts of food parenting practices. A Delphi study with an application to snacking behavior. *Appetite, 79* (pp. 51–57).
24	Guzman J., Tompa E., Koehoorn M., de Boer, H., Macdonald, S. & Alamgir, H. (2015). Economic evaluation of occupational health and safety programmes in health care. *Occupational Medicine, 65(7)* (pp. 590–597). https://doi.org/10.1093/occmed/kqv114.
25	Haluza, D. & Jungwirth, D. (2015). ICT and the future of health care: aspects of health promotion. *International Journal of Medical Informatics, 84* (pp. 48–57). https://doi.org/10.1016/j.ijmedinf.2014.09.005.
26	Han, H., Ahn, D.H., Song, J., Hwang, T.Y. & Roh, S. (2012). Development of mental health indicators in Korea. *Psychiatry Investigation, 9(4)* (pp. 311–318).
27	Harris, N. & Sandor, M. (2013). Defining sustainable practice in community-based health promotion: a Delphi study of practitioner perspectives. *Health Promotion Journal of Australia, 24(1)* (pp. 53–60).
28	Hatamabadi, H.R., Sum, S., Tabatabaey, A. & Sabbaghi, M. (2016). Emergency department management of falls in the elderly: A clinical audit and suggestions for improvement. *International Emergency Nursing – Journal, 24* (pp. 2–8). https://doi.org/10.1016/j.ienj.2015.05.001.
29	Hawk, C., Schneider, M., Evans, M.W. Jr. & Redwood, D. (2012). Consensus process to develop a best-practice document on the role of chiropractic care in health promotion, disease prevention, and wellness. *Journal of Manipulative and Physiological Therapeutics, 35(7)* (pp. 556–567).
30	Holtzhausen, L.J., van Zyl, G.J. & Nel, M.M. (2014). Developing a strategic research framework for sport and exercise medicine. *British Journal of Sports Medicine, 48(14)* (pp. 1120–1126).
31	Jander, A., Crutzen, R., Mercken, L. & De Vries, H. (2015). Web-based interventions to decrease alcohol use in adolescents: a Delphi study about increasing effectiveness and reducing drop-out. *BMC Public Health, 15(340)*. https://doi.org/10.1186/s12889-015-1639-z.
32	Jones, M.L. & Boyd, L.D. (2012). Interdisciplinary approach to care: the role of the dental hygienist on a pediatric feeding team. *Journal of Allied Health, 41(4)* (pp. 190–197).
33	Junne, F., Ziser, K., Mander, J., Martus, P., Denzer, C., Reinehr, T., Wabitsch, M., Wiegand, S., Renner, T., Giel, K.E., Teufel, M., Zipfel, S. & Ehehalt, S. (2016). Development and psychometric validation of the 'Parent Perspective University of Rhode Island Change Assessment-Short' (PURICA-S) Questionnaire for the application in parents of children with overweight and obesity. *BMJ Open, 6(11)*. https://doi.org/10.1136/bmjopen-2016-012711.

ID	*Note: Missing numbers are sources that did not meet the inclusion criteria.
34	Junod Perron, N., Cerutti, B., Picchiottino, P., Empeyta, S., Cinter, F. & van Gessel, E. (2014). Needs assessment for training in interprofessional skills in Swiss primary care: a Delphi study. *Journal of Interprofessional Care, 28(3)* (pp. 273–275).
35	Kelly, B., King, L., Bauman, A. E., Baur, L. A., Macniven, R., Chapman, K. & Smith, B. J. (2014). Identifying important and feasible policies and actions for health at community sports clubs: a consensus-generating approach. *Journal of Science and Medicine in Sport, 17(1)* (pp. 61–66).
36	Kelly, M., Wills, J., Jester, R. & Speller, V. (2016). Should nurses be role models for healthy lifestyles? Results from a modified Delphi study. *Journal of Advanced Nursing, 73(3)* (pp. 665–678). https://doi.org/10.1111/jan.13173.
38	Lauriks, S., de Wit, M. A., Buster, M. C., Arah, O. A. & Klazinga, N. S. (2014). Composing a core set of performance indicators for public mental health care: a modified Delphi procedure. *Administration and Policy in Mental Health and Mental Health Services Research, 41(5)* (pp. 625–635).
39	Li, Y., Ehiri, J., Hu, D., Oren, E., & Cao, J. (2015). Framework of behavioral indicators evaluating TB health promotion outcomes: a modified Delphi study of TB policymakers and health workers. *Infectious Diseases of Poverty, 4(56).* https://doi.org/10.1186/s40249-015-0087-4.
40	Li, Y., Ehiri, J., Hu, D., Zhang, Y., Wang, Q., Zhang, S. & Cao, J. (2014). Framework of behavioral indicators for outcome evaluation of TB health promotion: a Delphi study of TB suspects and Tb patients. *BMC Infectious Diseases, 14(268).* https://doi.org/10.1186/1471-2334-14-268.
41	Liu, X., Erasmus, V., Sun, X., Cai, R., Shi, Y. & Richardus, J.H. (2014). Preventing HIV transmission in Chinese internal migrants: a behavioral approach. *The Scientific World Journal.* https://doi.org/10.1155/2014/319629.
42	Maijala, V., Tossavainen, K. & Turunen, H. (2016). Primary health care registered nurses' types in implementation of health promotion practices. *Primary Health Care Research & Development, 17(5)* (pp. 453–563). https://doi.org/10.1017/s1463423615000547.
43	Maijala, V., Tossavainen, K. & Turunen, H. (2015). Identifying nurse practitioners' required case management competencies in health promotion practice in municipal public primary health care. A two-stage modified Delphi study. *Journal of Clinical Nursing, 24* (pp. 2554–2561). https://doi.org/10.1016/j.ienj.2015.05.001.
44	Maijala, V., Tossavainen, K., & Turunen, H. (2016). Health promotion practices delivered by primary health care nurses: Elements for success in Finland. *Applied Nursing Research, 30* (pp. 45–51). https://doi.org/10.1016/j.apnr.2015.11.002.
45	Manavi, S., Olyaee Manesh, A., Yazdani, S., Shams, L., Nasiri, T., Shirvani, A. & Emami Razavi, H. (2013). Model for implementing evidence based health care system in Iran. *Iranian Journal of Public Health, 42(7)* (pp. 758–766).
46	Mao, F., Han, Y., Chen, J., Chen, W., Yuan, M., Hong, A.Y. & Fang, Y. (2016). Development of a Multidimensional Functional Health Scale for Older Adults in China. *Community Mental Health Journal, 52(4)* (pp. 466–471). https://doi.org/10.1007/s10597-015-9945-6.

ID	*Note: Missing numbers are sources that did not meet the inclusion criteria.
47	McGladrey, B.W., Hannon, J.C., Faigenbaum, A.D., Shultz, B.B. & Shaw, J.M. (2014). High school physical educators' and sport coaches' knowledge of resistance training principles and methods. *Journal of Strength and Conditioning Research, 28(5)* (pp. 1433–1442).
48	McKenna, H., McDonough, S., Keeney, S., Hasson, F., Lagan, K., Ward, M., Kelly, G. & Duffy, O. (2014). Research priorities for the therapy professions in Northern Ireland and the Republic of Ireland: a comparison of findings from a Delphi consultation. *Journal of Allied Health, 43(2)* (pp. 98–109).
49	McVeigh, J., MacLachlan, M., Gilmore, B., McClean, C., Eide, A.H., Mannan, H., Geiser, P., Duttine, A., Mji, G., McAuliffe, E., Sprunt, B., Amin, M. & Normand, C. (2016). Promoting good policy for leadership and governance of health related rehabilitation: a realist synthesis. *Global Health, 12(1)*. https://doi.org/10.1186/s12992-016-0182-8.
50	Melnyk, B.M., Gallagher-Ford, L., Long, L.E. & Fineout-Overholt, E. (2014). The establishment of evidence-based practice competencies for practicing registered nurses and advanced practice nurses in real-world clinical settings: proficiencies to improve healthcare quality, reliability, patient outcomes, and costs. *Worldviews on Evidence-Based Nursing, 11(1)* (pp. 5–15).
51	Milat, A.J., King, L., Bauman, A.E. & Redman, S. (2013). The concept of scalability: increasing the scale and potential adoption of health promotion interventions into policy and practice. *Health Promotion International, 28(3)* (pp. 285–298).
54	Morgan, A.J., Chittleborough, P. & Jorm, A.F. (2016). Self-help strategies for sub-threshold anxiety: A Delphi consensus study to find messages suitable for population-wide promotion. *Journal of Affective Disorders, 206* (pp. 68–76). https://doi.org/10.1016/j.jad.2016.07.024.
55	Morgan, D.J., Croft, L.D., Deloney, V., Popovich, K.J., Crnich, C., Srinivasan, A., Fishman, N.O., Bryant, K., Cosgrove, S.E. & Leekha, S. (2016). Choosing Wisely in Healthcare Epidemiology and Antimicrobial Stewardship. *Infection Control & Hospital Epidemiology, 37(7)* (pp. 755–760). https://doi.org/10.1017/ice.2016.61.
56	Mostert-Phipps, N., Pottas, D. & Korpela, M. (2013). Guidelines to encourage the adoption and meaningful use of health information technologies in the South African healthcare landscape. In C.U. Lehmann, E. Ammenwerth & C. Nøhr (eds), *MEDINFO 2013: Proceedings of the 14th World Congress on Medical and Health Informatics* (pp. 147–151). IOS Press.
57	Moynihan, S., Paakkari, L., Välimaa, R., Jourdan, D. & Mannix-McNamara, P. (2015). Teacher Competencies in Health Education: Results of a Delphi Study. *PLoS ONE, 10(12)*. https://doi.org/10.1371/journal.pone.0143703.
58	Nematollahi, M., Khalesi, N., Moghaddasi, H. & Askarian, M. (2012). Second Generation of HIV Surveillance System: A Pattern for Iran. *Iranian Red Crescent Medical Journal, 14(5)* (pp. 309–312).
59	Norris, S.A., Anuar, H., Matzen, P., Cheah, J.C., Jensen, B.B. & Hanson, M. (2014). The life and health challenges of young Malaysian couples: results from a stakeholder consensus and engagement study to support non-communicable disease prevention. *BMC Public Health, 14(2)*. https://doi.org/10.1186/1471-2458-14-s2-s6.

ID	*Note: Missing numbers are sources that did not meet the inclusion criteria.
60	Pinto, R.O., Pattussi, M.P., Fontoura Ldo, P., Poletto, S., Grapiglia, V.L., Balbinot, A.D., Teixeira, V.A. & Horta, R.L. (2016). Validation of an instrument to evaluate health promotion at schools. *Revista de Saúde Pública, 50(2)*. https://doi.org/10.1590/s01518-8787.2016050005855.
61	Pollack, L.A., Plachouras, D., Sinkowitz-Cochran, R., Gruhler, H., Monnet, D.L., Weber, J.T. & Transatlantic Taskforce on Antimicrobial Resistance (TATFAR) Expert Panel on Stewardship Structure and Process Indicators (2016). A Concise Set of Structure and Process Indicators to Assess and Compare Antimicrobial Stewardship Programs Among EU and US Hospitals: Results From a Multinational Expert Panel. *Infection Control & Hospital Epidemiology, 37(10)* (pp. 1201–1211). https://doi.org/10.1017/ice.2016.115.
62	Poole, N., Schmidt, R.A., Green, C. & Hemsing, N. (2016). Prevention of Fetal Alcohol Spectrum Disorder: Current Canadian Efforts and Analysis of Gaps. *Substance Abuse and Rehabilitation, 10(1)* (pp. 1–11). https://doi.org/10.4137/sart.s34545.
63	Porcheret, M., Grime, J., Main, C. & Dziedzic, K. (2013). Developing a model osteoarthritis consultation: a Delphi consensus exercise. *BMC Musculoskeletal Disorders, 14(25)*. https://doi.org/10.1186/1471-2474-14-25.
64	Quecedo Gutiérrez, L., Ruiz Abascal, R., Calvo Vecino, J.M., Peral García, A.I., Matute González, E., Muñoz Alameda, L.E., Guasch Arévalo, E. & Gilsanz Rodríguez, F. (2016). 'Do not do' recommendations of the Spanish Society of Anaesthesiology, Critical Care and Pain Therapy. 'Commitment to Quality by Scientific Societies' Project. *Revista Española de Anestesiología y Reanimación, 63(9)* (pp. 519–527). https://doi.org/10.1016/j.redar.2016.05.002.
65	Quinn, C. & Bonuck, K. (2012). Identifying breastfeeding-sensitive conditions by expert consensus. *Journal of Human Lactation, 28(4)* (pp. 535–542). https://doi.org/10.1177/0890334412456603.
66	Rangraz, J.F. & Rezaiimofrad, M.R. (2013). Development of Common Data Elements to Provide Tele self-Care Management. *Acta Informatica Medica, 21(4)* (pp. 241–245).
67	Ridde, V. & Sombie, I. (2012). Street-level workers' criteria for identifying indigents to be exempted from user fees in Burkina Faso. *Tropical Medicine and International Health, 17(6)* (pp. 782–791).
68	Rogozinska, E., D'Amico, M.I., Khan, K.S., Cecatti, J.G., Teede, H., Yeo, S., Vinter, C.A., Rayanagoudar, G., Barakat, R., Perales, M., Dodd, J.M., Devlieger, R., Bogaerts, A., van Poppel, M.N., Haakstad, L., Shen, G.X., Shub, A., Luoto, R., Kinnunen, T.I., Phelan, S., Poston, L., Scudeller, T.T., El Beltagy, N., Stafne, S.N., Tonstad, S., Geiker, N.R., Ruifrok, A.E., Mol, B.W., Coomarasamy, A., Thangaratinam, S. & International Weight Management in Pregnancy (iWIP) Collaborative Group (2015). Development of composite outcomes for individual patient data (IPD) meta-analysis on the effects of diet and lifestyle in pregnancy: a Delphi survey. *BJOG: An International Journal of Obstetrics, 123(2)* (pp. 190–198). https://doi.org/10.1111/1471-0528.13764.

ID	*Note: Missing numbers are sources that did not meet the inclusion criteria.
69	Rubinstein, S.M., Bolton, J., Webb, A.L. & Hartvigsen, J. (2014). The first research agenda for the chiropractic profession in Europe. *Chiropractic & Manual Therapies, 22(1)*. https://doi.org/10.1186/2045-709x-22-9.
70	Salehi, A., Hashemi, N., Saber, M. & Imanieh, M.H. (2015). Designing and conducting MD/MPH dual degree program in the Medical School of Shiraz University of Medical Sciences. *Journal of Advances in Medical Education & Professionalism, 3(3)* (pp. 105–110).
71	Schaffalitzky, E., Leahy, D., Cullen, W., Gavin, B., Latham, L., O'Connor, R., Smyth, B.P., O'Dea, E. & Ryan, S. (2015). Youth mental health in deprived urban areas: a Delphi study on the role of the GP in early intervention. *Irish Journal of Medical Science, 184(4)* (pp. 831–843). https://doi.org/10.1007/s11845-014-1187-z.
72	Schneider, F., van Osch, L. & de Vries, H. (2012). Identifying factors for optimal development of health-related websites: a delphi study among experts and potential future users. *Journal of Medical Internet Research, 14(1)*. https://doi.org/10.2196/jmir.1863.
73	Setiyawati, D., Colucci, E., Blashki, G., Wraith, R. & Minas, H. (2014). International experts' perspectives on a curriculum for psychologists working in primary health care: implication for Indonesia. *Health Psychology & Behavioural Medicine, 2(1)* (pp. 770–784).
75	Syed, A.M., Camp, R., Mischorr-Boch, C., Houÿez, F. & Aro, A.R. (2015). Policy recommendations for rare disease centres of expertise. *Evaluation and Program Planning, 52* (pp. 78–84). https://doi.org/10.1016/j.evalprogplan.2015.03.006.
76	Taymoori, P. & Moshki, M. (2014). A Delphi study to curriculum modifying through the application of the course objective and competencies. *Journal of Education and Health Promotion, 3(124)*. https://doi.org/10.4103/2277-9531.145936.
77	Ter Haar, M., Aarts, N. & Verhoeven, P. (2015). Finding common ground in implementation: towards a theory of gradual commonality. *Health Promotion International, 31(1)* (pp. 214–230). https://doi.org/10.1093/heapro/dau077.
78	Teyhen, D.S., Aldag, M., Edinborough, E., Ghannadian, J.D., Haught, A., Kinn, J., Kunkler, K.J., Levine, B., McClain, J., Neal, D., Stewart, T., Thorndike, F.P., Trabosh, V., Wesensten, N. & Parramore, D.J. (2014). Leveraging technology: creating and sustaining changes for health. *Telemedicine and e-Health, 20(9)* (pp. 835–849).
79	Tomasik, T., Gryglewska, B., Windak, A. & Grodzicki, T. (2013). Hypertension in the elderly: how to treat patients in 2013? The essential recommendations of the Polish guidelines. *Polish Archives of Internal Medicine, 123 (7–8)* (pp. 409–416).
80	Tompa, E., de Boer, H., Macdonald, S., Alamgir, H., Koehoorn, M., & Guzman, J. (2016). Stakeholders' Perspectives About and Priorities for Economic Evaluation of Health and Safety Programs in Healthcare. *Workplace Health & Safety, 64(4)* (pp. 163–174). https://doi.org/10.1177/2165079915620201.
81	Uribe Guajardo, M.G., Slewa-Younan, S., Santalucia, Y. & Jorm, A.F. (2016). Important considerations when providing mental health first aid to Iraqi refugees in Australia: a Delphi study. *International Journal of Mental Health Systems, 10(1)*. https://doi.org/10.1186/s13033-016-0087-1.

ID	*Note: Missing numbers are sources that did not meet the inclusion criteria.
82	Van Hasselt, F.M., Oud, M.J. & Loonen, A.J. (2015). Practical recommendations for improvement of the physical health care of patients with severe mental illness. *Acta Psychiatrica Scandinavica, 131(5)* (pp. 387–396). https://doi.org/10.1111/acps.12372.
83	Van Scheppingen, A.R., ten Have, K.C., Zwetsloot, G.J., Kok, G. & van Mechelen, W. (2015). Determining organisation-specific factors for developing health interventions in companies by a Delphi procedure: Organisational Mapping. *Journal of Health Psychology, 20(12)* (pp. 1509–1522). https://doi.org/10.1177/1359105313516030.
84	Vankova, D., Kerekovska, A., Kostadinova, T. & Todorova, L. (2016). Researching health-related quality of life at a community level: results from a population survey conducted in Burgas, Bulgaria. *Health Promotion International, 31(3)* (pp. 534–541). https://doi.org/10.1093/heapro/dav016.
85	Vanmeerbeek, M., Govers, P., Schippers, N., Rieppi, S., Mortelmans, K. & Mairiaux, P. (2016). Searching for consensus among physicians involved in the management of sick-listed workers in the Belgian health care sector: a qualitative study among practitioners and stakeholders. *BMC Public Health, 16(164).* https://doi.org/10.1186/s12889-016-2696-7.
86	Vantamay, N. (2015). Using the delphi technique to develop effectiveness indicators for social marketing communication to reduce health-risk behaviors among youth. *The Southeast Asian Journal of Tropical Medicine and Public Health, 46(5)* (pp. 949–957).
87	Vasudevan, V., Rmmer, J.H. & Kviz, F. (2015). Development of the Barriers to Physical Activity Questionnaire for People with Mobility Impairments. *Disability and Health Journal, 8(4)* (pp. 547–556). https://doi.org/10.1016/j.dhjo.2015.04.007.
88	Vermandere, M., Lepeleire, J. D., Van Mechelen, W., Warmenhoven, F., Thoonsen, B. & Aertgeerts, B. (2013). Spirituality in palliative home care: a framework for the clinician. *Supportive Care in Cancer, 21(4)* (pp. 1061–1069).
89	Vestjens, L., Kempen, G.I., Crutzen, R., Kok, G. & Zijlstra, G.A. (2015). Promising behavior change techniques in a multicomponent intervention to reduce concerns about falls in old age: a Delphi study. *Health Education Research, 30(2)* (pp. 309–322). https://doi.org/10.1093/her/cyv003.
90	Walpole, S.C., Shortall, C., van Schalkwyk, M.C., Merriel, A., Ellis, J., Obolensky, L., Casanova Dias, M., Watson, J., Brown, C.S., Hall, J., Pettigrew, L.M. & Allen, S. (2016). Time to go global: a consultation on global health competencies for postgraduate doctors. *International Health, 8(5)* (pp. 317–323). https://doi.org/10.1093/inthealth/ihw019.
91	Wright, M.T., Lüken, F. & Grossmann, B. (2013). Quality in prevention and health promotion. Developing a common framework for quality development for members of the Federal Association for Prevention and Health Promotion in Germany. *Bundesgesundheitsblatt, 56(4)* (pp. 466–472). https://doi.org/10.1007/s00103-012-1628-7.

Literature

Aengenheyster, S., Cuhls, K., Gerhold, L., Heiskanen-Schüttler, M., Huck, J., & Muszynska, M. (2017). Real-time Delphi in practice – A comparative analysis of existing software-based tools. *Technological Forecasting and Social Change, 118*, 15–27.

Bogner, A., Littig, B., & Menz, W. (2014). *Interviews mit Experten. Eine praxisorientierte Einführung*. Springer. https://doi.org/10.1007/978-3-531-19416-5

Boulkedid, R., Abdoul, H., Loustau, M., Sibony, O., & Alberti, C. (2011). Using and reporting the Delphi method for selecting healthcare quality indicators: A systematic review. *PLoS One, 6*(6), 1–9. https://doi.org/10.1371/journal.pone.0020476

Cuhls, K. (2012). Zu den Unterschieden zwischen Delphi-Befragungen und "einfachen" Zukunftsbefragungen. In R. Popp (Ed.), *Zukunft und Wissenschaft: Wege und Irrwege der Zukunftsforschung* (pp. 139–158). Springer.

Cuhls, K., Blind, K., Grupp, H., Bradke, H., Dreher, C., Harmsen, D.-M., Hiessl, H., Hüsing, B., Jaeckel, G., Schmoch, U., & Zoche, P. (1998). Delphi '98. In *Studie zur globalen Entwicklung von Wissenschaft und Technik*. Fraunhofer Institut für Systemtechnik und Innovationsforschung.

Diamond, I. R., Grant, R. C., Feldman, B. M., Pencharz, P. B., Ling, S. C., Moore, A. M., & Wales, P. W. (2014). Defining consensus: A systematic review recommends methodologic criteria for reporting of Delphi studies. *Journal of Clinical Epidemiology, 67*(4), 401–409. https://doi.org/10.1016/j.jclinepi.2013.12.002

Evidenzbasierung. (2018). In M. A. Wirtz (eds), *Dorsch – Lexikon der Psychologie*. https://portal.hogrefe.com/dorsch/evidenzbasierung/. Accessed 7 May 2018.

Häder, M. (2014). *Delphi-Befragungen: Ein Arbeitsbuch*. Springer.

Hart, M. L., Jorm, A. J., Kanowski, L. G., Kelly, C. M., & Langlands, R. L. (2009). Mental health first aid for indigenous Australians: Using Delphi consensus studies to develop guidelines for culturally appropriate responses to mental health problems. *BMC Psychiatry, 9*(47). https://doi.org/10.1186/1471-244x-9-47

Hasson, F., Keeney, S., & McKenna, H. (2000). Research guidelines for the Delphi survey technique. *Journal of Advanced Nursing, 32*(4), 1008–1015. https://doi.org/10.1046/j.1365-2648.2000.t01-1-01567.x

Jirwe, M., Gerrish, K., & Keeney, S. (2009). Identifying the core components of cultural competence: Findings from a Delphi study. *Journal of Clinical Nursing, 18*(18), 2622–2634.

Jorm, A. (2015). Using the Delphi expert consensus method in mental health research. *Australian & New Zealand Journal of Psychiatry, 49*(10), 887–897. https://doi.org/10.1177/0004867415600891

Jung, M., & Bleyer, T. (2017). *Technologien in einer Altenpflege der Zukunft – Eine Delphi-Studie*. Bundesanstalt für Arbeitsschutz und Arbeitsmedizin.

Jünger, S., Payne, S. A., Brine, J., Radbruch, L., & Brearley, S. G. (2017). Guidance on conducting and reporting Delphi studies (CREDES) in palliative care: Recommendations based on a methodological systematic review. *Palliative Medicine, 31*(8), 684–706. https://doi.org/10.1177/0269216317690685

Keeney, S., Hasson, F., & McKenna, H. (2001). A critical review of the Delphi technique as a research methodology for nursing. *International Journal of Nursing Studies, 38*(2), 195–200.

Keeney, S., Hasson, F., & McKenna, H. (2006). Consulting the oracle: Ten lessons from using the Delphi technique in nursing research. *Journal of Advanced Nursing, 53*, 205–212.

Keeney, S., Hasson, F., & McKenna, H. (2011). *The Delphi technique in nursing and health research*. Wiley-Blackwell.

Linstone, H. A., & Turoff, M. (Eds.). (1975). *The Delphi method: Techniques and applications*. Addison-Wesley.

Linstone, H. A., & Turoff, M. (2002). *The Delphi method: Techniques and applications*. New Jersey Institute of Technology.

Linstone, H. A., & Turoff, M. (2011). Delphi: A brief look backward and forward. *Technological Forecasting and Social Change, 78*, 1712–1719.

Moher, D., Liberati, A., Tetzlaff, J., Altman, D. G., & The PRISMA Group. (2009). Preferred reporting items for systematic reviews and meta-analyses: The PRISMA statement. *PLoS Medicine, 6*(6). https://doi.org/10.1371/journal.pmed1000097

Niederberger, M., & Kuhn, R. (2013). Das Gruppendelphi als Evaluationsinstrument. *Zeitschrift für Evaluation, 1*, 53–77.

Niederberger, M., & Renn, O. (2018). *Das Gruppendelphi-Verfahren. Vom Konzept bis zur Anwendung*. Springer. https://doi.org/10.1007/978-3-658-18755-2_3

Nowack, M., Endrikat, J., & Guenther, E. (2011). Review of Delphi-based scenario studies: Quality and design considerations. *Technological Forecasting and Social Change, 78*, 1603–1615.

Ramm, M. (2014). Response, Stichprobe und Repräsentativität: Zwei Dokumente zum Deutschen Studierendensurvey (DSS). *Hefte zur Bildungs- und Hochschulforschung, 72*, 14–21.

Rowe, G., & Wright, G. (2011). The Delphi technique: Past, present, and future prospects – Introduction to the special issue. *Technological Forecasting and Social Change, 78*, 1487–1490.

Steurer, J. (2011). The Delphi method: An efficient procedure to generate knowledge. *Skeletal Radiology, 40*(8), 959–961. https://doi.org/10.1007/s00256-011-1145-z

Vidgen, H., & Gallegos, D. (2011). *What is food literacy and does it influence what we eat: A study of Australian food experts*. Queensland University of Technology.

Von der Gracht, H. A. (2012). Consensus measurement in Delphi studies: Review and implications for future quality assurance. *Technological Forecasting and Social Change, 79*(8), 1525–1536.

Witt, R. R., & de Almeida, M. C. P. (2008). Identification of nurses' competencies in primary health care through a Delphi study in southern Brazil. *Public Health Nursing, 25*(4), 336–343.

World Health Organization (WHO). (1986). *Ottawa charter for health promotion*. http://www.euro.who.int/__data/assets/pdf_file/0006/129534/Ottawa_Charter_G.pdf. Accessed 3 May 2018.

The manufacturer's authorised representative in the EU is Springer Nature Customer Service Centre GmbH, Europaplatz 3, 69115 Heidelberg, Germany. If you have any concerns regarding our products, please contact ProductSafety@springernature.com

Printed and bound by CPI Group (UK) Ltd, Croydon, CR0 4YY
28/09/2026
02224076-0004